Topics in Anaesthesia and Critical Care

H.K.F. VAN SAENE, L. SILVESTRI, M.A. DE LA CAL (EDS)
Infection Control in the Intensitive Care unit
1998, 380 pp, ISBN 3-540-75043-6

J. MILIC-EMILI (ED)
Applied Physiology in Respiratory Mechanics
1998, 246 pp, ISBN 3-540-75041-X

G. GUARNIERI, F. ISCRA
Metabolism and Artificial Nutrition in the Critically Ill
1999, 130 pp, ISBN 88-470-0042-4

J. MILIC -EMILI, U. LUCANGELO, A. PESENTI, W.A. ZIN
Basics of Respiratory Mechanics and Artificial Ventilation
1999, 268 pp, ISBN 88-470-0046-7

M. TIENGO, V.A. PALADINI, N. RAWAL
Regional Anaesthesia, Analgesia and Pain Management
1999, 362 pp, ISBN 88-470-0044-0

I. SALVO, D. VIDYASAGAR
Anaesthesia and Intensive Care in Neonates and Children
1999, 324 pp, ISBN 88-470-0043-2

G. BERLOT, H. DELOOZ, A. GULLO
Trauma Operative Procedures
1999, 210 pp, ISBN 88-470-0045-9

Anestesia e Medicina Critica

G. SLAVICH
Elettrocardiografia Clinica
1997, 328 pp, ISBN 3-540-75050-9

G.L. ALATI, B. ALLARIA, G. BERLOT, A. GULLO, A. LUZZANI,
G. MARTINELLI, L. TORELLI
Anestesia e Malattie Concomitanti - Fisiopatologia e clinica del
periodo perioperatorio
1997, 382 pp, ISBN 3-540-75048-7

B. ALLARIA, M.V. BALDASSARE, A. GULLO, A. LUZZANI,
G. MANANI, G. MARTINELLI, A. PASETTO, L. TORELLI
Farmacologia Generale e Speciale in Anestesiologia Clinica
1997, 312 pp, ISBN 88-470-0001-7

A. GULLO
Anestesia Clinica
1998, 506 pp, ISBN 88-470-0038-6

Anaesthesia and Intensive Care
in Neonates and Children

Springer-Verlag Italia Srl.

I. Salvo
D. Vidyasagar (Eds)

Anaesthesia and Intensive Care in Neonates and Children

Series edited by
Antonino Gullo

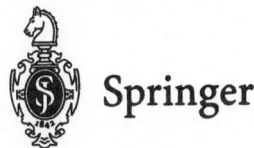 Springer

I. Salvo, MD
Department of Anaesthesia and Intensive Care
Buzzi Children Hospital, Milan - Italy

D. Vidyasagar, MD
Department of Pediatrics, College of Medicine at Chicago
University of Illinois, Chicago - USA

Series of *Topics in Anaesthesia and Critical Care* edited by
A. Gullo, MD
Department of Anaesthesia, Intensive Care and Pain Therapy
University of Trieste, Cattinara Hospital, Trieste - Italy

© Springer-Verlag Italia 1999
Originally published by Springer Verlag Italia, Milano in 1999

ISBN 978-88-470-0043-8   ISBN 978-88-470-2282-9 (eBook)
DOI 10.1007/978-88-470-2282-9

Library of Congress Cataloging-in-Publication Data: Applied for.

Cover design: Simona Colombo, Milan
Typesetting and layout: Compostudio, Milan

SPIN:10697744

Foreword

The anaesthesia and intensive care of neonates and children have assumed positions of primary importance in contemporary medicine. In these delicate fields of medicine, clinical research activities must be continually supported by interdisciplinary cooperations. Neonatal and pediatric intensive care requires that all involved physicians, including the surgeon and anesthesiologist, be willing to work together as a team. However, coordination of the various pathophysiological and clinical aspects of neonatal and pediatric critical medicine is highly complex. A complete and current review of anesthesia and intensive care of infants and children must include discussions of morbidity rates, so as to guide the clinician in choosing the diagnostic approach, as well as of monitoring techniques appropriate to support the therapeutic decision.

Much experience has been amassed regarding the management of critical clinical situations in the neonate requiring intensive care interventions. The use of surgery is particularly delicate: optimization of the perioperative period has become the "gold standard" for efficient and successfull management of critically ill neonates. Thus, preoperative evaluation, airway control, choice of fluid therapy and anesthesia protocols, and a thorough understanding of the various anesthesia routes represent fundamental issue for all members of the medical team involved in the care of such patients.

Local-regional anaesthesia is being increasingly and successfully used in this field of medicine, even though it had been previously contraindicated. Now that neonatal and pediatric surgery has overcome the limitations it faced in the 1960s and 1970s, anaesthesia has assumed an increasingly important role in the perioperative period for both general and specialty surgery. Heart surgery and organ transplantation represent two categories of intervention which depend upon team strategy and advanced technology.

Developments in methods of sedation and in the treatment of post-operative pain, together with new contributions from biotechnology and pharmacology, now permit sophisticated surgical interventions on both fetus and neonate. Of particular significance in this regard has been the development of the so-called "fetal anaesthesia".

Continuing education in these fields of medicine should include: a review of classic arguments such as respiratory distress syndrome and the techniques of respiratory support, including that of high frequency ventilation; the discussion of careful monitoring for sepsis and the application of all measures for the pre-

vention and treatment of eventual systemic infections; the overview of experimental therapies such as liquid ventilation, and the use of surfactants or modified respiratory gases containing nitric oxide for the treatment of refractory hypoxemia; and the consideration of experimental medical support techniques
such as hemopurification (i.e. CAVH and plasmapheresis) to eliminate toxins
and reactive metabolites from the blood stream. This last application, although
a fascinating area of research, is limited in that it is unable to offer any cure. The
successfull employment of such technology requires a deeper understanding of
the pathophysiological factors involved, a directed medical therapy, and often-
times an aggressive surgical intervention.

Recent progress in intensive care medicine for infants and children has been
significant. Members of the medical team caring for critically ill pediatric patients must remain up-to-date in both the pathophysiological and clinical aspects of the ailing and healing processes.

November 1998   *Antonino Gullo, MD*

Contents

MOTHER AND CHILD

PERIOPERATIVE SEDATION AND ANALGESIA

PAEDIATRIC INTENSIVE CARE UNIT (PICU)

Contributors

Arnold J.H.
Department of Anaesthesia, Paediatrics, Children's Hospital and Harvard Medical School, Boston, USA.

Baines P.
Intensive Care Unit, Royal Liverpool Children's Hospital, Liverpool, UK.

Borrometi F.
Department of Paediatric Anaesthesia and Intensive Care, Santobono Hospital, Naples, Italy.

Busoni P.
Department of Anaesthesia and Intensive Care, Meyer Hospital, Florence, Italy.

Calamandrei M.
Department of Anaesthesia and Intensive Care, Meyer Hospital, Florence, Italy.

Carpino V.
Department of Paediatric Anaesthesia and Intensive Care, Santobono Children's Hospital, Naples, Italy.

De Negri P.
Department of Anaesthesia, IRCCS Casa Sollievo della Sofferenza, San Giovanni Rotondo (FG) Italy.

Dotta A.
Department of Neonatology, Bambino Gesù Hospital, Rome, Italy.

Fedele L.
Department of Obstetrics and Gynaecology, University of Verona, Verona, Italy.

Fischer J.
Department of Neonatal and Paediatric Intensive Care, University Children's Hospital, Zürich, Switzerland.

Gagliardi L.
Department of Neonatology, Buzzi Children Hospital, Milan, Italy.

Gradnitzer E.
Universitätsklinik für Kinder und Jugendheilkunde, Graz, Austria.

Hamza J.
Department of Anaesthesia and Intensive Care, Hospital St-Vincent de Paul, Paris, France.

Hatch D.J.
Department of Paediatric Anaesthesia, Institute of Child Health, University of London, London, UK.

Introvini P.
Department of Neonatology, Buzzi Children Hospital Milan, Italy.

Ivani G.
Department of Anaesthesia and Intensive Care, Regina Margherita Children's Hospital, Turin, Italy.

Lönnqvist P.A.
Department of Paediatric Anaesthesia and Intensive Care, Astrid Lindgrens Children's Hospital, Karolinska Hospital, Stockholm, Sweden.

Marraro G.A.
Department of Anaesthesia and Intensive Care, Fatebenefratelli & Oftalmico Hospital, Milan, Italy.

Meursing A.E.E.
Department of Anaesthesiology, Sophia Kinderziekenhuis, Academisch Ziekenhuis, Rotterdam, The Netherlands.

Moores C.
Department of Anaesthetics, Royal Liverpool Children's Hospital, Liverpool, UK.

Morton N.S.
Department of Anaesthesia, Royal Hospital for Sick Children, Glasgow, UK.

Motta G.
Department of Neonatology, Buzzi Children Hospital, Milan, Italy.

Müller W.
Universitätsklinik für Kinder und Jugendheilkunde, Graz, Austria.

Natale A.
Department of Anaesthesia and Intensive Care, Santobono Children's Hospital, Naples, Italy.

Neidecker J.
Department of Anaesthesia and Intensive Care, Cardiovascular and Pneumological Hospital, Lyon, France.

Orzalesi M.
Department of Neonatology, Bambino Gesù Hospital, Rome, Italy.

Peluso V.
Department of Paediatric Anaesthesia and Intensive Care, Santobono Hospital, Naples, Italy.

Petros A.J.
Paedriatric Intensive Care Unit, Hospital for Sick Children, London, UK.

Resch B.
Universitätsklinik für Kinder und Jugendheilkunde, Graz, Austria.

Ring E.
Department of Paediatric, University of Graz, Austria.

Rödl S.
Department of Neonatology, University of Graz, Austria.

Sacquin P.
Department of Anaesthesia and Intensive Care, Hospital St-Vincent de Paul, Paris, France.

Salvo I.
Department of Anaesthesia and Intensive Care, Buzzi Children Hospital, Milan, Italy.

Seganti G.
Division of Neonatology, Bambino Gesù Hospital, Rome, Italy.

Simon L.
Department of Anaesthesia and Intensive Care, Hospital St-Vincent de Paul, Paris, France.

Urlesberger B.
Universitätsklinik für Kinder und Jugendheilkunde, Graz, Austria.

Vidyasagar D.
Department of Neonatology, Chicago Medical Center, University of Illinois, Chicago, USA.

Vonderweid U. de
Department of Neonatalogy and Intensive Care, IRCCS Burlo Garofalo, Trieste, Italy.

Wolf A.R.
Department of Paediatric Anaesthesia and Intensive Care, Royal Hospital for Sick Children, Bristol, UK.

Zakowski M.
Department of Anaesthesiology, Cedars-Sinai Medical Center, Los Angeles, USA.

Zanconato G.
Department of Obstetrics and Gynaecology, University of Verona, Verona, Italy.

Zobel G.
Department of Paediatrics, University of Graz, Austria.

Zoia E.
Department of Anaesthesia and Intensive Care, Buzzi Children Hospital, Milan, Italy.

PERIOPERATIVE MANAGEMENT

Chapter 1

Preoperative evaluation

V. Carpino, F. Borrometi, A. Natale, V. Peluso

Preoperative anaesthesiologic evaluation is generally considered an important phase of anaesthesiologic management and strictly related to anaesthesiologic procedure and postoperative care [1]. For this reason, the anaesthesiologist can be defined the "perioperative doctor". Today, progress in diagnostic tests and improved patient monitoring may sometimes result in less emphasis on preoperative evaluation, being considered less important than the actual anaesthesiologic activity.

Thanks to a correct and complete preoperative assessment, a young patient's conditions can be precisely evaluated and the optimal preoperative and anaesthesia management chosen [2, 3]; underestimating the preoperative evaluation can potentially increase the risk of unexpected and dangerous complications.

Only after this preliminary visit, will the anaesthesiologist decide whether additional laboratory tests are required and if there is a need to consult other specialists.

It is important to bear in mind that the anaesthesiologic evaluation is the first occasion to meet the little patient and his parents and this instance provides the opportunity to prepare them adequately for the hospitalization experience. Very often, they have not received an adequate explanation of the procedure, and gaining their confidence can be considered the first step to patient cure. Parents might have more fears about anaesthesia than surgery. Parents and child experience a psychological interaction, i.e., when a situation is reassuring for the child, it will be the same for his parents and vice versa [4].

The child (if old enough) should be involved in the examination, in order to gain his confidence. While speaking to him, the anaesthesiologist should adapt words and gestures and avoid threatening attitudes. He will have to describe to operating room environment to the patient, and the possible discomfort (blowing air into a mask or bearing a venepuncture): in such cases, a lie may be useful in the short term but might cause long-term mistrust.

At the end of the assessment, parents should be informed about the type of anaesthesia and the monitoring and the estimated anaesthesiologic risk the patient will have to face. Parents should feel free to ask questions. Their written informed consent is then requested. Parents should also be informed of the possibility to assist their child during induction, at institutions that allow it, and counseled on required behavior.

A psychological evaluation of the child will help to determine whether pre-anaesthesia is required and, in such a case, which drug, dosage, and route of administration should be used.

History

In most cases the patient is not able to tell his own history and generally his parents do that for him. If a child is old enough, his collaboration can be elicited. The anaesthesiologist must very carefully gather the information provided in the history. Frequently, he must elicit exhaustive answers from the parents. They often fail to declare some pathologies because they may not be perceived as such (for example, to have thalassemia minor Mediterranean anemia is usually considered as an "inherited trait" instead of a real pathology) or because they are uncomfortable or unwilling to acknowledge them (AIDS, mental retardation).

During the interview there are some common questions to be asked of all patients, while other questions vary according to the individual and the surgery planned. A preoperative form, usually included in the anaesthesiologic chart, may be used as a guideline for interviewing the child's parents so that the questions can follow a precise logical order and no information is disregarded.

In gathering the family history details, the anaesthesiologist must seek for anaesthetic-related complications or accidents, serious allergic reactions, or hereditary pathologies relevant from an anaesthesiologic point of view.

The past medical history must be scrupulously collected: it is important to record any previous hospitalization or surgery and related data accurately examined; in the anaesthesiological records, it is necessary to seek for information related to difficulties encountered (such as airway anomalies, intubation difficulties, adverse reaction). The paediatrician caring for the child may give an important contribution, especially in the setting of elective procedures largely prepared on an outpatient basis, by preoperative medical evaluations, and by introducing the child to anaesthesia and postoperative events. Consulting him or reading his report on the patient's clinical status could be useful, in particular, to understand the severity of pre-existing pathologies (asthma, hemoglobinopathies) or for the definition of complex pathologies that parents are unable to explain [5-7]. Particularly in the outpatient setting, an appropriate evaluation by the paediatrician may help avoid last-minute delays or cancellation of scheduled surgery [8].

For paediatric patients, the medical history begins during the mother's pregnancy: problems during gestation and birth can be relevant especially in the neonatal period. For this reason, the anaesthesiologist needs to verify whether the child is born at term 38-42 weeks), if the pregnancy was uncomplicated, if there were any perinatal complications, and if it was necessary to admit the baby to a neonatal ICU. Then, the anaesthesiologist needs to know the birth weight and whether it is appropriate for the gestational age, so that he may anticipate problems that could occur during and after anaesthesia.

It is necessary to obtain a detailed history of allergies caused by environmental allergens or by drugs. The anaesthesiologist has to obtain specific information regarding any possible allergy to latex in a high-risk patients; actually, in recent years, many studies have proven there to be an increase in the incidence of severe allergic reactions to latex and that most of the children who have had intraoperative reactions to latex-containing devices have meningomyelocele, extrophy of the bladder, or other urinary tract anomalies or frequent latex exposure. Parents of the children who are at risk are asked to remember children's reactions after touching latex-containing objects (adhesive bandages, catheter) or toys (balloons, bath-mats) [9-11].

Also, the anaesthesiologist must collect information about the kind of drugs that the patient is taking and consider their possible interaction with anaesthesia (bronchodilators) or with surgery (anticoagulants, anti-inflammatories).

Additional questions will be asked to obtain information about the history of any recent upper respiratory infection (see below) and to collect details suggesting a clotting disorder (hematomas, frequent and prolonged epistaxis, unusual bleeding after minor trauma).

For emergency surgery patients and for outpatients, it is necessary to record the time of last oral intake, bearing in mind that the pre-operative fasting (usually 6-8 h) may be shorter for newborns and children up to 6 months of age and that clear fluids are allowed until 2-3 h before anaesthesia [12, 13]; on the other hand, some intestinal pathologies or trauma can decrease gastrointestinal motility.

Physical examination

A child's examination should be different from that of an adult. The environment should be "reassuring" and there should not be any frightening objects or instruments. During the visit, the availability of little toys could be useful to entertain the child and get his collaboration.

Initially, the child may be observed without separating him from his parents: the signs of a regular respiratory activity, the presence of nasal congestion, nutritional status, and of a normal, age-related growth and behavior may be appreciated without involving the little patient.

At first, the anaesthesiologist can examine the child while in his parent's arms and, next, on a cot, avoiding, if possible, the recumbent position, because, in this position, the child feels threatened. The visit should follow a series of criteria to avoid stress to the child, beginning with the use of gestures which children are familiar with (cardiac and pulmonary auscultation) and leaving at the end the most unpleasant (oral inspection with tongue depressor) or painful procedures.

Special attention should be paid to the inspection of the oral cavity, highlighting the deciduous dentition status and the presence of orthodontic braces, recording whether they are fixed or mobile. If a very loose tooth were accidentally removed during anaesthesia, this event should be recorded in the chart and the tooth attached to it. Moreover, the anaesthesiologist should record additional conditions which may interfere with intubation (limitations in mouth opening, tonsillar hypertrophy, trachea deviations, cleft lip, micrognathia), beararing in mind that a congenital malformation is often associated with other abnormalities which might be less evident.

In the younger patients, the state of hydration (moistness of mucous membranes, unelastic skin, sunken anterior fontanel) must be checked very carefully, especially when patients have been fasting for many hours or when they have significant vomit and diarrhea.

It is useful to remember that babies and children dissipate heat quickly and, for this reason, they should stay undressed for as short as possible; moreover, it is important to consider children's sense of modesty and to let them undressed only for the strictly necessary time. The place where the examination is conducted should be respectful of the patient's privacy. If an operation has a generic definition (for example, removal of a foreign body or of a cutaneous lesion), it is advisable to perform a quick but careful examination of the lesion to be treated: its characteristics and its size and location may significantly affect the anaesthesiologic procedure (the length of the operation, possible blood loss, patient decubitus, etc.).

In particular cases, the examination will be addressed to specific apparatuses or organs according to the results emerging from medical history, evaluating possible anaesthetic implications (Table 1).

Table 1. Medical history and review of systems: anaesthetic implications. (Modified from [14])

System	History	Possible anaesthetic implication
Central nervous and neuromuscular systems	• Seizures	Medications: drug interactions, possible inadequate serum levels, valproate-induced hepatitis
	• Head trauma	Elevated intracranial pressure; anemia
	• Hydrocephalus	Possible elevated intracranial pressure
	• CNS tumor	Possible elevated intracranial pressure; chemotherapeutic drugs and interactions
	• Developmental delay	Bulbar dysfunction and risk of aspiration
	• Neuromuscular disease	Altered response to relaxants
	• Muscle disease	Risk of malignant hyperthermia; hyperkalemia after succinylcholine
	• Muscular dystrophy	Possible risk of malignant hyperthermia
Cardiovascular system	• Heart murmur	Septal defect; avoid i.v. air bubbles; hemoconcentration; endocarditis prophylaxis
	• Cyanosis	Right-to-left cardiac shunt: i.v. air bubbles; hemoconcentration; endocarditis prophylaxis
	• History of Squatting	Possible tetralogy of Fallot
	• Diaphoresis with feedings	Congestive heart failure

(cont.)

Table 1. (cont.)

	• Hypertension	Possible coarctation of the aorta; renal disease; pheochromocytoma
	• Transplant recipient	Fixed heart rate; insensitivity to anticholinergic drugs
Respiratory system	• Prematurity	Increased risk of postoperative apnea; possible lower respiratory tract illness
	• Bronchopulmonary dysplasia	Lower airway obstruction; reactive airways; possible subglottic stenosis; possible postoperative hypoxia and apnea; pulmonary hypertension
	• Lower respiratory infection, cough	Reactive airways; bronchospasm medication history; drug interactions
	• Croup	Possible subglottic stenosis/anomaly
	• Snoring, sleep apnea	Perioperative airway obstruction; hypoxia
	• Asthma	β-agonist or theophylline drugs; pulmonary hypertension or cor pulmonale; steroid use: adrenal insufficiency, postoperative hypoxia
	• Cystic fibrosis	Drug interactions; pulmonary toilet; pulmonary dysfunction; reactive airways
	• Recent cold	Possible lower respiratory tract infection; reactive airways
Gastrointestinal/ hepatic system	• Vomiting, diarrhea	Electrolyte abnormality; dehydration; full stomach
	• Growth failure	Possible anemia
	• Gastroesophageal reflux	Risk of aspiration; reactive airways; hypoxia
	• Jaundice	Altered drug metabolism; risk of hypoglycemia
	• Frequency, nocturia	Unrecognized diabetes; urinary tract infection
	• Renal failure/dialysis	Electrolyte abnormality; hyper- or hypovolemia; anemia; medication history
Endocrine/ metabolic system	• Hypoglycemia	Hypoglycemia
	• Diabetes	Insulin requirement; intraoperative hypoglycemia
	• Steroid therapy	Adrenal insufficiency
Haematologic system	• Anemia	Transfusion requirements
	• Bruising, excessive bleeding	Coagulopathy
	• Sickle cell disease	Anemia; transfusion; hydration; oxygenation; orthopedic tourniquet use
	• AIDS	Susceptibility to infection; infectious risk to medical personnel
Allergies	• Medication history	Drug reactions; drug interactions
Dental	• Loose teeth	Dental trauma; aspiration of tooth

Laboratory data

Laboratory procedures should be performed based on clinical examination and patient history [15]. The uselessness of routine preoperative examinations has been highlighted by many international studies [16-19]. Though in our country there is a trend in medical practice to omit routine blood tests in healthy children scheduled for minor surgery [20, 21], some paediatric anaesthesiologists remain rather "conservative", feeling that a larger number of examinations is necessary and might provide better medicolegal protection.

It is important to remember that routine laboratory testing exposes the child to painful procedures to detect clinically irrelevant abnormalities that do not modify the anaesthesiologic procedure. The clinically relevant elements can usually be determined by a careful assessment based on the patient's history and physical examination.

It is desirable that in the near future "consensus conferences" convene which might reduce the distance between the two positions to standardize paediatric anaesthesiologist practice.

Routine chest X-rays are not always necessary either, but may be useful when a serious pulmonary illness is suspected [22].

Special problems

Upper respiratory tract infection

The anaesthesiologist must often evaluate patients affected by an upper respiratory tract infection (URI). Numerous studies report a higher incidence of laryngismus, bronchospasm, and intra- or post-operative hypoxia among these patients [23-25] and, for this reason, elective surgery should be postponed for 2-4 weeks for patients with URI.

A different decision could be taken in patients constantly suffering from URI for otolaryngologic surgery (adenotonsillectomia, myringotomy) [26] and, generally for patients whose pathologic condition is a cause or aggravation of a URI (cleft palate). In some cases scheduled surgery cannot be postponed for long and, consulting the surgeon, the anaesthesiologist will decide the best timeframe.

Whatever decision is made, it should be discussed with the child's parents, who should be informed of potential risks and benefits.

Asthma

Elective surgery must be postponed when asthmatic patients present with even slight wheezing upon auscultation or if they had an acute asthmatic crisis during the last 4 weeks.

The asthmatic patient must be accurately examined and in most serious cases baseline ECG, chest X-rays and blood gas analysis should be obtained; normally, medication should be maintained up to the morning of the surgery and the theophylline blood level should be monitored (10-20 µg/ml provides the optimal therapeutic effect). Supplemental steroid therapy and/or nebulized β-adrenergic agents before induction can be used to reduce the risk of bronchospasm. For anaesthesia drugs with a strong bronchodilator effect such as halotane (interaction with theophylline and β-stimulants!) should be prefered and those with more histamine-releasing effects avoided.

Heart murmur

During the medical examination the paediatric anaesthesiologist frequently finds that the patient is affected by a heart murmur not noticed before. Some general rules can be used to examine such a patients. If the patient is completely asymptomatic and the heart murmur is soft, systolic, and variable, this will probably not cause haemodynamic effects and will not interfere significantly with anaesthesia. Loud, constant, transmitted diastolic heart murmurs are likely due to relevant heart defects [27]. In such cases, the cardiologist must be consulted and, possibly an echocardiogram performed. Appropriate antibiotic therapy must be prescribed for prophylaxis of subacute bacterial endocarditis in patients with ascertained defects [28].

Preterm infant

Former preterm infants are patients at risk of apnea in the first 12-24 h after general anaesthesia. The main risk factor is their postconceptual age: apnea occurs in about 10% of infants younger than 60 weeks of postconceptual age and this percentage rises to about in 25% of cases for infants younger than 44 weeks [29]. Additional risk factors are prior history of apnea at home, respiratory distress, intubation and mechanical ventilation, or anemia [30]. The use of regional anaesthesia techniques may reduce the incidence of postoperative apnea [31]. Apnea monitoring is absolutely necessary during the first postoperative 24 h for any infant considered at risk.

Seizures

The patient suffering from a seizure disorder will be appropriately assessed, recording the type of seizures, their frequency, the kind of anticonvulsant drugs that the child is taking and checking their possible interaction with anaesthetic drugs. Elective surgery is postponed in children whose seizure disorders are not under adequate pharmaceutical control. In contrast, it is necessary to bear in mind that patients with well-controlled epilepsy may present breakthrough seizures caused by hospitalization stress, protracted fasting, or surgical trauma. In the most complex cases, serum concentration of anticonvulsant drugs should be measured to assure therapeutic level. The scheduled medication should be taken up to the morning of surgery, although because of the long plasma half-life of anticonvulsants allows a dose can be missed without significant consequences. If there will be a prolonged postoperative fasting, an appropriate i.v. or i.m. therapy should be instituted (scheduled).

References

1. Roizen MF (1990) Preoperative evaluation. In: Miller RD (ed) Anaesthesia, 3rd ed. Churchill Livingstone, New York, pp 763-798
2. Krane EJ, Davis PJ, Smith RM (1996) Children preoperative praparation. In: Motoyama Davis (ed) Smith's anaesthesia for infants and children, 6th ed. Mosby, St Louis, pp 213-228
3. Stewart DJ (1994) Preoperative valuation and preparation for surgery. In: Gregory GA (ed) Paediatric anaesthesia, 3rd ed. Churchill Livingstone, New York, pp 179-195
4. Pusch F, Wilding E, Grabner CM (1998) Principles in peri-operative paediatric medicine. Anaestesia 53:69-71
5. Fisher QA, Feldman MA, Wilson MD (1994) Paediatric responsabilities for preoperative evaluation. J Pediatr 125:675-684
6. Means LJ, Ferrari LR, Fishe QA et al (1996) Evaluation an preparation of paediatric patients undergoing anaesthesia. Paediatrics 98:502-507
7. Maxwell LG, Deshpande JK, Wetzel RC (1994) Preoperative evaluation in children. Ped Clin North Am 41:93-110
8. Macarthur AJ, Macarthur C, Bevan JC (1995) Determinants of paediatric day surgery cancellation. J Clin Epidemiol 48(4):485-489
9. Setlock MA, Cotter TP, Rosner D (1993) Latex allergy: failure of prophylaxis to prevent severe reaction. Anaesth Analg 76:650-652
10. Birnbaum J, Porri F, Pradal M et al (1994) Allergy during anaesthesia. Clin Exp Allerg 24:915-921
11. Means LJ, Fescorla FJ (1995) Latex anaphylaxis: report of occurrence in two paediatric surgical patients and review of the literature. J Pediatr Surg 30:748-751
12. Schreiner MS, Tribwasser A, Keon TP (1990) Ingestion of liquids compared with preoperative fasting in paediatric outpatients. Anaesthesiology 72:593-597
13. Splinter WM, Schaefer JD, Zunder IH (1990) Clear fluids three hours before surgery do not affect the gastric fluid contents of children. Can J Anaesth 36:55-58
14. Motoyama EK, Davis PJ (1996) Smith's Anaesthesia for infants and children, 6th ed. Mosby, St-Louis, p 217
15. MacPherson (1993) Preoperative laboratory testing: should any tests be "routine" before surgery? Med Clin North Am 77:289-308
16. O' Connor ME, Drasner K, (1990) Preoperative laboratory testing of children undergoing elective surgery. Anaesth Analg 70:176-180
17. Steward DJ (1991) Screening tests before surgery in children. Can J Anaesth 38:693-695
18. Narr BJ, Warner ME, Schroeder DR et al (1997) Outcomes of patients with no laboratory assessment before anaesthesia and a surgical procedure. Mayo Clin Proc 72(6):505-509
19. Patel RI, Dewitt L, Hannallah RS (1997) Preoperative laboratory testing in children undergoing elective surgery: analysis of current practice. J Clin Anaesth 9(7):569-575
20. Borrometi F, Peluso V, Carpino V (1997) Esami di laboratorio preoperatori di routine in chirurgia paediatrica d'elezione: studio retrospettivo su 3000 casi. First National SARNePI Congress

21. Meneghini L, Zadra N, Zanette G et al (1998) The usefulness of routine preoperative laboratory test for one-day surgery in helthy children. Pediat Anaesth 8:11-15
22. Wood RA, Hoekelman RA (1981) Value of the chest x-ray as a screening test for elective surgery in children. Paediatrics 67:447-449
23. Liu LMP, Ryan JF, Cote CJ et al (1988) Influence of upper respiratory infections on critical incidents in children during anaesthesia. Abstracts World Congress of Anaesthesiology
24. Cohen MM, Cameron CB (1991) Should you cancel the operation when a child has an upper respiratory tract infection? Anesth Analg 72:282-288
25. Rolf N, Coté CJ (1992) Frequency and severity of desaturation events during general anaesthesia in children with and without upper respiratory infections. J Clin Anaesth 4:200-203
26. Levy L, Pandit UA, Randel GI et al (1992) Upper respiratory tract infections and general anaesthesia in children. Anaesthesia 47:678-682
27. Rosenthal A (1984) How to distinguish between innocent and pathologic murmurs in childhood. Pediatr Clin North Am 31:1229
28. Dajani AS, Bisno AL, Chung KJ et al (1990) Prevention of bacterial endocarditis recommendations by the American Heart Association. JAMA 264:2919-2922
29. Malviya S, Swartz J, Lerman J (1993) Are all preterm infants younger than 60 weeks postconceptual age at risk for postanaesthetic apnea? Anaesthesiology 78:1076-1081
30. Coté CJ, Zaslavsky S, Downes JJ et al (1986) Postoperative apnea in former preterm infants after inguinal herniorrharphy. Anaesthesiology 82:809-822
31. Kurth CD, Spitze AR, Broennle AM et al (1987) Postoperative apnea in preterm infants. Anaesthesiology 66:483-488

Chapter 2

Clinical approach, monitoring and decision making in paediatric intensive care

P. Baines, C. Moores

Clinical approach

Organisation

Critically ill children are best cared for in specialised paediatric intensive care units, not, as is sometimes practised, on general paediatric wards, or on adult intensive care units. Though it seems reasonable to accept that the care of critically ill children by specialised medical, nursing and technical staff with more regular experience of the care of critically ill children will improve the quality of care, this is not accepted by all.

Research from other areas of medicine shows clear benefits from concentrating the management of less common disease in particular centres [1]. This is supported by work specifically on paediatric intensive care. Pollack et al. [2], in a study in the USA, found that although the mortality rate in tertiary centres was higher than in nontertiary centres; once allowance was made for disease severity (PRISM) [3], there was an eightfold higher risk of dying when more severely ill patients were cared for in nontertiary than in tertiary centres. Gemke et al. [4] studied paediatric intensive care admissions in the Netherlands, finding an odds ratio of 2.5 for mortality in nontertiary centres. Shann et al. [5] compared the mortality of children in Victoria, Australia, a region with centralised paediatric intensive care, with a region in the UK where PICU was more fragmented. Adjusting for severity of illness using the PIM [6] score, they found an odds ratio for risk of death of 2.1 in the UK compared with Victoria. Regionalisation of intensive care allows ready access to support from other paediatric specialities (cardiology, nephrology and surgical, amongst others), which is important in the management of critically ill children.

Which of these factors is more important in improving the care of critically ill children is uncertain. Pollack's group has attempted to tease out some factors, finding that the presence of an intensivist reduced the odds ratio for dying to 0.65 in the USA [7].

Accepting a clear case for centralisation of critical care facilities for children presents further requirements. Clinicians in the nontertiary hospitals must maintain adequate skills to resuscitate and stabilise children prior to transfer to the tertiary paediatric centre, even though their paediatric clinical caseload may decline as paediatric services are centralised. Transport services to ensure the timely and safe transfer of critically ill children need to be developed or formalised and funded. The relationship of the tertiary paediatric centre to other tertiary centres, such as cardiac or neurological, will need to be clarified.

A dedicated paediatric transport service would seem to improve the quality of care during transport. Although the issue has not been subjected to a randomised trial, all the published case series suggest fewer problems when children are transferred by dedicated teams (Table 1).

A developing concept is the idea that a critical care transport team transports the intensive care to the child rather than transferring the child to the intensive care. These approaches are contrasted as "scoop and run" contrasted with "stay and play". Stabilisation prior to transport is vital, and transfer should be delayed until the child is stabilised. Transfer is then safer.

Recommendations for the composition and requirements for retrieval teams have been made for the UK [13].

Table 1. Quality of care during transport

Specialised team	Nonspecialised team	Reference
	117 children: 21% physiological deterioration or equipment failure in 21%	Kanter 1989, USA [8]
25 errors in 96 children	64 errors in 34 transfers	McNab 1991, Canada [9]
	56 children: 75% incidence of complications	Barry 1994, UK [10]
49 children: equipment errors, 2%; physiological deterioration, 12%	92 children: equipment errors, 20%; physiological deterioration, 11%	Edge 1994, USA [11]
51 transfers: 2 had preventable deterioration		Britto 1995, UK [12]

Resuscitation and stabilisation

Resuscitation of children is important prior to any attempts at definitive management.

This is best guided by a structured approach, prioritising the steps to be performed sequentially, which is described as the ABC approach to resuscitation. The approach ensures basic cardiorespiratory stability prior to concentrating on management appropriate to the specific diagnosis in that child. Courses (APLS in the UK and the PALS course in the USA, which has extended to other countries) have been developed to familiarise doctors who rarely encounter critically ill children with practical aspects of paediatric resuscitation and stabilisation. These courses combine both theoretical lectures and the tuition of specific skills such as airway management and tracheal intubation. Obviously, practical skills are vital in the resuscitation of critically ill children, and there is concern that retention of skills taught on these short courses may be suboptimal [14].

There are some important differences in the resuscitation of children and adults [15]; most importantly, although adults commonly collapse from a cardiac cause, this is less common in children, collapse more commonly being a consequence of airway or respiratory disease.

The normal values for heart rate and blood pressure are different in children of different ages and need to be considered as appropriate targets for resuscitation [16].

Blood glucose should be determined early in resuscitation as critically ill children are prone to hypoglycaemia.

Before concentrating on the more advanced areas of paediatric critical care practice it is vital to ensure the basic aspects of clinical care are correct. These include areas such as temperature homeostasis and adequate but not overwhelming fluid resusucitation.

Endotracheal tube misplacement following poor taping technique, endotracheal tube obstruction following poor endotracheal tube toilet, and poor humidification potentially cause major morbidity, from easily avoidable causes. Good basic clinical care by both medical and nursing staff is a prerequisite of good critical care medicine.

Specific conditions

Diaphragmatic hernia

Classically the neonate with a congenital diaphragmatic hernia (CDH) was recognised by the combination of scaphoid abdomen, respiratory distress, and absent breath sounds over one hemi-thorax, more usually the left side. The characteristic chest radiographic findings of bowel in the chest are usually recognised after intubation. Fifteen to twenty percent of hernias will occur on the right, these having a worse prognosis. A nasogastric tube should be placed to drain the bowel. Feeds should be avoided to prevent bowel distension and further compression of the lung. Increasingly, these hernias are diagnosed antenatally, with delivery close to the surgical unit a consideration.

These children will usually be promptly transferred to a paediatric surgical unit, though it must be recognised that stabilisation prior to safe transfer is more important than speed. Some children only have minimal respiratory distress, and indeed some are not diagnosed until some years later.

Outcome is related best to development of the lung. The lung on the side of the diaphragmatic hernia is obviously underdeveloped. The lung on the contralateral side is also underdeveloped. As well as being small, the lungs are also abnormal, with changes in the pulmonary vasculature. The heart is abnormal, with poor development of the left ventricle. Several theories to explain this have been proposed, though it may reflect the reduced blood flow through the lung during fetal life. Other abnormalities may be present in children with CDH, some of these being associated with certain syndromes.

Initially therapy involved emergency surgical correction of the hernia as soon as the diagnosis was made, in the belief that the lung was collapsed by the hernia. As it is now appreciated that what determines outcome is pulmonary hypoplasia, and that operation usually worsens respiratory function [17], there is a trend to later correction. Operation is delayed until the child is stable [18].

The initial approach was one of aggressive ventilation maintaining a low $PaCO_2$, high pH, and good oxygenation (based on values which defined survivors). Alkalosis served to reduce the pulmonary arterial pressures. Operation was contemplated once ductal shunting resolved. Since the determinant of outcome is lung growth, and as aggressive ventilation promotes lung fibrosis by damaging the lungs, a more relaxed approach is now taken. Hypercapnia is tolerated, providing preductal oxygenation saturation is maintained. Through most of these changes overall mortality remained relatively constant [19].

Novel techniques have been used in the management of children with CDH. The success of high frequency oscillation (HFOV) in other forms of neonatal respiratory failure led to its use in CDH, where the ability to ventilate with less ventilator-induced lung injury whilst stabilising the child is appealing. As always with the use of HFOV, if there is no improvement within the first few hours, a significant improvement is unlikely [20].

Inhaled nitric oxide (iNO) has been used in infants with CDH, though there are no formal trials of this therapy. In cases reports iNO has improved oxygenation, though the response seems unreliable.

Extracorporeal membrane oxygenation (ECMO) is used as rescue therapy for other forms of neonatal respiratory distress [21] and has been applied to children with diaphragmatic hernias. The use of ECMO in children with CDH is controversial. If outcome is determined by the degree of pulmonary hypoplasia, there may not be adequate time for lung growth during an acceptably short course of ECMO. However, if pulmonary hypertension is the principle concern, ECMO may be appropriate. Children with diaphragmatic hernia tend to be on longer ECMO runs than those with other causes of respiratory failure. A comparison of two centres, one of which routinely uses ECMO, the other of which rarely uses ECMO, has been reported [19] with no difference in mortality. Data from the UK ECMO trial showed that of 18 children with CDH who achieved the entry criteria, four survived following treatment with ECMO (compared with no survivors of 17 children allocated to conventional mangement). However, at 1 year only one of the four survivors was normal [22].

All the usual steps to maintain physiological stability, attention to thermoregulation, maintenance of normal blood glucose levels, and ensuring an appropriate fluid balance, amongst other features, are important in the management of infants with CDH.

Cardiac disease

In babies who collapse at birth or shortly there after the question of the presence of cardiac disease may be raised. It is difficult to refute a diagnosis of cardiac disease outwith a cardiac centre, as exclusion of cardiac disease is more difficult than confirming a cardiac diagnosis. Some conditions, particularly total anomalous pulmonary venous drainage, are very difficult to exclude.

The important steps remain the initial resuscitation of the child, again ensuring cardiorespiratory stability. Intubation may be required, along with adequate venous access and maintenance of a normal blood sugar.

Exclusion of noncardiac disease is important. Neonatal pulmonary vasculature is well developed, and respiratory disease producing pulmonary hypertension may cause desaturation following shunting through the patent foramen ovale.

If there is concern regarding cardiac disease following immediate resuscitation, it is important to obtain a chest radiograph and electrocardiograph (ECG). The chest radiograph may demonstrate lung disease of sufficient severity to account for the desaturation or may show features suggestive of cardiac disease (including a large cardiac shadow, or abnormal cardiac silhouette or abnormal pulmonary vascularity). The normal neonatal ECG differs from the normal ECG of older children, being of faster rate and having relative right ventricular dominance. Again, specific cardiac conditions are associated with specific features on the ECG [23].

Children who collapse shortly after birth as a result of cardiac disease usually have predominantly either cyanosis or heart failure, though once severely ill, the inciting event may become difficult to recognise.

In children with cyanosis the hyperoxia test may be useful. The child is exposed to 100% oxygen, either in a headbox, or more easily if intubated. If there is cyanotic heart disease, the PaO_2 will usually remain below 100 mmHg. If the problem is one of pulmonary disease, the PaO_2 will usually exceed 100 mmHg. Blood for PaO_2 should be taken from the right arm to exclude right to left shunting at the ductal level. The test requires some interpretation. In the presence of severe lung disease (which would be obvious on the chest radiograph) the PaO_2 may not exceed 100 mmHg. If the child is hypoventilating, even though 100% oxygen may be administered, the alveolar PO_2 may be much lower than predicted, and so the interpretation of the hyperoxia test also depends on a relatively normal $PaCO_2$. A normal $PaCO_2$ is all the more important in neonates as the pulmonary vasculature is more sensitive to acidosis and a rise in $PaCO_2$ will causes pulmonary vasoconstriction with hypoxia as a consequence of shunting.

One of the commoner pulmonary causes of desaturation which may be confused with cardiac disease is persistent fetal circulation (PFC), also called persistent pulmonary hypertension of the newborn (PPHN). In these children the pulmonary vascular resistance decreases as the child is made alkalotic, either by administration of bicarbonate or by hyperventilation, which may be combined with the hyperoxia test as a hyperoxia hypocarbia test. There is a sudden change in saturation as the pH rises, with fall of PVR, not a gradual change. In these children the chest radiograph are usually relatively normal, though there may be minor changes.

If the diagnosis of cyanotic heart disease is made, the child's condition can often be improved by intravenous infusion of prostaglandin E1. This opens the ductus arteriosus and improves flow by allowing supply of the pulmonary circulation from the systemic circulation, or in case of transposition of the great arteries, by allowing mixing. Prostaglandin should be started at 10-20 ng/kg/ per minute and can be escalated, depending on the response, to 100-200 ng/kg/ per minute. At higher doses apnoeas, fever and vasodilation producing hypotension are more common.

In these circumstances the child should be transferred to a cardiac centre for diagnosis, usually by echocardiography, and further management.

If the symptoms are more those of congestive cardiac failure, the differential diagnoses include coarctation, the hypolastic left heart syndrome, patent ductus arteriosus (PDA), cardiomyopathy and disturbances of cardiac rhythm.

Coarctation is recognised by the features of heart failure with a marked difference between the femoral pulses and the upper limb pulses. Symptoms develop as the duct closes, so children present from a few days of age. A pressure gradient may be demonstrated between the lower limb and upper limb. Hypoplastic left heart syndrome (HLHS, the commonest cause of death from cardiac cause in under 1-year-old children) presents at a similar age, with similar features, though without the disparity in pulses. On the contrary, the femoral pulses may be better than the upper limb pulses.

These conditions are usually diagnosed by echocardiography. In both initial treatment is with prostaglandin, as described for cyanotic heart disease, to open the ductus arteriosus and allow perfusion of the sytemic circulation by blood from the pulmonary circulation. Once the child is stable, operative repair of the coarctation can be performed. The management of HLHS is more controversial, but operation (the Norwood procedure) is usually offered.

PDA is more often a complication of prematurity. If the duct remains open, then, as the pulmonary vascular resistance falls with age, blood flow to the lungs increases and heart failure develops. This usually occurs some days after birth. The clinical features are those of wet lung fields, hepatomegaly and a systolic murmur. Again, the diagnosis is usually confirmed by echocardiography. If the PDA causes symptoms, a course of indomethacin may be used to close it, and should this prove unsuccessful, surgery may be necessary.

Disturbances of rhythm, both bradycardia and tachycardia, may cause cardiovascular symptoms. A diagnosis of bradycardia may have been made antenatally, often being confused with the bradycardia of fetal distress. Maternal systemic lupus erythematosus predisposes to fetal heart block. Isoprenaline to accelerate the rate, or pacing, may be necessary.

Tachycardia may cause heart failure as well as diagnostic confusion. It is necessary to separate an appropriate acceleration of heart rate in an ill child from tachycardia causing heart failure as the primary illness. Tachycardias may be caused by specific diseases, such as the long QT syndrome. The treatment is to slow the heart rate. If supraventricular tachycardia is the problem, therapy will include adenosine or cardioversion. Other agents may be required to control the heart rate should sinus rhythm be unstable. Control of neonatal tachycardias is often difficult.

Decision making

In many cases children have single system disease. Operative management should be deferred until the child is resuscitated, ensuring perioperative stability. Important examples include the management of CDH as discussed above and children with pyloric stenosis. These children present with hypochloraemic alkalosis as a consequence of electrolyte losses in the vomit. Operation should not be contemplated until the child is appropriately resuscitated and blood biochemistry returns towards normal.

In recent years it has been recognised that the performance of nonelective procedures after hours, often by junior surgeons and anaesthetists, is not optimal management [24]. Increasingly, the need for urgent surgery to be performed during routine operating lists, with space maintained for urgent cases, is being recognised. There are some true emergencies, where stability will not be assured until the operation is performed, and operation and resuscitation are carrried out at the same time. Examples include penetrating trauma and bleeding oesophageal varices.

In children with multisystem disease, some priorities must be established, concentrating on the problems which need immediate management, the others being delayed for later correction.

Scoring systems

Scoring systems designed to predict outcome were developed for critically ill adults and have been extended to paediatric intensive care. It might be hoped that they would guide clinical management.

Two "all comer" scores are used to determine disease severity in paediatric critical care practice, PRISM [3] and PIM [6]. A newer version of PRISM, PRISM III, has recently been produced [25] though it is less commonly used than PRISM. PRISM is used more commonly than PIM and considers 14 variables over a variable time period (from 8 to just under 32 h), generating a predicted risk of mortality for each patient. PIM, a more recently described score, uses fewer variables and is a point of the ICU first contact score. This makes PIM easier to collect. A concern of allowing data collection up to 32 h, given that many of the deaths occur in the first 24 h, is that PRISM merely recognises death is occurring rather than predicting it.

Separate from "all comer" scores are those which relate to specific disease. As an example, many scores are described for meningococcal disease [26] with more described each year.

It is important to appreciate the common limitations of these scores. They describe the outcome of groups of patients, rather than making useful predictions for individual patients. Overall, three of ten patients with an average predicted mortality of 30% will die, and one of ten patients with an average predicted mortality of 90% will survive. Scores produce a predicted risk of mortality and do not produce categorical outcomes: this patient will survive/this patient will not. The scores, then, are more useful for assessing unit performance, either against other units or through time. The scoring sytems are not useful in predicting the outcome of individual patients, though there are attempts to produce scoring systems for this purpose.

Variance in actual mortality from mortality predicted by a score, whether higher or lower, may not reflect the performance of the ICU. A difference in patient population may alter the calibration of the score. This has been well described for adult scoring systems. Similarly, a difference in referral pattern or pre-ICU management may alter the performance of any scoring system.

It has been suggested that scoring sytems such as PIM which use point of first contact data may be used for triage, to decide the need for ICU admission.

A child who has multiple diseases, each of which on their own would be treatable, may be one of the more difficult cases to consider. It is important to consider the interaction of disease in the child, accepting that the presence of two or more diseases may have a more than additive effect. For example, the survival of children with tracheoesophageal fistula of birth weight >1 500 g without major cardiac abnormality is 97%. With birth weight less than 1 500 g or major cardiac abnormality it declines to 59%, and with both, in addition to tracheoesophageal fistula, the survival is 22% [27].

Approach to withdrawal of treatment

On occasion, it is apparent that children will not survive their time on the intensive care unit, or, should they survive, will be left with such severe damage that withdrawal of therapy is contemplated. In these instances it is the likelihood of cerebral recovery which is the most important consideration.

These are obviously difficult decisions. It is important to act in the best interests of the child. Decisions should be made jointly by doctors, nurses and parents. The wishes and concerns of the child should be considered when decisions are made, should they be known, though this is more relevant for older children.

At times controversy is inevitable, reflecting differences in belief and experience amongst those who need to reach agreement. Although the parents obviously have a large input into the decision, the principle concern must remain the child's interests [28].

The way in which treatment is withdrawn will depend on the circumstances. Although the approach is described as withdrawal of therapy, it is more usually a change in direction of therapy from one with the aim of cure to one where the prime aim is relief of discomfort or suffering. The provision of adequate sedation and analgesia are vital. In some units all-invasive therapy (intubation and inotropes) are withdrawn. In other units a limit is placed on escalation of therapy.

Monitoring

Anaesthesia

In recent years the use of monitoring in the operating theatre has increased, in response to attempts to reduce anaesthetic mortality and morbidity, which are higher in children than in adults, and highest in neonates [29].

The most important monitor in the operating theatre is the presence of a trained and vigilant anaesthetist. In the absence of an adequately skilled anaesthetist to respond to data or alarms generated by a monitor, the monitor is useless. Furthermore, if the monitoring is overly complex or awkward to use, by distracting the anaesthetist's attention from the patient, monitoring may be harmful.

Various groups have defined minimal monitoring which should be used for all patient groups [30]. These emphasise the importance in all patients of the presence of an appropriately trained anaesthetist. For monitoring, they suggest which parameter or physiological system should be monitored rather than describing precise ways of monitoring. Monitoring may be continuous (the display of the ECG on a monitor) or intermittent (intermittently feeling a patient's radial pulse).

Two major groups of monitors may be described: those which monitor the patient and those which monitor the delivery of anaesthesia.

Monitors of the delivery of anaesthesia

The anaesthetic machine should be checked carefully prior to the start of anaesthesia.

Monitors commonly used include FiO_2 monitoring and ventilator alarms. Both are obviously important.

An important feature of equipment monitors is that they alert the anaesthetist to the problem before that problem causes physiological perturbation. For example, a ventilator disconnect alarm set at an appropriate delay will warn of the disconnect before the saturation starts to fall, which is a later and more dangerous mode of detection of ventilation disconnection.

More proximal monitors, such as those which monitor the pipeline supplies of gases, are also important in the delivery of safe anaesthesia.

Patient monitors

The degree of monitoring depends on several factors amongst which are the condition of the patient and the procedure being performed. For some short, simple procedures the only monitor used may be a pulse oximeter. For most cases, however, monitoring will usually include pulse oximeter, end-tidal capnography and noninvasive blood pressure measurements. In young babies temperature is more commonly monitored and this is often done with an oesophageal temperature probe, which may also be used as a stethoscope.

The more complex the procedure and the younger and iller the child is, the more monitoring will be used.

Intensive care monitoring

In general, monitoring on the intensive care unit resembles monitoring used in operating theatres. It facilitates safe transfer of patients between theatre and intensive care if the monitoring used on intensive care and theatres is the same.

Again monitors on the intensive care unit may be separated into those which monitor the patient and those which monitor the delivery of care.

The equipment used on the intensive care unit is becoming increasingly complex and has inbuilt monitoring sytems. Such systems include the ventilators and syringe or infusion pumps. The more complex the equipment, the more training is required before its use and the more opportunities are present for equipment malfunction or misuse. Staff must be experienced and familiar with the equipment used on the intensive care unit.

Patient monitoring

Most ventilated patients in intensive care will be continuously monitored by ECG and pulse oximetry. Depending on their condition, blood pressure monitoring will be either by invasive arterial line, which also allows sampling of blood, or by intermittent cuff blood pressure measurements. End-tidal carbon dioxide monitoring is becoming increasingly common.

Apart from the general monitors used on the intensive care unit, specific monitors may be used for specific conditions. Examples of these include intracranial pressure monitoring for the management of head injuries and the various monitors used for patients with shock: PAOP measurements with a ballon-tipped flow-directed catheter, measurements of cardiac output, measurements of SvO_2, and gastric tonometry, amongst others. These specific monitors are not discussed further in this review.

Most of the monitors have alarms. For these alarms to have any value, appropriate limits need to be set and reviewed as the patient's condition changes.

Monitoring during transport should be of the same standard as that practised on the intensive care unit. This is facilitated by the development of portable multi-modal monitors of small size with a good battery life.

Audit of practice

To ensure that quality of care is maintained it is important to audit practice on the intensive care unit. Exactly how this is achieved varies between units. Most units will review their practice over time. In addition, individual cases may be studied further in regular morbidity and mortality meetings. An important mode of review is the use of critical incident reporting.

References

1. Jenkins KJ, Newburger JW, Lock JE, Davis RB, Coffman GA, Iezzoni LI (1995) In-hospital mortality for surgical repair of congenital heart defects: preliminary observations of variation by hospital caseload. Paediatrics 95:323-330
2. Pollack MM, Alexander SR, Clarke N, Ruttiman UE, Tesselaar HM, Bachulis AC (1991) Improved outcomes from tertiary centre paediatric intensive care: statewide comparison of tertiary and nontertiary care facilities. Crit Care Med 19:150-159
3. Pollack MM, Ruttiman UE, Getson PR (1988) Paediatric risk of mortality (PRISM) score. Crit Care Med 16:1110-1116
4. Gemke RJBJ, Bonsel GJ (1995) Paediatric intensive care assessment of outcome study group. Comparative assessment of paediatric intensive care: a national multicentre study. Crit Care Med 23:238-245
5. Pearson G, Shann F, Barry P, Vyas J, Thomas D, Powell C, Field D (1997) Should paediatric intensive care be centralised? Trent versus Victoria. Lancet 349:1213-1217
6. Shann F, Pearson G, Slater A, Wilkinson K (1997) Paediatric index of mortality (PIM): a mortality prediction model for children in intensive care. Intensive Care Med 23:201-207
7. Pollack MM, Cuerdon TT, Patel KM (1994) Impact of quality of care factors on paediatric intensive care mortality. JAMA 272:941
8. Kanter RK, Tompkins JM (1989) Adverse events during interhospital transport: physiologic deterioration associated with pretransport severity of illness. Paediatrics 84:43-48
9. McNab AJ (1991) Optimal escort for interhospital transport of paediatric emergencies. J Trauma 31:205-209
10. Barry PW, Ralston C (1994) Adverse events occurring during interhospital transfer of the critically ill. Arch Dis Child 71:8-11
11. Edge WE, Kanter RK, Weigle CGM, Walsh RF (1994) Reduction of morbidity in interhospital transport by specialised paediatric staff. Crit Care Med 22:1186-1191
12. Britto J, Nadel S, Maconchie I, Levin M, Habibi P (1991) Morbidity and severity of illness during interhospital transfer: impact of a specialised paediatric retrieval team. Br Med J 311:836-839
13. Standards for paediatric intensive care (1996) Produced by a working party under the auspices of the Paediatric Intensive Care Society. Pub Saldatore, Hertfordshire
14. McHale SP, Brydon CW, Wood MLB, Liban JBL (1994) A survey of nasotracheal intubating skills among advanced trauma life support course graduates. Br J Anaesth 72:195-197
15. Advanced Life Support group (1993) BMJ, pp 7-12
16. The National heart, lung and blood institute (1987). Report of the second task force on blood pressure control in children Paediatrics 79:1-25
17. Sakai H, Tmura M, Bryan AC et al (1987) The effect of surgical repair on respiratory mechanincs in congenital diaphragmatic hernia. J Paediatr 11:432
18. Bohn DJ, Pearl R, Irish MS, Glick PL (1996) Postnatal management of congenital diaphragmatic hernia. Clin Perinatol 23:843-872
19. Azarow K, Messineo A, Pearl R, Filler R, Barker G, Bohn D (1997) Congenital diaphragmatic hernia – a tale of two cities: the Toronto experience. J Paediatr Surg 32:395-400
20. Paranka MS, Clark RH, Bradley AY, Null DM (1995) Predictors of failure of high frequency oscillatory ventilation in term infants with severe respiratory failure. J Paediatr 95:400-404
21. UK collaborative ECMO trial group (1996) UK collaborative randomised trial of neonatal extracorporeal membrane oxygenation. Lancet 348:75-82
22. The UK collaborative ECMO group (1998) Abstract the collaborative UK ECMO trial: follow up to one year of age. Paediatrics 101:690

23. Park MK (1995) Paediatric cardiology for practitioners. Mosby, St. Louis, pp 367-373
24. Lunn JN (1992) Implications of the national confidential enquiry into perioperative deaths for paediatric anaesthesia. Paediatr Anaesth 2:69-72
25. Pollack MM, Patel KM, Ruttiman UE (1997) The paediatric risk of mortality III-Acute physiology score (PRISM III)-APS: a method of assessing physiologic instability for paediatric intensive care unit patients. J Paediatr 131:575-581
26. Derkx HHF, van den Hoek J, Redekop WK, Bijlmer RPGM, Bossuyt PMM (1996) Meningococcal disease: a comparison of 8 severity scores in 125 children. Intens Care Med 22:1433-1441
27. Spitz L, Kiely E, Moorcraft JA, Drake DP (1994) At risk groups in oesophageal atresia. J Paediatr Surg 29:723-725
28. Fleischman AR, Nolan K, Dubler NN, Epstein MF, Gerben MA, Jellinek MS, Litt IF, Miles MS, Oppenheimer S, Shaw A, van Eys J, Vaughan VC (1994) Caring for gravely ill children. Paediatrics 94:433-439
29. Cohen MM, Cameron CB, Duncan PG (1990) Paediatric anaesthesia morbidity and mortality in the perioperative period. Anaesth Analg 70:160-167
30. Association of Anaesthetists (1988) Recommendations for standards of monitoring during anaesthesia and recovery. Association of Anaesthetists of Great Britain and Ireland

Chapter 3

The choice of paediatric anaesthesia system

A.E.E. Meursing

The airway and ventilation of the infant and child give rise to the most frequent complications in paediatric anaesthesia, i.e. problems in the oxygenation. An understanding of this pathology rests upon a knowledge of normal development in anatomy, physiological function and the specific differences between the adult and the paediatric airway. With this understanding and knowledge, an appropriate choice of anaesthesia system (circuit) can be made.

Airway in paediatrics

The highly vascular mucosa of the mouth is continuous with that of the larynx and trachea. The mucosa is loosely adherent to the underlying structure in most areas, but highly adherent to the vocal cords and laryngeal surface of the epiglottis. The submucosa consists of loose fibrous stroma, except on the tracheal surface of the epiglottis and the vocal cords. For this reason, most inflammatory processes of the airway above the level of the vocal cords are limited by the barrier formed by the firm adherence of the mucosa to the vocal cords.

Therefore, the epiglottitis is usually confined to the supraglottic structures and laryngo-tracheo-bronchitis does not spread above the level of the vocal cords.

Developmental anatomy

There are five major differences between the neonatal and adult airway [1-3, 5].
1. *Tongue*: the infant tongue is relatively large in proportion to the rest of the oral cavity, thus more easily obstructs the airway, especially in the neonate. The tongue is more difficult to manipulate and stabilize with a laryngoscope blade.
2. *Position of larynx*: the infant larynx is higher in the neck (C3-4) than in the adult (C4-5). The tongue is closer to the roof of the mouth and easily obstructs the airway. The more rostral location also creates difficulty in visualization of laryngeal structures; a straight laryngoscope blade better facilitates visualization of the larynx.
3. *Epiglottis*: the adult epiglottis is broad and its axis is parallel to that of the tracheal. Because the infant epiglottis is narrower, shorter and angled away from

the axis of the trachea, it is more difficult to lift the epiglottis with the tip of a laryngoscope blade.
4. *Vocal folds*: the infant vocal folds have a lower attachment anteriorly than posteriorly (angled), whereas in the adult, the axis of the vocal folds is perpendicular to that of the trachea. This anatomical feature occasionally leads to difficulty in intubation, i.e. the tip of the endotracheal tube is caught at the anterior commissure of the vocal folds.
5. *Subglottic area*: the narrowest portion of the infant larynx is the non-distensible cricoid cartilage; in the adult, it is the rima glottidis. In the adult, therefore, an endotracheal tube which traverses the glottis will pass freely into the trachea, because the airway beyond is of a larger diameter. In the child, however, an endotracheal tube might easily pass through the vocal folds but not through the subglottis. A tightly fitting endotracheal tube that compresses tracheal mucosa may cause oedema in subglottic structures (cricoid cartilage), leading to a significant increase in airway resistance upon extubation.

As the child matures (by approximately 10-12 years of age) the cricoid and thyroid cartilages grow, thus eliminating both the angulation of the vocal cords and the narrow subglottic area.

In infants and children younger than 3 years of age, the head is large in proportion to the trunk.

Airway selection

The infant's tongue is relatively large in proportion to the oropharynx and often obstructs the airway during induction of anaesthesia or loss of consciousness from any cause. It is important, therefore, to select an oropharyngeal airway of proper size to achieve unobstructed air exchange. The laryngeal mask airway (LMA) is a mask shaped to cover the entrance of the larynx (hence its name) with a tube coming out of the mouth. After insertion, air is blown into the cuff of the mask so that it seals optimally. Although primarily shaped to fit the adult larynx, it has found wide application in infancy and childhood; it is not intended for long-term use. Artificial ventilation has been used with LMA but, especially in the young infant, is recommended only for primary resuscitation purposes.

An appropriately sized uncuffed tracheal tube may be chosen according to age. In general, it is desirable to select an uncuffed tube which would result in an air leak around the 20-30 cm H_2O peak inflation pressure (PIP) in children under 10 years of age.

Preoperative preparation

The ability of the child to open the mouth must be assessed (Mallampati). Subsequently, the entrance size of the mouth, the size of the tongue, loose or missing teeth, size and configuration of palate, size and configuration of mandible, and location of larynx are verified. Is there a stridor: in- or expiratory? Are there obvious congenital anomalies which may fit a recognizable syndrome? The finding of one anomaly mandates a search for other anomalies; if a congenital syndrome is diagnosed, all anaesthetic implications must be considered.

Proper equipment must be prepared and it is advisable to have an alternative plan ready.

Choice of drugs

For a "normal" airway, anaesthesiologists will choose to use a non-depolarizing relaxant (mivacron, atracurium, rocuronium, vecuronium or pancuronium) after the administration of a sedative in an appropriate dose. Often a small dose of analgetic (fentanyl, sufentanil, alfentanil or remifentanil) to obtund airway reflexes is added. The choice of the relaxant will depend on the type of the procedure, condition of the patient, or the preference of the anaesthesiologist. In the case of a full stomach or difficult airway, most anaesthesiologists will still prefer to use suxamethonium chloride (1-2 mg·kg^{-1}). This may cause increased intracranial and ocular pressure as well as a dramatic increase in potassium chloride, leading to arrhythmia. The use of methylatropine (0.01-0.02 mg·kg^{-1}) is recommended.

As mentioned above, it is advisable to maintain spontaneous ventilation in the initial phases of management of a difficult airway. This is best achieved by using inhalational anaesthetics in either oxygen or with oxygen-enriched air by face mask or slowly titrating short-acting anaesthetics such as propofol (2-3 mg·kg^{-1}), etomidate (0.25 mg·kg^{-1}) or midazolam (0.5 mg·kg^{-1}).

Pathology

The most frequently encountered congenital abnormalities are the Pierre Robin syndrome, cricoid stenosis, hypoplasia or agenesis of bronchi or trachea, hygroma or lymphoma.

Infections necessitating anaesthesia or intensive care include abscesses, epiglottitis, Jackson tracheobronchitis and bronchopneumonia.

Our anaesthesia colleagues often support the paediatricians or ear, nose, throat specialists in removing from the airway all sorts of foreign bodies: peanuts, marbles, toys and sticks, etc.

In the emergency room, trauma or burns of the airway confront the attending physicians with a problem of managing the airway.

Metabolic diseases of infancy and childhood may cause infestation of submucous tissues such as the mucopolysaccharidoses [4].

Anaesthetic management

The components of proper preparation consist of the use of a drying agent, titrated anaesthesia, vasoconstriction of mucous membranes, preparation of patient and parents, and adequate assistance and equipment. Also, the surgeon should be made well aware of the anticipated problems.

After securing intravenous access, it is preferred to preserve spontaneous ventilation. It is imperative that the anaesthetist in charge makes an optimal attempt at laryngoscopy as multiple repeated attempts may cause laryngeal oedema and bleeding. The position of the patient is such that the longitudinal axes come as close as possible. Fortunately, the larynx of the child can rather easily be moved externally by hand. The two-anaesthetist-three hands technique as described by Brown and coworkers may be extremely useful. Prior to these steps, an alternative plan should be available: laryngeal mask, fibreoptic intubation, retrograde intubation, or a surgical airway. Risks, advantages and disadvantages should be well considered in advance and the rule "get out or get help" should never be forgotten.

Circuits [6]

Children, having higher oxygen consumption, carbon dioxide production, and minute ventilation, require higher fresh gas flows per kilogram than adults. The design of a breathing system should meet certain criteria: it should be lightweight, have a minimum number of connections, and be easy to assemble and use without error. It should reliably deliver oxygen, nitrogen, nitrous oxide, and anaesthetic vapours and should eliminate carbon dioxide. Conservation of heat and humidity are of paramount importance. By reducing water and heat loss from the patient, the system should protect the airway mucosa and reduce the risk of pulmonary complications after prolonged surgery. In addition, dead space and resistance to breathing should be minimized. In children, the monitoring of airway pressure is very important. If anaesthesia is administered, concentration of inspired gases is strongly recommended. In centres where flammable agents are still in use, non-conductivity is essential.

The most commonly used breathing system for neonates is some version of the Mapleson E or D system. Ayre's original T-piece was modified by Rees, who added an expiratory limb to prevent air dilution and an open-ended 500 ml reservoir bag to allow respiration to be monitored and positive pressure to be applied. The recently introduced ADE breathing system has never gained much popularity in Europe, despite its obvious attractions. The T-piece remains the least cumbersome breathing circuit for infants and young children, with the Magill attachment or Bain system being popular for older children.

In spontaneous respiration in infants and children, some continuous positive airway pressure (CPAP) – in intermittent positive pressure ventilation (IPPV) positive end expiratory pressure (PEEP) – is recommended up to 3 cm H_2O to prevent collapse of the smaller airways.

References

1. Davenport H (1980) The newborn patient. In: Paediatric anaesthesia, 3rd ed. Heinemann, London, pp 113-115
2. Cote CJ, Todres ID (1993) Pediatric airway. In: A practice of anaesthesia for infants and children, 2nd ed. Grune and Stratton, New York
3. Shorten GD, Armstrong DC, Roy WI, Brown L (1995) Assessment of the effect of head and neck position on upper airway anatomy in sedated paediatric patients using magnetic resonance imaging. Paediatr Anaesth 5:243-248
4. Walker RW, Darowski M, Morris P, Wraith JE (1994) Anaesthesia and mucopolysaccharidoses. A review of airway problems in children. Anaesthesia 49:1078-1084
5. Berry FA, Yemen TA (1994) Pediatric airway in health and disease. Pediatr Clin North Am 41:153-180
6. Friesen RH, McIlvaine WB (1989) Basic techniques of paediatric anaesthesia. In: Sumner E, Hatch DJ (eds) Textbook of paediatric anaesthetic practice. Bailliere Tindall, London, pp 113-139

Chapter 4

Update on inhalation anaesthesia

D.J. Hatch

Despite the introduction of topical analgesic creams, inhalational induction of anaesthesia is still widely practised in young children, especially those below the age of 3-5 years. Around 30% of anaesthetists responding to a survey in August 1995 used inhalational more frequently than intravenous induction in this age group where uptake of inhaled agents is particularly rapid.

In children the induction characteristics of the ideal inhalational agent are particularly important (Table 1) though, clearly, recovery profile, cardiovascular stability, minimal metabolism, stability in soda lime and lack of central nervous system excitation are as important as they are in adults. Cyclopropane was an agent which had many of these characteristics, giving rapid smooth induction. However, because of its explosive properties halothane was widely accepted as the least pungent of the other inhalational agents available, giving the smoothest induction with minimal risk of laryngospasm and hypoxaemia. Its disadvantages are well known and include myocardial irritability, especially in the presence of adrenaline, depression of myocardial and respiratory function, cerebral vasodilatation, biotransformation, and, rarely, hepatotoxicity. Since it is rapidly disappearing from adult anaesthetic practice, lack of familiarity with its use by younger anaesthetists will soon have to be added to this list of disadvantages.

Two new inhalational agents have recently become available in this country: sevoflurane, a fluorinated methyl isopropyl ether, and desflurane, a fluorinated methyl ethyl ether (Fig. 1). Fluorine has 0.001% of the ozone depleting activity of chlorine, so both these new drugs should be more environmentally friendly. Their physical prosperties suggest rapid uptake and elimination, especially in children (Tables 2 and 3). Desflurane, however, is extremely pungent and causes severe irritation of the upper respiratory tract if used for induction of anaesthesia. In one study, approximately half the children induced with des-

Table 1. Ideal inhalational anaesthetic for children

- Non-pungent
- Rapid induction and recovery
- Cardiovascular stability
- Minimal metabolism
- Stable in soda lime
- CNS stability

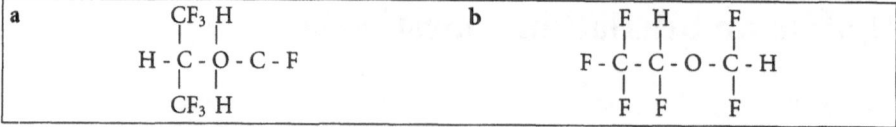

Fig. 1a,b. *Sevoflurane*, a fluorinated methyl isopropyl ether (a); *desflurane*, a fluorinated methyl ethyl ether (b)

Table 2. Sevofluorane

Molecular weight	200
Boiling point	58.5°C
Saturated vapour pressure	160 mmHg
Blood/gas	0.68
Fat/blood	48

Table 3. Desflurane

Molecular weight	168
Boiling point	22.8°C
Saturated vapour pressure	669 mmHg
Blood/gas	0.42
Fat/blood	27

flurane developed laryngospasm so that is not recommended for inhalational induction.

Sevoflurane is relatively insoluble in blood, giving it the potential for rapid induction and recovery. It is relatively non-pungent and non-irritant with a higher potency and is very useful for induction in children. It can be given from a standard vaporiser whilst a specially designed, heated, pressurised vaporiser is required for administration of desflurane. Minimum alveolar concentration (MAC) falls with age with the newer agents as it does with the older ones though interestingly data from Lerman's group in Toronto [1-4] suggest that MAC of sevoflurane does not increase over the first few months of life in the way that it does with most other agents (Table 4).

Table 4. Minimum alveolar concentrations in sevoflurane and desflurane

Age	Sevoflurane	Desflurane
Under 1 month	3.3	9.16
1-6 months	3.2	9.42
6-12 months	2.5	9.92
3-5 years	2.5	8.62
Adult	2.0	6.0

This group has also demonstrated that the MAC-sparing effect of nitrous oxide is less with the newer insoluble agents than with the more soluble predecessors. The absolute MAC values of sevoflurane at different ages are shown in Table 5.

Table 5. MAC-sparing effect of nitrous oxide

Halothane	60%
Isoflurane	40%
Sevoflurane	24%
Desflurane	20%

Pharmacodynamics

Cardiovascular system

There is fairly clear evidence that sevoflurane does not activate the sympathetic nervous system, does not cause coronary steal, and produces less myocardial sensitisation to adrenaline than halothane. Johanneson Reported 61% arrhythmias in ENT surgery with halothane, 5% with sevoflurane. There have been similar reports in dental anaesthesia. Sevoflurane produces less tachycardia than isoflurane and similar myocardial depression, which means that it is less of a myocardial depressant than halothane [5].

Nervous system

Sevoflurane has an effect similar to that of isoflurane on intracranial pressure and a minimal effect on cerebral blood flow, cerebral metabolic oxygen consumption, and autoregulation of the cerebral blood supply.

Respiratory system

Since much of the early work was carried out in countries where spontaneous breathing is less frequent during anaesthesia than in this country, there is naturally concern about the respiratory effects of this new anaesthetic agent [6]. An early paper from Japan in 1987 suggested that it might have a greater depressant effect on respiration than halothane, though this study was poorly controlled. More recently, Yamikage [7], using a respiratory inductive plethysmograph, has suggested that sevoflurane is more a respiratory depressant than halothane at high values of MAC. However, no mention is made in this paper of any attempt to validate the plethysmograph for quantitative measurements. Work by Karen Brown [8] from Montreal showed that minute ventilation and respiratory frequency were lower in infants during 1 MAC sevoflurane than during halothane anaesthesia, which may reflect different effects of these anaesthetic agents on ventilatory control. Anaesthetic management included the use of a laryngeal mask. Flow, airway pressure and $P_{et,CO2}$ were measured during spontaneous ventilation and airway occlusions. Respiratory inductive plethysmography was used to assess chest wall motion. Measurements were obtained in 30 infants and young children, randomised to receive 1 MAC halothane or sevoflurane in $N_2O:O_2$. Some respiratory depression, evidenced by a $P_{et,CO2}$ of 45 mmHg (6 kPa), was present in both groups. Minute ventilation and respiratory frequency were significantly lower during sevoflurane than halothane anaesthesia. There was no difference in respiratory drive, but the shape of the flow waveform differed according to anaesthetic agent, with peak inspiratory flow being reached later, and peak expiratory flow earlier, in the sevoflurane group. There was also significantly less thoraco-abdominal asynchrony during sevoflurane anaesthesia.

Toxicity

Although as much as 5% of sevoflurane may be metabolised, trifluoroacetic acid, one of the main hepatotoxic breakdown products of halothane metabolism, is not produced during hepatic metabolism of this agent [9-10]. Metabolism occurs by defluorination via cytochrome P450-2E1 to hexafluoroisopropanol and inorganic fluoride, which is then conjugated with glucuronic acid and excreted in the urine. Peak fluoride levels are approximately half of the widely accepted nephrotoxic level of 15 μmol and the area under the curve is significantly less than with known nephrotoxic agents such as methoxyflurane (metabolised by P450-31+P450-2E1). Although higher levels have been reported in a few studies, there have been no clinical reports of renal toxicity even in renally impaired patients or after prolonged administration of anaesthetics, despite the fact that 2 million patients worldwide have received sevoflurane. Kharash has recently suggested that intrarenal metabolism may be more important than hepatic metabolism, and it is interesting to note that the cytochrome P450 required for metabolism is not found in the human kidney.

Sevoflurane is partially degraded by carbon dioxide absorbents to produce small amounts of compound A (fluoromethyl-2,2-difluoro-1-(trifluoromethyl) vinyl ether), which causes mild renal changes in rats at concentrations above those found clinically. However, these changes depend on a β-lyase, of which rats possess more than humans. (LC50 of compound A in rats is 1 h at 1 000 ppm and 3 h at 400 ppm; 3 days per week over 8 weeks has virtually no effect up to 120ppm in rats. In humans the maximum reported concentration peaking after 9 h is 37 ppm apart from one report of 60 ppm with baralyme. Maximum reported in children at 2 l/min is 15 ppm). Levels of compound A are increased with increase in temperature and with decrease in flow rate and are higher in the presence of baralyme and fresh soda lime. Paediatric patients produce less carbon dioxide so that a given fresh gas flow rate will produce a lower concentration of compound A in a child than in an adult. However, this may be offset by the increased MAC in children and the fact that many paediatric anaesthetists may rely more heavily on inhaled anaesthetics alone rather than a balance with intravenous agents. Eger has recently suggested that compound A is genotoxic, at least in Chinese hamster ovary cells, and this may be of concern in the early stages of pregnancy. The American FDA currently does not recommend the use of sevoflurane with flow rates less than 2 l/min though the Committee on Safety of Medicines in this country has not issued a similar restriction. Further research is clearly needed to support or refute the FDA's somewhat arbitrary restriction.

Fang and co-workers in 1995 [11] pointed out that the combination of dry soda lime or baralyme with some anaesthetics agents could produce carbon monoxide, particularly if the absorber was not flushed after standing overnight. This problem is greatest with desflurane and least with halothane and sevoflurane.

Sevoflurane in clinical practice

My colleagues and I took part in the multicentre Phase III randomly controlled trials of the drug [12]. A total of 81 patients were studied, 42 randomly assigned to receive sevoflurane, and 39 to receive halothane. The groups were similar with respect to age, weight, sex, premedication and type of surgery. When the inhaled agent concentration was increased incrementally by equi-MAC steps according to a stictly defined protocol, Sevoflurane induction resulted in statistically significantly quicker ($p<0.05$) loss of eyelash reflex and end of induction (defined as regular breathing, central fixed pupils). The incidence of complications was similar in the two groups, with no serious complications in either group and no serious desaturation. Blood pressures were also similar during induction in the two groups.

Recovery characteristics were studied in 40 daycases, none of whom had sedative premedication. Recovery scores (Aldrete system) were statistically significantly lower in the sevoflurane group than with halothane. The Hannallah pain score was, however, higher in the earlier recovery period with sevoflurane, suggesting that when this drug is used, even more care must be taken to provide children with adequate analgesia [13].

Sevoflurane appears to provide a smooth rapid induction in children. The results of the early studies comparing the speed of induction of sevoflurane with halothane in children have been inconclusive, some finding sevoflurane to be more rapid than halothane as we did, and others finding no difference when inhaled concentrations are increased incrementally. In a further randomly controlled study in our own department we compared induction times using the maximum available concentration of each agent from the outset, that is to say 8% sevoflurane with 5% halothane, and found no statistically significant difference in the time to loss of eye lash reflex or end of induction between the two agents. Induction was rapid and smooth with both agents though voluntary movements before loss of consciousness (struggling) were significantly greater than halothane. A significantly larger number of parents of children who had previously had a halothane anaesthetic, when questioned, indicated a preference for sevoflurane [10, 14]. Involuntary movements after induction of anaesthesia are minimal when rapid induction with high inspired concentration is used [15].

Although neither sevoflurane or desflurane are ideal anaesthetic agents, sevoflurane in particular seems to have significant advantages over its predecessors, certainly for induction. Both sevoflurane and desflurane have advantages during maintenance and recovery, though whether these advantages justify their cost remains to be seen.

References

1. Lerman J, Oyston JP, Gallagher TM, Miyasaka K, Volgyesi GA, Burrows FA (1996) The minimum alveolar concentration (MAC) and hemodynamic effects of halothane, isoflurane and sevoflurane in newborn swine. Anaesthesiology 73:717-721
2. Lerman J, Sikich N, Kleinman S, Yentis S (1994) The pharmacology of sevoflurane in infants and children. Anaesthesiology 80:814-824
3. Lerman J (1995) Sevoflurane in paediatric anaesthesia. Anaesth Analg 81:S4-S10
4. Piat V, Dubois MC, Johanet S, Murat I (1994) Induction and recovery characteristics and hemodynamic responses to sevoflurane and halothane in children. Anaesth Analg 79:840-844
5. Ebert TJ, Harkin CP, Muzi M (1995) Cardiovascular responses to sevoflurane: a review. Anaesth Analg 81:S11-S22
6. Doi M, Takahashi T, Ikeda K (1994) Respiratory effects of sevoflurane used in combination with nitrous oxide and surgical stimulation. J Clin Anaesth 6:1-4
7. Yamakage M, Tamiya K, Horikawa D, Sato K, Namiki A (1994) Effects of halothane and sevoflurane on the paediatric respiratory pattern. Paediatr Anaesth 4:53-56
8. Brown K, Aun C, Stocks J, Jackson E, Mackersie A, Hatch D (1998) A comparison of the respiratory effects of sevoflurane and halothane in infants and young children. Anaesthesiology 89:86-92
9. Frink EJ (1995) The hepatic effects of sevoflurane. Anaesth Analg 81:S46-S50
10. Frink EJ, Green WB, Brown EA, Malcomson M, Hammond LC, Valencia FG et al (1996) Compound A concentrations during sevoflurane anaesthesia in children. Anaesthesiology 84:566-571
11. Fang ZX, Eger EI II (1995) Factors affecting the concentration of compound A resulting from the degradation of sevoflurane by soda lime and baralyme in a standard anaesthetic circuit. Anaesth Analg 81:564-568
12. Black A, Sury MJ, Hemington L, Howard R, Mackersie A, Hatch DJ (1996) A comparison of the induction characteristics of sevoflurane and halothane in children. Anaesthesia 51:539-542
13. Sury MRJ, Black A, Hemington L, Howard R, Hatch DJ, Mackersie A (1996) A comparison of the recovery characteristics of sevoflurane and halothane in children. Anaesthesia 51:543-546
14. Kataria B, Epstein R, Bailey A, Schmitz M, Backhus WW, Shoeck D et al (1996) A comparison of sevoflurane to halothane in paediatric surgical patients: results of a multicentre international study. Paediatr Anaesth 6:283-292
15. Sigston PE, Jenkins AMC, Jackson EA, Sury MRJ, Mackersie AM, Hatch DJ (1997) Rapid

inhalational induction in children: 8% sevoflurane compared with 5% halothane. Br J Anaesth 78:362-365

Chapter 5

Choice of perioperative fluids and transfusion

I. Salvo, E. Zoia

This article gives a practical approach to the perioperative fluid management of infants and children undergoing surgical procedures. Understanding disorders of the body fluids and complicated systems controlling volume, distribution, tonicity, and composition of the fluids requires a knowledge of the normal body water compartments and their chemical composition as well as the normal function of the control mechanism. Therefore, we will start briefly by discussing the normal anatomy of the body fluids.

Changes in body fluid composition and distribution

Water is the most abundant component of the body, constituting approximately 55% of the body weight of an adult and as high as 75%-80% of the normal neonate and the premature infant, respectively. Changes in total body water occur as the child grows. There is a rapid decrease in total body water as a percentage of body weight during the first year of life: from 75% at birth to approximately 70% at 6 months and 60% at 1 year of age. Thereafter, the percentage of total body water gradually decreases until the child reaches puberty, when, in boys, the percentage is greater because of the differences in body fat content between boys and girls.

Total body water is distributed into two major compartments: extracellular (ECF) and intracellular (ICF) fluids. The anatomy of body water compartments from early fetal life throughout childhood has been studied by Friss-Hansen [1]. This author emphasizes the changes in the ratio ECF/ICF water from birth to the teenage years (Table 1). The preterm infant has a very high proportion of its total body weight as water, with two-thirds residing in the ECF. As the cells grow and multiply and organs develop, the intracellular proportion of the total body water increases with a corresponding reduction in the ECF.

The normal electrolyte composition of body fluids is shown in Table 2. The total cations and anions within a particular fluid space must be equal [2]. Because of the higher ECF volume in infants, there is more sodium and chloride per kilogram and less potassium in the infant than in the adult.

The ECF is further divided into plasma volume (intravascular fluid which represents from 4% to 5% of body weight, not much higher than in adults) and interstitial fluid (fluid within the interstices of the cells and partly in the con-

Table 1. Distribution of body water between extracellular and intracellular fluids (ECF/ICF) as per cent of body weight. (Modified from[1])

Age	Total water %	Extracellular water %	Intracellular water %	ECF/ICF
0-1 day	79	43.9	35.1	1.25
1-10 days	74	39.7	34.3	1.14
1-3 months	72.3	32.2	40.1	0.80
3-6 months	70.1	30.1	40	0.75
6-12 months	60.4	27.4	33	0.83
1-2 years	58.7	25.6	33.1	0.77
2-3 years	63.5	26.7	36.8	0.73
3-5 years	62.2	21.4	40.8	0.52
5-10 years	61.5	22	39.5	0.56
10-16 years	58	18.7	39.3	0.48

nective tissue) separated by the capillary membrane, which is passively permeable to all, except cells and protein, following pressure gradients. The cellular membrane, which separates ECF from ICF is passively permeable, only to water, following osmotic pressure gradients.

The fluid compartments do not exist as fixed spaces with identical composition but rather are in constant interchange with each other and have strikingly different composition. Methods of movement of solutes and water include diffusion along electrochemical gradients, by hydrostatic pressure, osmotic forces, bulk flow, active transport, capillary blood flow, and oncotic pressure. Complex feedback control mechanisms exist to ensure homeostasis and involve the kid-

Table 2. Normal electrolyte composition of body fluids

Electrolytes	Plasma (mEq/L)	Interstitial fluid (mEq/L)	Intracellular fluid (mEq/L)
Cations			
• Sodium	140	143	±10
• Potassium	4	4	160
• Calcium	5		3.3
• Magnesium	2		26
Total cations	151		
Anions			
• Chloride	104	114	±2
• Bicarbonate	25	29	±8
• Phosphate	2		95
• Sulfate	1		20
• Organic acids	6		
• Protein	13		55
Total anions	151		

neys, lungs, circulatory, and endocrine systems and the CNS. The maintenance of extracellular volume is centered around the control of the balance of sodium (renin-angiotensin-aldosterone system), while the most important determinant of the osmolarity of the body fluids is the excretion or retention of water by the kidneys, thirst mechanisms, and the intake of water (antidiuretic hormone).

Which compartments are affected when a patient gains or loses fluid depends on the nature of the fluid and the rate at which it is gained or lost. The intravascular compartment is the most accessible one because it serves as the interface between the outside environment (through skin, lungs, kidneys, and gastrointestinal tract). It can also lose fluid directly to the outside (hemorrhage) or receive fluid directly from the outside (i.v. fluids). Next in line is the interstitial fluid, a sort of storage area where excessive fluid can be stored or drawn from very easily. Beyond that, there is the ICF, which can only be reached through the other two compartments and is protected by the cellular membrane from all fluid shifts except those generated by osmotic gradient.

Thus, a patient who loses isotonic fluid rapidly will develop shock (the loss is borne primarily by the intravascular compartment). A patient who loses isotonic fluid slowly will become dehydrated (participation of the fluids of the interstitial fluid). A patient who losses pure water will develop CNS symptoms in addition to dehydration (participation of the ICF) and will rarely develop shock because his entire body water is participating in the volume loss. In the opposite direction we have circulatory overload, peripheral edema, and cellular swelling, depending on the rate and nature of the fluid gain.

Development of renal function

Development of renal function occurs throughout the first 12 months of postnatal life. In many respects, the newborn kidney is similar to the newborn lung. Both have a high vascular resistance, resulting in a low blood flow. This low blood flow leads to a low glomerular filtration rate (one fourth that of the adult). Concentrating ability is limited so lack of fluid intake or loss of fluids leads to problems much more rapidly. In premature babies, excessive fluid administration delays closure of the arterial duct.

Sodium balance is dependent on sodium intake in neonates and daily sodium intake increases with degree of prematurity. Giving sodium free liquids will more rapidly produce hyponatremia, and sodium excretion after a sodium load is not very efficient in neonates. Shortly after birth, the transition of fetal circulation to that of the neonate results in an increase in systemic pressure and a decrease in renal vascular resistance. These changes lead to a rapid improvement in renal blood flow, and by the time the neonate is 4-5 days old there is a marked improvement in the ability of the neonate kidney to conserve fluid as well as excrete an overload.

Basic fluid and electrolyte requirements

Maintenance fluid is the amount of liquids the body needs for replacement of basal daily losses from normal functions of the lungs, skin, kidneys, and gastrointestinal tract.

Insensible water is the term given to losses through the skin and lungs. About two thirds of an infant's daily insensible water loss is through the skin, and one third through the lungs. Insensible water is affected by several factors including clothing, body temperature, respiratory rate, sedation, anaesthesia, ambient humidity, and temperature. In the neonates also gestational age, the method used for controlling body temperature, and phototherapy affect insensible water.

Fever increases insensible water loss by 7 ml/kg body weight per 24 h for each degree of temperature above 37°C [3].

The volume of insensibile water losses in milliliters can be related to the energy expended in calories with 1 ml of water being lost for each calorie metabolized [4]. Calories expended, in turn, can be related to the body weight at all ages. The fluids lost from the lungs and skin are electrolyte-free. With sweating, considerable amounts of sodium and potassium may be lost. Under normal conditions insensible water loss is approximately 30 ml per 100 calories expended through the skin and 15 ml per 100 calories through the lungs [5] (Table 3). Total net fluid loss is about 100 ml/100 calories (=1 ml/kcal).

To simplify the calculation of fluid requirements in the perioperative period we can follow the suggestions of Holiday and Segar [4] (Table 4). The electrolyte requirement is for sodium 2-3 mEq/kg/per day, and potassium 1-2 mEq/kg/per day. Potassium is usually omitted in the intraoperative period.

Table 3. Maintenance water and electrolyte requirements based on caloric expenditure. (From [5] with permission)

Body weight (kg)	Calories expended (kcal/kg/day)	Water requirements (ml/100 kcal/day)	Electrolyte requirements (mEq/100 kcal/day)
3-10	100	Insensible	
10-20	1000+50 kcal/kg for each kg>10	Skin=30 Lung=15	Sodium=2.5-3.0 Potassium=2.0-2.5
>20	1500+20 kcal/kg for each kg>20	Renal=70 Stool=5	Chloride=4.5-5.5

Preoperative assessment

The preoperative assessment of fluid volume and state of hydration varies from elective surgery with no or slowly developing fluid deficit to the severely trau-

Table 4. Daily and hourly basal maintenance fluid requirements. (From [4])

Weight (kg)	Water (24 h)	Water (h)
3-10	100 ml/kg	4 ml/kg
10-20	1 000 ml+50 ml /kg	40 ml+2 ml/kg
>20	1 500 ml+20 ml/kg	60 ml+1 ml/7kg

matized patient who is undergoing a deficit in blood and interstitial volume (rapidly occurring fluid loss) and in whom it is difficult to evaluate fluid balance. After an accurate clinical history, the evaluation of water balance should consider clinical signs (blood pressure, heart rate, skin turgor, mucous membranes, fontanelle pressure, capillary refill, peripheral perfusion, core-peripheral temperature gradient), urine (volume, electrolytes, osmolarity, urea, creatinine, acid base status), serum (electrolytes, glucose, osmolarity, hematocrit, urea, creatinine, acid base status), and body weight.

Fasting and oral liquid intake

Maintenance fluids are provided to prevent dehydration before surgery. In elective procedures, there is almost always time for an appropriate period of fasting from solids, milk, and water. Prevention of pulmonary aspiration and the effort to decrease risk of dehydration or hypoglycemia from prolonged fasting is part of the overall process of preoperative evaluation and preparation of the patient. Published evidence shows no difference in gastric residual volume or pH in children who have a standard 8-h fast compared with those allowed to ingest unlimited amounts of clear liquids (water, apple juice, sugar water) up to 2 h before anaesthesia induction [6-8]. The guidelines for preoperative fasting of the ASA based on these studies, August 1997, are summarized in Table 5 [9].

As a practical rule, one may ask the parents to withhold all milk and solids after midnight and then offer the child clear liquids until 2 h before surgery.

Table 5. Summary of fasting recommendations. (From [9])

Ingested material	Minimum fasting period
Clear liquids*	2 h
Breast milk	4 h
Solids, nonhuman milk and infant formula	8 h

* Examples of clear liquids include water, fruit juice without pulp, carbonated beverages, clear tea, and black coffee

Intraoperative fluid replacement

The aim of intraoperative fluid replacement is to provide fluid and electrolytes to prevent the kidney having to conserve or excrete large amounts of either component. Intraoperative fluid replacement is made up by *maintenance fluids* and *replacement fluids*.

1. *Maintenance fluids*: the daily and hourly basal maintenance fluid requirements are shown in Table 4. The combination of basal maintenance fluid requirements and basal electrolyte requirements results in a *hypotonic electrolyte solution*. Therefore, the usual intravenous maintenance fluids given to children by paediatricians in the ward is one fourth- to one third - strength saline. Sweat and diarrhea are hypotonic fluids as well.

2. *Replacement fluids*: losses secondary to trauma, burns, peritonitis, bleeding, and losses from the upper gastrointestinal tract are *isotonic fluids*. All these losses are very high in sodium and may all be considered as loss of ECF. Therefore every surgery, injury, or upper gastrointestinal tract loss should be replaced by an isotonic balance salt solution, that is, one that contains approximately 140 mEq/l of sodium, 100 mEq/l of chloride, and small amounts of other electrolytes.

However, for practical purposes, balanced solutions can be used to replace all types of intraoperative losses, both isotonic and hypotonic. The kidney is much better equipped to excrete overloads of sodium than it is to compensate for excess losses of sodium that are not appropriately replace [10] (Table 6).

Factors which reduce the maintenance fluid requirements by up to 70% are the use of humidified inspired gases, high antidiuretic levels (particularly after trauma), high room-humidity, and hypothyroidism. Sedation and anaesthesia also reduce basal metabolic rate and therefore fluid requirements. In renal failure restriction of fluid intake is more aggressive, down to 30% of basal plus the urine output. After cardiopulmonary bypass, fluid intake is often restricted to around 50% of basal levels and in hypothermia fluid input should be reduced by 12% per degree Celsius below 37°C.

Factors which increase the basal fluid needs up to 50% are surgery of the abdominal cavity, hyperthyroidism, radiant heaters, and phototherapy. Preterm neonates or children who are hyperventilating may need 20% above basal rates.

Table 6. Intraoperative fluid administration. (Modified from [10])

First hour
- 4 ml/kg for every hour of fluid deprivation prior to surgery

Basic hourly fluid
- Maintenance 4 ml/kg/h +
- Surgical trauma
  - mild trauma: 2-4 ml/kg/h
  - moderate trauma: 5-7 ml/kg/h
  - severe trauma: 8-12 ml/kg/h

Pyrexia increases the fluid requirements by 12% per degree Celsius and very hot ambient temperature over 31°C may mean the child needs 30% more fluid per degree Celsius above 31°C. Burn injuries result in an increased fluid requirement of about 4% per percentage of burn on the first day, decreasing to 2% per percent burn area on the second day. Much attention must be paid on gastrointestinal fluid losses. As a rule, fluid intake and output should always be charted in detail and the volume and composition of the fluid intake be titrated against losses and laboratory results.

Glucose

The sugar content of fluids should be high enough to spare breakdown of proteins and to prevent ketosis, while avoiding hyperglycemia.

It has long been thought that the paediatric patient might be at special risk for developing hypoglycemia. Hypoglycemia is defined as glycemia <30 mg/dl in neonates and glycemia <40mg/dl in older infants and children. Welborn et al. [11] reported fasting glucose levels for several hundred paediatric outpatients who had been fasting between 6 and 17 h. None of these patients had hypoglycemia. Therefore, in routine healthy patients who are well prepared (correct fasting time), it appears that there is no need for glucose in the intraoperative period, nor is there a need to monitor serum glucose in these patients. However, many authors still suggest using balanced fluids with low concentrations of glucose (from 1% to 2.5%) during surgery to avoid any possible risk of intraoperative and postoperative hypoglycemia [12, 13]. The mild hyperglycemia created by these low glucose solutions does not seem to cause any harm and disappears at the end of the first hour [14].

Concerning high-risk patients, many authors suggest that these patients do run the danger of hypoglycemia during surgery. Therefore patients receiving hyperalimentation or glucose solutions, neonates (especially those who are small for gestional age) infants of diabetic mothers, and children with heart disease should all have basal glucose infusions and their glucose carefully monitored during surgery.

In conclusion, even though there is no evidence, as of yet of harm caused by hyperglycemia (cerebral ischemia) in children, glucose levels in the blood must be kept within a reasonable range and much attention must be given to neurosurgical patients [15, 16].

Treatment of hypovolemia and blood loss

Measurements of blood loss during massive hemorrhage are usually unreliable. More reliable are clinical signs, such as capillary refill, temperature gradient (i.e., between rectum and skin), urine output, central venous pressure, or diastolic blood pressure, as a guide for estimating blood loss and volume status. In small infants blood pressure is an excellent reflection of blood volume. The

Table 7. Blood volume in children

Age	Volume (ml/kg)
Neonate	100
3 months	80-85
Adult	70

hematocrit is not a good reflection of volume status intraoperatively. Normal blood volumes for children are shown in Table 7.

Crystalloids or colloids

Administration of crystalloids or colloids may be considered for intravascular volume replacement when losses are in form of exudate, transudate, blood, or third-space losses especially when these are rapid and ongoing. For each 100 ml crystalloid given the intravascular volume is expanded by about 30 ml while the interstitial fluid volume increases by 70 ml. To replace blood loss, therefore, crystalloids need to be given in a volume of three times the measured blood lost. In contrast, colloids expand intravascular volume on a milliliter for milliliter basis and also have a much longer intravascular half-life.

Blood transfusion

The approach to blood replacement has changed greatly in past few years. The danger of blood-borne diseases, such as hepatitis and AIDS, has resulted in a much more balanced approach to the risk and benefits of blood transfusions. The concept of an acceptable hematocrit and a normal hematocrit can assist the clinician in determining both the adequate preparation of the patient as well as in recognizing an acceptable hematocrit in the intraoperative and postoperative period. Table 8 gives a list of normal and arbitrary acceptable hematocrits levels, where an acceptable level of hematocrit is defined as that tolerated by infants and children without the need for blood transfusion [10].

Although healthy children, or those with chronic anemia, may tolerate low hematocrit values, this is not true in neonates, children with cardiac disease or

Table 8. Indication for blood transfusion in children. (Modified from [10])

	Normal hematocrit level	Acceptable hematocrit level
Premature	40-45	35
Newborn	45-65	30-35
3 months	30-42	25
1 year	34-42	20-25
6 years	35-43	20-25

chronic pulmonary disease, and children with multisystemic trauma, who may have coexisting hypovolemia. In these patients hematocrit levels must be kept between 33% and 35%.

Postoperative fluids

As for the intraoperative period, fluid intake and output should also be carefully charted in detail in the postoperative period and the volume and composition of the fluid intake be titrated against losses and laboratory results. The use of hypotonic maintenance solution in the postoperative period is often cause of *dilutional hyponatremia*. Vomiting, the most common anaesthetic complication, causes loss of fluid high in sodium. Vomiting, together with low losses of blood or interstitial fluids and the release of antidiuretic hormone to maintain volume can result in acute dilutional hyponatremia [17]. When the extracellular fluid becomes hypotonic, water is transferred from the ECF to the ICF, resulting in cerebral edema (CNS irritability and depression, decreasing level of consciousness, disorientation, vomiting, and in severe cases, seizure activity). A very simple way to prevent acute dilutional hyponatremia is to maintain all children postoperatively on balanced salt solution until they begin to eat. After a minor surgical procedure, hunger more than thirst helps to indicate when alimentation can be started (usually from the third hour after extraperitoneal procedures).

After major surgical procedures, hourly urine output should be kept (0.5-1.0 ml/kg per hour) and daily weighing of the patient can help, together with a central venous line, in judging fluid balance. An arterial line can be useful for serial determination of blood pressure, serum tests, and blood gases. Gross abnormalities in plasma electrolytes should be corrected as shown in Table 9.

Children are less able to withstand starvation than adults. The smaller the child, the shorter his energy store will last, as nutrients are not only required to

Table 9. Correction of electrolytes abnormalities

Abnormalities	Calculation of deficit	Intervention
Low sodium	Na desired - Na actual $\cdot$ kg $\cdot$ 0.6	Slow correction (or diuretics if low sodium due to excess water)
High sodium		Restore intravascular volume and urine output; slow correction
Low potassium	K desired - K actual $\cdot$ kg $\cdot$ 0.3	Slow correction with frequent checks and ECG monitoring; correct concurrent low chloride
High potassium		Stop K i.v.; monitor ECG; alkalinize, calcium, dextrose+insulin; ion exchange resin

meet basal needs but also for incorporation into growing tissues. Therefore, provision of nutritional support after surgery is extremely important. Energy requirements for most patients may be calculated using the traditional maintenance water requirements (see previous paragraph "Basic fluid and electrolyte requirements") that derived from measurements of metabolic rate in normal children (Table 10). For short-term maintenance therapy in a previously well-nourished infant or child, however, a combination of some parenteral nutrition and the patient's own fat stores is adequate to prevent severe ketosis and tissue catabolism. This is accomplished by administering glucose equal to approximate 20% of the total caloric expenditure. In a more severe condition, expecially in the undernourished child, nutritional therapy should provide the required calories by parenteral or enteral administration of carbohydrate, fat, aminoacids, minerals, and vitamins.

Factors that increase energy requirements are fever (12% per degree Celsius above 37°C), cardiac failure (15%-25%), major surgery (20%-30%), sepsis (40%-50%), burns (up to 100%). The neonate appears to be different from the older children with regard to the stress response: energy requirements in neonate-seem to return to normal within 12 h after surgery.

It must be emphasized that these figures are only a general guideline: each critically ill patient must be assessed individually and his response to nutritional support should be constantly reassessed.

Table 10. Caloric requirements for parenteral nutrition

Weight	Calories kcal/kg/day
1-10 kg	100-120
10-20 kg	1 000+50 kcal for each kg>10
>20 kg	1 500+20 kcal for each kg>20 or
	1 500-1 700 kcal/m^2/day

References

1. Friss-Hansen BJ (1961) Body water compartments in children. Paediatrics 28:171
2. Gamble JL (1950) Chemical anatomy, physiology and pathology of extracellular fluid. Harvard University Press, Cambridge
3. Mirkin G (1962) Insensible weight loss in infants with fever. Paediatrics 30:279-284
4. Holiday MA, Segar WE (1957) Maintenance need for water in parenteral fluid therapy. Paediatrics 19:823-832
5. Boineau FG, Lewy JE (1990) Estimation of parenteral fluid requirements. Paediatr Clin N Am 37:257
6. Schreiner MS, Triebwasser A, Kenn TP (1990) Ingestion of liquids compared with preoperative fasting in paediatric outpatients. Anaesthesiology 72:593-597
7. Sandlar BK, Goresky GV, Maltby JR, Shaffer EA (1989) Effect of oral liquids and raniti-

dine on gastric fluid volume and pH in children undergoing outpatient surgery. Anaesthesiology 71:327-330

8. Splinter WM, Stewart JA, Muir JG (1989) The effect of preoperative apple juice on gastric content, thirst and hunger in children. Can J Anaesth 36:55-58

9. ASA (1997) Practice guidelines for preoperative fasting and use of pharmacologic agents. American Society of Anaesthesiology

10. Freid EB, Bagwell JM (1997) Perioperative fluid management. In: Badgwell JM (ed) Clinical paediatric anaesthesia. Lippincott-Raven, Philadelphia, pp 213-224

11. Welborn LG, McGill WA, Hannallah RS et al (1986) Perioperative blood glucose concentrations in paediatric outpatients. Anaesthesiology 65:543-547

12. Dubois MC, Gouyet L, Murat I et al (1992) Lactated ringer with 1% dextrose: an appropriate solution for perioperative fluid therapy in children. Paediatr Anaesth 2:89-104

13. Welborn LG, McGill WA, Hannallah RS et al (1987) Glucose concentration for routine intravenous infusion in paediatric outpatient surgery. Anaesthesiology 67:427-430

14. Murat I, Dubois MC, Gouyet L (1991) Apports hydroélectrolytiques en anaesthésie pédiatrique. In: Conférences d'actualisation. Congrès national d'anaesthésie réanimation. Masson, Paris, pp 339-357

15. Lanier WL, Stangland KJ, Scheinthauer BW et al (1987) The effects of dextrose infusion and head position on neurologic outcome after complete cerebral ischemia in primates: examination of a model. Anaesthesiology 66:39-48

16. Sieber FS, Smith DS, Traystman RJ et al (1988) Glucose: a reevaluation of its intraoperative use. Anaesthesiology 67:72-81

17. Burrows FA, Shutack JG, Crone RK (1983) Inappropriate secretion of antidiuretic hormone in a post surgical pediatric population. Crit Care Med 11:527-531

Chapter 6

Outpatient surgery in paediatric patients

P.A. LÖNNQVIST

As with spinal anaesthesia, outpatient surgery in paediatric patients has been practiced since the start of this century. It constituted a substantial part of paediatric anaesthesia even before the days of health care budget cuts, due both to the fact that most paediatric surgical procedures can be regarded as minor surgery and thus are well suited to be performed on an outpatient basis and also because of the psychological advantages for the child and parents when hospitalization can be avoided. Currently, outpatient surgery is very much "en vogue" mainly for financial reasons and more and sicker patients are now being treated as day cases. Although oupatient vs inpatient surgery represents true savings for the health care system and is also frequently viewed as an improvement by the patient, anaesthesiologists have to be very professional and careful not to be pressured into performing anaesthesia in patients that are not suitable as outpatients. The occasional complication that might occur due to the lack of postoperative supervision can dramatically affect the economic aspects of day care and, thus, quality control is essential. In the presently changing medicolegal climate one should also be very careful with the selection of patients that are to undergo outpatient surgery.

Here some important aspects of outpatient surgery and anaesthesia in paediatric patients are discussed. The texts by Morton and Lord [1] and Hannallah and Epstein [2] are recommended for more in-depth reviews of this topic.

Selection of patients

In numbers and costs, paediatric surgery generally make up a minor part of the total cost for surgery (adults and children combined). Thus, very little can be gained by trying to "squeeze" marginal paediatric cases into day care. As professionals we should therefore resist attempts to put less fit paediatric patients on the outpatient surgical list, both due to medical considerations and the relative lack of savings in a wider perspective. The author, thus, recommends a restrictive attitude towards an "it can be done" attitude by surgeons and hospital administrators.

Although there is currently no general consensus about patient selection some factors might merit more specific considerations.

Age

In Europe many hospitals do not accept children under 6 months of age for anaesthesia and surgery on an outpatient basis. This is considered to be too conservative by some physicians, especially American colleagues who are under pressure from insurance companies, but taking the numerically small number of such patients into consideration as well as the often relatively high anxiety of the parents to shoulder the postoperative responsibility following day surgery performed on their small babies, the author believes the 6-month limit to be a very good general principle. However, exceptions to this rule can obviously be made especially for very brief procedures or for anaesthesia/deep sedation in connection with radiographic examinations in children older than 1 month. In the author's personal opinion there is no place for outpatient care for neonatal patients for whatever reason.

A specific problem in this respect is the ex-premature NICU graduate. A lot of these patients will be disqualified due to various sequelae of their prematurity and neonatal intensive care, i.e., chronic lung disease/bronchopulmonary dysplasia or reactive airway disease. However, even patients who have had a fairly uneventful neonatal period will still be at risk for postoperative apnea for a prolonged period of time. After 60 gestational weeks (g.w.) the risk for postoperative apnea is only slightly less than 5%, a figure that obviously is absolutely unacceptable [3, 4]. Even after 60 g.w. a residual risk for apnea must exist, especially in the presence of concomitant anemia or hypoxic episodes. Thus, in the author's practice ex-premature (<36 g.w.) children are not accepted for outpatient surgery for the first 12 months of postnatal life.

Physical condition

The patients should be otherwise healthy or any chronic disease should be under asymptomatic control. Thus, the rule must be that only ASA (American Society of Anaesthesiologists) 1-2 patients should be accepted for ambulatory surgery. An exception to this rule might be patients who are only scheduled for radiographic examinations, i.e., CT or MRI scans. Children with obstructive apnea represent a group of patients that deserves special attention in this regard. Obstructive apnea is most often due to adenotonsillary hypertrophy but is also associated with certain craniofacial abnormalities. The prevalence is equal in boys and girls and the highest incidence is in the 3 to 7-year age group. Overall the incidence is approximately 1.5%-3.5 % in the paediatric population. Such patients not only have problems with upper airway patency but can also have other systemic symptoms, i.e., poor weight gain, hypertension, and right ventricular strain [5]. If these patients present for adenotonsillectomy, it is apparent to the anaesthesiologist that the patient should be admitted to the hospital for postoperative care. However, if the patient is scheduled for some other type of surgery, this syndrome can easily be missed and the patient can then accidentally be accepted for outpatient surgery. Since these patients have a very high incidence of

postoperative complications, it is vital that the preoperative screening procedure picks up patients with this syndrome so that they can be properly canceled
and re-scheduled.

ENT patients

Most ENT procedures, i.e., otologic examination, bilateral myringotomy and tube
placement, and adenoid-ectomy, can be performed on an outpatient basis. However, controversy exists regarding whether paediatric tonsillectomies can also safely be done in outpatients. The risk for significant, unnoticed postoperative bleeding is a serious and not infrequent phenomenon in these patients. Parents are not
qualified to check for this complication and it is, thus, not reasonable to put the responsibility on them for this demanding task. Centers where, despite this, tonsillectomies are performed on an outpatient basis are under the obligation to develop a very high quality protocol in order to prevent disastrous complication from
occurring following early discharge. A better option for this patient category is to
treat them on an "overnight" basis. In this context one should also appreciate the
substantial risks of using nonsteroidal anti-inflammatory drugs (NSAIDs) or potent antiemetics in tonsillectomy patients. NSAIDs increase the risk for postoperative bleeding and anti-emetics, i.e., ondansetron, may effectively mask nausea
and vomiting caused by swallowing of significant amounts of blood.

Premedication

With newer anaesthetics, better patient/parent information, better mental
preparation, and parental presence at induction it can be argued whether routine premedication still has a place in paediatric outpatient anaesthesia. The
availability of high-quality local anaesthetics, i.e., EMLA and AMETOP, which
allow almost pain-free venous cannulation also reduces the need for premedication. Avoiding a drug associated with potential unwanted side effects – i.e., opioids: postoperative nausea and vomiting (PONV), and midazolam: postoperative confusion and long-term adverse behavioral changes [6] – can obviously be
beneficial for the patient. However, not to give premedication just to avoid postoperative sedation and to get the patient alert quickly and "street fit" so that he
can be rapidly discharged is not really valid in paediatric patients. This is a good
example of when one cannot directly transpose adult experiences and practices
to the paediatric setting. First, paediatric patients, by definition, always have a
parent or guardian present. A child with slight but prolonged residual sedation is
often preferred by the parents since this will increase the ease of home transport
and also the handling of the child once back home. Second, the lack of such
residual sedation in combination with high-quality pain relief achieved by a peripheral regional block, for example, makes it very difficult for an unauthorita-
tive parent to restrict the mobility of very active children. At our institution we
have had two such outpatients. Inguinal hernia repair was performed in these

children, who where then re-admitted to the emergency room on the same evening because of significant scrotal hematoma from riding a bicycle and frank wound rupture after jumping and playing in a "pool of balls"! Slight residual postoperative sedation can, thus, in fact be viewed as a beneficial effect of premedication. In the author's experience clonidine, an α_2 agonist which can be delivered by the oral, rectal or intravenous route, is an attractive and inexpensive premedication in the setting of paediatric outpatient surgery. It reduces the need for general anaesthetics, potentiates analgesia, and provides a suitable degree of residual sedation for the afternoon and early evening of the day of surgery.

Drugs/techniques

Short-acting anaesthetic agents are preferable although older drugs such as halothane and thiopental should still be regarded as acceptable options for outpatient anaesthesia. Sevoflurane is a very useful drug in oupatients for a number of reasons. One of its major merits is the possibility to use it as a "single agent". Thus, induction, maintenance and, if necessary, endotracheal intubation can be performed with the use of only sevoflurane. The "single-agent" technique restricts the number of drugs to which the patient is exposed and limits the possibility for unknown and unwanted interactions of multiple drugs. With sevoflurane there have been reports of an increased incidence of agitation/confusion in the recovery room following anaesthesia and this should be taken into consideration [7]. This can be explained in part by insufficient analgesia since the recovery is very rapid after sevoflurane anaesthesia. Thus, good quality analgesia reduces the problem. It also appears as if the choice of premedication might have an affect. At our department early postoperative agitation/confusion is rarely observed after premedication with morphine or clonidine whereas it is not infrequently experienced following premedication with midazolam. If the anaesthesiologist is planning to use sevoflurane, the author recommends that the patient not be premedicated with midazolam but with another agent instead if indeed premedication is required. If intravenous induction is preferred by the patient or the anaesthesiologist, propofol is a good alternative. The only major drawback with propofol is that it frequently produces pain or discomfort on injection even if premixed with lidocaine. Propofol can also be used for maintenance as a part of a total intravenous technique but then requires the addition of some analgesic drug and if paralysis is necessary a muscle relaxant as well.

Regardless of the anaesthetic technique chosen, a very useful option is to use some local anaesthetic technique as an analgesic complement. This assures excellent intra- and postoperative analgesia and allows the use of a very light general anaesthetic, resulting in both a reduction of volatile or intravenous agent used (reduction of cost) and rapid recovery (increasing turnover). Peripheral nerve blocks (i.e., ilioinguinal, penile, various lower limb blocks) or local infiltration of local anaesthetics in the surgical wound might be preferable but caudal blocks can also be used successfully in subumbilical surgery.

Kokki and co-workers have recently described the use of bupivacaine spinal anaesthesia complemented by intravenous sedation for outpatient surgery in children. They report a very high success rate, no apparent delay in discharge, and a very low incidence of postdural puncture headache [8, 9]. Our own group has demonstrated better immediate postoperative pain relief with this technique than with sevoflurane alone and we also found similar discharge times in the two groups of patients, underscoring the much shorter duration of bupivacaine spinal anaesthesia in children than in adults [10]. Spinal anaesthesia complemented by intravenous sedation might, thus, be an interesting alternative to explore further in patients who are scheduled for subumbilical surgery.

Postoperative pain control

Adequate pain control is of paramount importance following any type of paediatric surgery. Lack of proper pain relief is maybe most problematic in outpatients since postoperative pain can cause PONV, may delay discharge, and can cause substantial suffering following the return home. The best way of handling this problem is to try to prevent pain by administering analgesics or by performing a nerve block (see discussion above) prior to the surgical intervention. Administration of paracetamol either orally as part of the premedication or rectally immediately following anaesthetic induction is now widely practiced. Recent publications indicate that previous dosage regimens have been too conservative and that an initial dose of 40 mg/kg of paracetamol is more effective without causing any pharmacokinetic concerns [11, 12]. Diclofenac (0.5-1 mg/kg) or other NSAIDs can also be useful in this regard and might be preferable to paracetamol for orthopedic surgery. Intravenous low-dose ketorolac (0.15 mg/kg) has also been found to be very useful in outpatients in the author's personal experience. If more severe pain is anticipated, a combination of paracetamol and codeine can be an effective alternative. Occasionally the intraoperative use of opioids might be indicated, in which case short-acting agents, i.e., alfentanil, might be preferable to the longer-acting agents. However, it is important to keep in mind the substantial emetic potential associated with the use of opioids. At our institution the incidence of postoperative vomiting was reduced from 25% to 10% when morphine was replaced by nonopioids in the premedication. Thus, opioids should not be a routine part of outpatient anaesthesia.

It is also important to instruct the parents how to handle the potential pain problem once they are home. Additional doses of paracetamol (immediately on arrival at home and also before bedtime) is usually satisfactory and better than on-demand administration. Parents should, however, be informed not to exceed 100-120 mg/kg of paracetamol during the first 24 h, including the doses given during the hospital stay, in order to avoid potential toxicity problems. If more severe pain can be expected the parents should be supplied with paracetamol-codeine suppositories to help the child during the evening and night after surgery. If pain still persists despite adequate administration of analgesics, the parents should be informed to contact the hospital for further advice since more severe pain might be a sign of a significant postoperative complication.

Postoperative nausea and vomiting (PONV)

This most distressing postoperative complication has received considerable attention in recent years. Apart from causing the patient substantial discomfort, PONV delays discharge from the day surgery unit [13] and is one of the most frequent causes of unexpected hospitalization following outpatient surgery [14]. The overall incidence of PONV is high in paediatric patients (25%-80%) [15]. In children under 2 years of age PONV appears to be a much less of a problem than in older children [16]. Certain types of surgery are associated with a very high incidence of PONV, i.e., strabismus surgery, tonsillectomies, and correction of prominent ears [15]. According to the quality assurance program at our outpatient surgical unit, parents conceive PONV to be a much greater problem than postoperative pain. Thus, in order to achieve a successful outpatient program one needs to develop an anaesthetic and postoperative protocol that will minimize the incidence of PONV and treat more significant or prolonged PONV reactions. Kokki and co-workers have reported a PONV incidence of <10% in a mixed outpatient population following spinal anaesthesia combined with intravenous sedation [8, 9]. Spinal anaesthesia or other regional techniques combined with intravenous sedation with propofol might, thus, be an attractive alternative in this context. Regarding the choice of other anaesthetics, no firm recommendations can be made apart from restrictivity concerning the administration of opioids [15]. A nitrous oxide-free anaesthetic based on propofol and/or sevoflurane combined with regional anaesthesia might, in the author's opinion, be worth considering over other techniques. The issue of PONV prophylaxis has not yet been clarified but it appears reasonable to give prophylaxis to patients who previously have had problems with PONV and to patients who are scheduled for surgery associated with a high incidence of PONV. A number of drugs have been tested and recommended as prophylaxis, making it difficult to give any more firm recommendations. However, a large (>2 000 patients) prospective, randomized, double-blind study in adults recently found low-dose droperidol to be as effective as ondansetron in preventing PONV [17]. Whether this is also true in children remains to be confirmed. For treatment of already established PONV, low-dose droperidol appears to be as effective as to the newer agents, i.e., ondansetron. Considering the high price of ondansetron, droperidol still appears to be defending its place as a first-line drug for the treatment of already established PONV.

Follow-up/Audit

As pointed out at the beginning of this text, follow-up and quality assurance are fundamental in the context of outpatient surgery. It is vital that various problems are identified that may arise from drifts in clinical practice or as a result of changes in the unit's protocol in order to prevent more serious complications from occurring. Follow-up is also greatly appreciated by the parents and is a very easy way of promoting goodwill for the unit and the hospital. Thus, it is recommended to phone all patients on the day after discharge in order to identify any problems, to answer any questions, and to get an idea of the parent's overall satisfaction. Medical audit is also very useful for obtaining outside views on the unit's organization and the different protocols. Audits represent a good opportunity to improve the quality and safety of the outpatient surgery program and networks between hospitals with similar patient populations and a general organization should be established to increase the possibility of such audits.

In conclusion, paediatric outpatient surgery can be very rewarding both from the patient's and from an economical point of view. However, in order to harvest these benefits from paediatric outpatient surgery one has to very careful not to be pressured into accepting unsuitable patients and also to pay meticulous attention to all the details from start to finish. Awareness of the necessity for follow-up and audit of the program is also fundamental to a successful outpatient practice.

References

1. Morton NS, Lord D (1994) Paediatric anaesthesia. In: Whitwam JG (ed) Day-case anaesthesia and surgery. Blackwell, Oxford, pp 303-346
2. Hannallah RS, Epstein BS (1994) Outpatient anaesthesia. In: Geregory G (ed) Paediatric anaesthesia, 3rd ed. Churchill Livingstone, New York, pp 773-792
3. Malviya S, Swartz J, Lerman J (1993) Are all preterm infants younger than 60 weeks postconceptual age at risk for postanaesthetic apnea? Anaesthesiology 78:1076-1081
4. Coté CJ et al (1995) Postoperative apnea in premature infants after inguinal herniorraphy. Anaesthesiology 82:809-822
5. Warwick JP, Mason DG (1998) Obstructive sleep apnea syndrome in children. Anaesthesia 53:571-579
6. McGraw T, Kendrick A (1998) Oral midazolam premedication and postoperative behaviour in children. Paediatr Anaesth 8:117-121
7. Lerman J et al (1996) Induction, recovery, and safety characteristics of sevoflurane in children undergoing ambulatory surgery – a comparison with halothane. Anaesthesiology 84:1332-1340
8. Kokki H, Hedolin H (1995) Comparison of spinal anaesthesia with epidural anaesthesia in paediatric surgery. Acta Anaesthesiol Scand 39:896-900
9. Kokki H, Hedolin H (1996) Comparison of 25 G and 29 G Quincke spinal needles in paediatric day case surgery. A prospective randomized study of the puncture characteristics, success rate and postoperative complaints. Paediatr Anaesth 6:115-119
10. Oddby E et al (1998) Postoperative nausea and vomiting in paediatric outpatients: sevoflurane vs spinal anaesthesia with propofol sedation. Reg Anaesth Pain Med 23:A15
11. Anderson B, Kanagasundarum S, Woolard G (1997) Analgesic efficacy of paracetamol in children using tonsillectomy as a pain model. Anaesth Intensive Care 24:669-673
12. Birmingham PK et al (1997) Twenty-four-hour pharmacokinetics of rectal acetaminophen in children. Anaesthesiology 87:244-252
13. Splinter WM, Roberts DJ, Rhine EJ, MacNeill HB, Komocar L (1995) Nitrous oxide does not increase vomiting after myringotomy. Can J Anaesth 42:274-276
14. Splinter WM, Paradis V (1995) Unexpected admissions after paediatric ambulatory surgery – a 4 year review. Anaesth Analg 84:S26

15. Baines D (1996) Postoperative nausea and vomiting in children. Paediatr Anaesth 6:7-14
16. Karlsson E, Larsson LE, Nilsson K (1990) Postanaesthetic nausea in children. Acta Anaesthesiol Scand 34:515-518
17. Fortney JT et al (1998) A comparison of the efficacy, safety, and patient satisfaction of ondansetron versus droperidol as antiemetics for elective outpatient surgical procedures. Anaesth Analg 86:731-738

Chapter 7

Locoregional anaesthesia in paediatrics

P. Busoni, M. Calamandrei

The risks and complications related to regional anaesthesia in paediatrics include inadvertent dural puncture, total spinal block, toxic phenomena, and infections. However, proper pain management is important in the care of a child after surgery. It allows the patient to breathe deeply and walk earlier, it decreases the magnitude of the postoperative stress response, and it improves the overall quality of patient care. Multiple modalities exist for administering medications to such children, including intramuscular, intravenous, patient-controlled analgesia, and epidural, spinal, and nerve blocks.

Paediatric patients often are very sensitive to the respiratory depressive effects of agents used for analgesia and sedation. These should be used with particular caution in nonintubated infants under 3-6 months of age, patients with haemodynamic or airway instability, patients with evolving neurologic conditions, or patients with altered ventilatory control. In the patient with pain, however, in whom sedation is contraindicated, regional anaesthesia offers analgesia without the concern of masking an evolving neurologic examination.

The severely injured child becomes chemically dependent when receiving continuous infusion of opioids or benzodiazepines. The stress response associated with withdrawal can have adverse effects, including increased catabolism and poor wound healing. Regional anaesthesia may be effective when parenteral narcotics are inadequate or lead to undesired effects.

Peripheral blocks

Subcutaneous infiltration of the skin with a local anaesthetic solution is the most commonly used technique of administering a local anaesthetic in children [1]. However, local anaesthetic infiltration of traumatic lacerations requires special attention. Commonly, the wound is dirty and requires extensive scrubbing and irrigation. Our practice is to apply the local anaesthetic topically, using simple wound irrigation with 1% lidocaine. Alternatively, the peripheral nerve supplying the injured area may be blocked more proximally.

Because local anaesthetics are manufactured at a pH of 4-5 and are administered by injections, they are as painful as bee stings (pH 1.5-3). The pain of local anaesthetic injections can be minimized by using buffered anaesthetic solutions. Local anaesthetics are not manufactured with buffer because the buffering affects the shelf-life of the drug. Buffering a local anaesthetic solution, such as lidocaine, with sodium bicarbonate (9 ml of lidocaine combined with 1 ml of 1 mEq/ml bicarbonate) immediately before administration may make the injection painless and hasten the onset of analgesia.

Bier block, a technique of i.v. regional anaesthesia using low-dose lidocaine (1.5 mg/kg) has been demonstrated to be safe and efficacious for the management of children's upper-extremity fractures and dislocations [2]. Trauma or operations of the upper extremity can also be managed with techniques such as interscalene, infraclavicular, and axillary blocks performed by bolus or infusion. Possible complications and side effects associated with regional anaesthetic techniques of the upper extremity include total spinal, pneumothorax, Horner's syndrome, hemidiaphragmatis paralysis, neuropraxia, seizures, and pleural effusion. Some of these complications can cause the patients to develop pulmonary insufficiency or can result in neurologic alterations .

Many patients with lower-extremity trauma, especially those with sharp femoral fractures, may benefit from a femoral nerve block prior to being moved from their hospital bed to the operating table, since they are in excruciating pain any time motion occurs. In fact, some traumatologists administer low-dose femoral nerve blocks in the field to provide pain relief prior to painful movement. Although many lower-extremity procedures can be performed with combined femoral-sciatic and lateral femoral cutaneous nerve block, with the sciatic nerve block performed with the hip flexed and the knee flexed at 90°, a patient with an open tibula or fibular fracture will not be able to move his or her leg into this position without extreme pain. These children present the ideal situation for a sciatic block via the anterior approach [3]. This can be accomplished with the nerve stimulator technique. The anatomic landmarks are the anterior superior iliac spine, the pubic tubercle, and the great trochanter. A line is drawn between the anterior superior iliac spine and the pubic tubercle. This line is divided into thirds. A second line is drawn parallel to the first, passing through the greater trochanter. At the junction of the middle and medial thirds of the first line, a perpendicular line is drawn until it crosses the second line. This is the entry point for the insulated needle and identifies the surface marking for the point at which the sciatic nerve courses into the lower extremity. This is also the level of the lesser trochanter of the femur. An insulated needle is inserted perpendicular to the skin and advanced while twitches are sought in the lower leg. If the lesser trochanter is encountered, the needle is moved slightly medial and then advanced further. Once adequate twitches are obtained at a low rate (0.1 to 0.4 mA) and aspiration is negative, medication can be injected with intermittent aspiration to obtain adequate nerve block. A lateral femoral cutaneous nerve block can also be performed to ensure analgesia to the entire lower extremity, having already performed the femoral nerve block prior to moving the child. A simple technique to provide continuous femoral nerve block can be employed in some circumstances [4].

A Tuohy needle can be passed through the fascia lata and then the fascia iliaca, immediately lateral to the femoral artery distal to the inguinal ligament. If the needle is inserted too deeply it enters the iliopsoas muscle, giving a characteristic "woody" feeling. Easy passage of the catheter 5-8 cm cephalad confirms correct positioning. A nerve stimulator is not required. An infusion of bupivacaine 0.125% at a rate of 0.3 ml/kg/per hour controlled by a volumetric infusion pump is appropriate for an average of 3-5 days pain control. Local infection at the site of the catheter insertion could present a possible complication. It is also worth noting that one must be careful about applying limb tourniquets in patients who have suffered head trauma, since tourniquet use can increase intracranial pressure.

Pain therapy for rib fractures includes intercostal and interpleural blocks. Intercostal nerve blocks result in the highest local anaesthetic blood level. Interpleural analgesia is administered by inserting a Tuohy needle into the pleural space 5-8 cm from the spinous process. The hanging drop technique is used. When the needle is moved between the parietal and visceral pleura, the drop is aspirated, indicating the correct positioning. A single dose of local anaesthetic can be administered or a catheter placed. Advancing the needle further can result in pneumothorax. Local anaesthetic administered at this level can track cephalad and result in hemidiaphragmatic paralysis as well as Horner's syndrome.

Peripheral blocks for common paediatric operations

Circumcision is probably the most common operation carried out in the paediatric population. After a light general anaesthesia is induced, local anaesthetic is infiltrated subcutaneously in a ring at the base of the penis in a volume sufficient to produce an obvious weal. This subcutaneous ring technique is easy and effective and probably the safest. Other techniques which require a deeper insertion of the needle could cause bleeding, usually from the dorsal vascular structures. A hematoma confined within the penile fascia may compress the arterial supply to the penis and cause gangrene. This block is also useful for distal hypospadias repair.

The combined ilioinguinal and iliohypogastric nerve block (inguinal field block) is one of the most useful and commonly performed blocks in paediatric anaesthesia. Herniotomy and orchidopexy are the main indications. Only the cutaneous innervation is blocked and, therefore, supplementary general anaesthesia is required. The needle is inserted one (child's) fingerbreadth medial to the anterior superior iliac spine and directed posterolaterally until it strikes bone. It is then withdrawn slightly and the injection made as the needle is withdrawn to a subcutaneous position. The needle is then reinserted through the external oblique aponeurosis (a "click" should be felt) and further solution injected both above and below the aponeurosis as the needle is withdrawn. Dosages of bupivacaine 0.5% without epinephrine range between 2 and 10 ml according to age and body weight.

Central (perimedullar) blocks

In performing central blocks in children there are several anatomic peculiarities to be borne in mind:

- in early postnatal life, the sacrum consists of five distinct vertebrae. As ossification proceeds, fusion occurs between the sacral segments, beginning with the two lowest about the age of 18 years, and extending cephalad until the process is complete between the 25th and 30th years of life;
- the spinous processes of the sacral vertebrae are rudimentary;
- the L5-S1 interspace is the largest in the vertebral column;
- in children, the sacral angle is open widely;
- special fluidity of the epidural fat tissue;
- the intercristal line crosses the midline at the level of the fifth lumbar vertebra in children, and even lower, at the L5-S1 interspace, in neonates.

Continuous technique is based on the introduction of a catheter into the epidural space. A convenient approach is one that allows the catheter tip to run parallel to the dura (i.e. caudal and Taylor approach, lumbar epidural paramedian approach, etc.). The distal opening of the catheter inside the epidural space should be facing upward. It is well known that, in children, a catheter can be made to run upward (or downward) as desired due to the particular dimension of the epidural space, i.e. not as large as in adults. Therefore, catheters cannot bend or curl up, but they are forced to run upward instead.

A catheter passed into the epidural space by the caudal route can reach almost any level [5]. This is almost always true for the newborn and small infants up to about 6 kg. In older children, catheters are often arrested at L2-L3, L3-L4 or even L4-L5. Indications are prolonged operation on the limbs, external genitalia, and lower abdomen. Muscle relaxants can often be avoided and the postoperative period is favorable. Children are often impressively calm, opiates are unnecessary, and the incidence of nausea, vomiting, and urinary retention is therefore greatly reduced.

- *Dosage.* A dose of 1.5% mepivacaine (or 1.5% lidocaine or 0.5% bupivacaine) in plain solution 0.1 × n.dermatomes × years of age is given. Top-up dosages comprise one half the initial dosage.
- *Technique.* The child is turned into the lateral position, legs flexed. An intravenous cannula is inserted through the sacrococcygeal ligament as for the single-shot technique. The complete cannula is advanced 1 cm into the sacral canal and then the metal stylet withdrawn and the plastic sheat advanced an additional 1 cm. This allows the epidural catheter to pass more easily. An epidural catheter is measured against the back of the child from the end of the cannula to the desired spinal level. The catheter is then inserted through the plastic cannula and carefully advanced. The catheter can usually be advanced easily as far as the lumbar region. However, in premature babies, neonates, and small children, the catheter may reach the upper lumbar and even the thoracic or cervical regions.

In a study of 30 children, aged 1-12 years, the authors measured the length of catheters in the epidural space from the tip to the skin insertion. In only one case did the catheter reach as high as T6, and usually it was arrested at levels between T12 and L5. Thus, the height to which a catheter can be threaded in the inside of the epidural space depends on the age of the child. An advantage of the caudal route for epidural anaesthesia is that large-gauge catheters can be inserted even in the youngest children.

In older children, of course, the epidural space can easily be catheterized through the lumbar interspaces. If this is the case, it is suggested that a paramedian approach be used in order to incline the needle as appropriate. In fact, the inclined needle offers the rounded part of its tip to the dura, thus making any perforation more difficult. Additionally, any upward progression of the catheter inside the epidural space is easier as it is made to run parallel to the dura.

In children, a downward direction of the catheter is possible as well. In fact, at a sacral level, due to the rudimentary spinous processes, the needle can be inclined downward [6].This downward inclination is also possible at the L5-S1 interspace, due to the large intervertebral space, and at a lumbar level as well, provided a paramedian approach is used.

Any inclination of the needle, upward or downward, is therefore possible in children and thus the subsequently introduced catheter will follow a downward or an upward direction accordingly. If the catheter has been threaded easily (without meeting any important resistance) and if there is no resistance to injection, it can be confidently assumed that the catheter is well positioned in the epidural space, that is, without any kink and with the tip-opening facing cephalad or caudad. Every effort should be made to achieve this position(s), as only then will the desired level of anaesthesia be obtained with the minimum volume of local anaesthetic. The size of the catheter should be large enough to allow the drug to be injected at a rate of 0.5-0.7 ml/s. If the rate is slower, larger doses of drug will be probably required to achieve the desired levels of anaesthesia. Dosages are shown in Table 1.

Top-up injections are required soon after the first hour when 1.5% mepivacaine is used. Half of the initial dose can be given and repeated hourly. In the postoperative period continuous infusion through the catheter is obviously possible epidural patient-controlled analgesia (EPCA) (Table 2).

Table 1. Dosing guideline for regional blockade

Doses	Mepivacaine	Bupivacaine
Single dose (mg/kg)		
• Without epinephrine	5	2-2.5
• With epinephrine	7	2-2.5
Prolonged infusion (mg/kg/h)		
• Older infants and children	1.5-2	0.4
• Neonates	1	0.2

Table 2. Epidural patient-controlled analgesia (EPCA): dosage guidelines (morphine 0.02%)

EPCA doses	Basal rate	Lockout
1.25 µg/kg/hr	15 µg/kg/hr	15 min

In conclusion, caudal or lumbar epidural blocks are safe and advantageous. However, it is evident that:
1. children must be selected carefully; preoperative evaluation must be thorough, and coagulopathies and dehydration must be corrected;
2. the anaesthetist must be experienced and fully trained in regional block technique in children;
3. close monitoring of the pupils, heart rate, blood pressure, and respiration is essential.

References

1. Yaster M, Tobin JR, Quentin A et al (1994) Local anaesthetics in the management of acute pain in children. Paediatrics 124:165-176
2. Bolte RG, Stevens PM, Scott SM et al (1994) Bier block. J Paediatr Orthop 14:534-537
3. Beck GP (1983) Anterior approach to the sciatic nerve. Anaesthesiology 24:222-225
4. Jonson CM (1994) Continuous femoral nerve blockade for analgesia in children with femoral fractures. Anaesth Intens Care 22:281-283
5. Bosenberg AT, Bland BAR, Schulte-Steinberg O, Downing JW (1989) Thoracic epidural anaesthesia via caudal route in infants. Anaesthesiology 69:265-269
6. Busoni P, Sarti A (1987) Sacral intervertebral epidural block. Anaesthesiology 67:993-995

Chapter 8

Complications of regional analgesia in paediatric anaesthesia

A.R. WOLF

In recent years regional analgesia has become popular in paediatric anaesthetic practice. This enthusiasm for regional analgesia is due at least in part to the potential to deliver complete analgesia without major systemic side effects. Many of the techniques, such as caudal block, are simple to perform and their benefits are immediately obvious to clinicians, parents and patients. Critical evaluation has confirmed the practical advantages of regional analgesia over other techniques in the appropriate settings, but has also highlighted side-effects, disadvantages and risks [1-4]. Regional anaesthesia generally necessitates an additional invasive procedure, and this additional risk, however small, must be justified through the delivery of proven benefits [5]. It is therefore necessary to have a clear understanding of risk and benefit before looking at the complications of regional anaesthesia in more specific situations.

Risk and benefit

Assessment of risk and benefit have remarkable similarities when viewed schematically (Fig. 1).

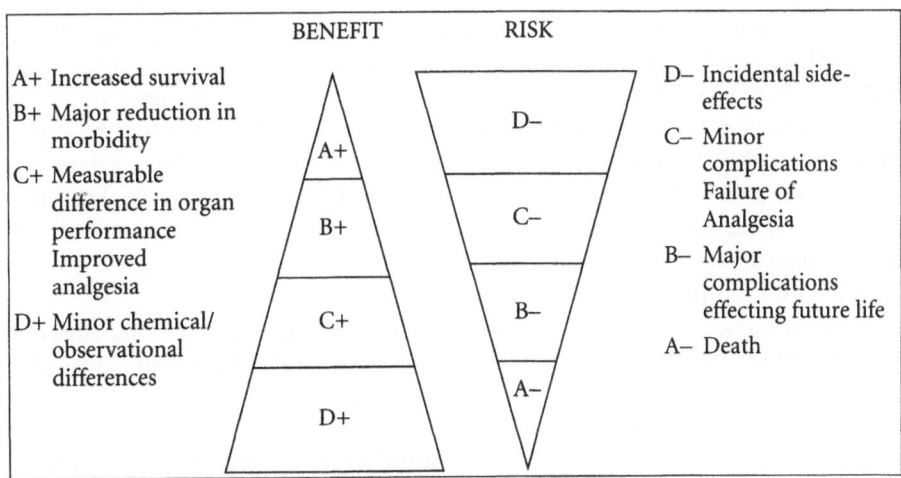

Fig. 1. Stratification of risk and benefit

The ultimate benefit (A+) is one where the frequency of survival is increased by using that technique, whereas the ultimate risk (A–) can be assessed by the frequency of mortality. Benefits can also be stratified under the headings of: B+, major reduction in morbidity (length of intensive care unit (ITU) stay, time on the ventilator, length of hospital stay and frequency of life-threatening complications); C+, measurable improvement in organ performance or quality of analgesia; and D+, minor chemical or observational differences that have no impact on morbidity.

Risks can be stratified under the headings of: B–, major complications affecting future life (i.e., tetraplegia, epidural abscess etc.); C–, minor complications of the technique that have no long-lasting effects (dural tap, haematoma, failure of the technique etc.), and D–, incidental variations or side effects compared to other techniques (vomiting, numbness etc.).

While minor risks and benefits (groups C and D) have a higher incidence and are easier to measure, it is the life-threatening and major risks and benefits (groups A and B) that are of most importance. The retrospective report in 1995 on accidents following paediatric extradural analgesia in which five cases of severe neurological damage occurred (two in 10 000) is clearly of concern in this respect [3]. While central blocks are rarely associated life death or severe mishaps (group A and B critical events), it is disturbing that human error or use of inappropriate equipment account for more than half the minor complications reported [4].

Categories of complications from regional analgesia

It is often assumed that a complication from regional analgesia represents a failure of care or of technique, but this is not usually the case. It has to be accepted that invasive procedures carry a finite risk, but familiarity with the technique and being aware of the most common pitfalls can help to minimise the risk. However, some categories of complications are avoidable by taking appropriate precautions and failure to take these steps could be regarded as negligent. For example, failure to insert an intravenous cannula prior to performance of a local block could be regarded as adding an unnecessary hazard to a procedure. If that child subsequently has a cardiovascular collapse following the block and no vascular access is available, the complications are likely to be more severe. Therefore all the categories of complications listed below can be regarded as either acceptable or unacceptable.

– Acceptable complications:
  • consequences of a properly performed block: for example, the onset of pneumothorax after a regional blockade or dural tap during an epidural or caudal injection.
– Unacceptable complications:
  • unforced errors due to inadequate knowledge or faulty technique: for example, failing to check the contents of the ampoule about to be injected, or

failing to be aware of the major effects of the particular block, or not knowing how to treat them;

- failure to provide a safe environment for regional blockade: for example, opioid epidural infusions have a potential to cause major ventilatory depression. While this represents an acceptable complication of regional blockade, failure to provide adequate monitoring both in terms of personnel and equipment is dangerous. An adverse event under these circumstances is unacceptable.

With these subclassifications in mind, complications can be categorised under the hereunder headings.

Complications due to the administration of the local block.

There is a finite risk of complications from local or general effects of the block. The risks of these can be reduced by experience [4], the use of appropriate equipment and safe technique [6].

- Local:
  - damage to nerves or blood vessels;
  - focal neurological events such as temporary blindness after a stellate ganglion block or apnoea after caudal block;
  - regional effects such as Horner's syndrome after stellate ganglion block;
  - undesired nerve block such as an additional femoral nerve block after ilioinguinal/iliohypogastric nerve block.
- General:
  - unexpected high block, hypotension, ventilatory failure, urinary retention, vomiting, etc.
- Technical:
  - incorrect placement: total spinal anaesthesia, intravascular injection or subdural injection.

Complications due to the analgesic agent.

These include the known effects of agents such as hypotension from local anaesthetics or ventilatory depression from opioids. It also includes unforced errors such as unsafe technique for injection [6] or injection of the wrong solution or of the incorrect amount of solution.

- Local:
  - local toxicity of the agent.
- General:
  - systemic drug absorption of local anaesthetics: hypotension, cardiotoxicity;
  - systemic drug absorption of opioids: ventilatory depression.
- Allergies.
- Methaemaglobinaemia.

Complications due to the equipment.

- Catheter migration, blockage, knotting, etc.
- Infusion pump error or failure.

Failure of the block.

- Partial failure.
- Total failure.

Perioperative complications.
- Ventilatory failure during epidural infusion.
- Epidural haematoma or epidural abscess.
- Pressure sores due to numbness.
- Delayed recovery after block.

Long-term complications.
- Backache, dermoid cyst, failure of repeat epidural.

How safe is paediatric regional anaesthesia?

Given the large potential for complications in paediatric regional anaesthesia, how safe is it? In the ADARPEF study [4] it was found that of the 24 409 cases involved, there were only 23 critical incidents reported. None of these included death or major neurological sequelae (Table 1).

Complications reported included dural penetration (eight cases), intravascular injection (six cases), technical problems, apnoea, cardiac arrhythmia and transient neurological sequelae. The major conclusions from this study was that.

1. Peripheral blocks are very safe and may be preferred to central blockade if feasible [5] They appear, from the literature, to be underused and undervalued. Given their safety profile they should be used more often.
2. Caudal blocks are safe but the potential for disaster is always present [3]. This central block should be treated with great care despite the routine nature of the procedure. Simple precautions such as sterility, confirming safe placement before injection, slow injection and avoiding air injection are mandatory.
3. The low incidence of complications in the youngest age group may reflect that only the most experienced paediatric anaesthetists are involved in these cases.
4. Similarly, the absence of complications in the patients receiving thoracic epidurals compared with those receiving lumbar epidurals may also be due in part to the experience of the anaesthetists involved in those procedures.

Table 1. Incidence of complications from regional anaesthesia

Type of anaesthesia	Cases (%)	Complications
Total regional/local cases	24 409	0.9/1 000
Total central blocks	15 013 (61.5)	1.5/1 000
Caudal epidural	12 111 (49.6)	0.7/1 000
Lumbar epidurals	1 732 (7.1)	3.7/1 000
Thoracic epidurals	135 (0.6)	0
Spinals	506(2.1)	2.0/1 000
Peripheral blocks	4 090 (16.8)	0

This aspect is highlighted in the British National Confidential enquiry into postoperative deaths [7], which showed that, although general anaesthesia is relatively safe (0.9/10 000 deaths exclusively related to general anaesthesia), several deaths in infants undergoing minor surgery occurred which had been managed by anaesthetists not used to providing routine anaesthesia in paediatric patients

The ADARPEF study also reported 11 cases of improper equipment being used and two cases of overdose of local anaesthetic. They concluded that the incidents would not have occurred had the appropriate guidelines been adhered to. In a separate Australian study on complications of regional anaesthesia [8], of the 160 complications examined, the commonest problem was cardiovascular incidents, but there were 24 drug errors, including the wrong drug (ten cases) or an inappropriate drug (four cases) being delivered. Clearly, it is the avoidable or unacceptable complications that need to be eliminated from paediatric practice while at the same time striving to reduce the incidence and treating the consequences of unavoidable or acceptable complications.

Risk/benefit ratio for some individual procedures

Given the published data on risks of regional analgesia , it is necessary for the paediatric anaesthetist to approach the risk benefit ratio of a particular procedure within the context of his or her individual experience and the environment in which he or she works. Below are some of the more common dilemmas which highlight the risk/benefit ratio for particular procedures.

1. Paediatric hernia repair. Herniorrhaphy is usually carried out as a day stay procedure. If the patient receives general anaesthesia alone, only 50% of patients will require postoperative analgesia. Local techniques that have been studied include caudal, ilioinguinal/iliohypogastric block, local infiltration and local instillation into the wound. These techniques appear to provide equally effective analgesia. Major disadvantages (risk) in this context include hospital admission due to vomiting or prolonged lower limb block. Caudal analgesia or systemic opioids may be hard to justify in this context.
2. Re-implantation of ureters and other major abdominal procedures. Epidural analgesia in this context is associated with improved analgesia, improved postoperative recovery [9], avoidance of the pain of bladder spasm, and earlier discharge from hospital. The alternative of opioid infusion may be safer in institutions that have limited experience of postoperative epidural infusion. Both techniques have limited group A/B risks (Fig. 1).
3. Spinal anaesthesia for hernia repair in ex-premature infants. Despite a relatively high failure rate, spinal anaesthesia has been advocated in this group based on a reduction of postoperative apnoeas and measured differences in ventilation [10]. However, recently the benefits of this technique over an ap-

propriate general anaesthetic/caudal technique have been questioned [11]. Infants tolerate awake spinal anaesthesia with minimal cardiovascular changes [12] although occasionally these infants may require ventilatory support if the local block becomes too high. Additional sedation for these infants can cause severe apnoeas and bradycardia [13]

References

1. Wolf AR, Hughes D (1993) Pain relief for infants undergoing abdominal surgery: comparison of infusions of iv morphine and extradural bupivacaine. Br J Anaesth 70:10-16
2. McGown RG (1982) Caudal analgesia in children. Five hundred cases for procedures below the diaphragm. Anaesthesia 37:806-818
3. Flandin-Blety C, Barrier G (1995) Accidents following extradural analgesia in children. The results of a retrospective study. Paediatr Anaesth 5:41-46
4. Giaufre E, Dalens B, Gombert A (1996) Epidemiology and morbidity of regional anaesthesia in children: a one-year prospective survey of the French-language society of paediatric anaesthesiologists. Anaesth Analg 83:904-912
5. Berde C (1996) Regional anaesthesia in children: what have we learned? Anaesth Analg 83:897-900
6. Jaffe RA, Siegel LC, Schnittger I et al (1995) Epidural air injection assessed by transesophageal echocardiography. Reg Anaesth 20:152-155
7. Campling EA (1989) Report of the National Confidential Enquiry into Perioperative Deaths. NCEPOD, London
8. Fox MA, Webb RK, Singleton R et al (1993) The Australian incident monitoring study. Problems with regional anaesthesia: an analysis of 2 000 incident reports. Anaesth Intensive Care 21:646-649
9. McNeely JK, Farber NE, Rusy LM et al (1997) Epidural analgesia improves outcome following paediatric fundoplication. A retrospective analysis. Reg Anaesth 22:16-22
10. Krane EJ, Haberkern CM, Jacobson LE (1995) Postoperative apnoea, bradycardia, and oxygen desaturation in formerly premature infants: prospective comparison of spinal and general anaesthesia. Anaesth Analg 80:7-13
11. Wolf AR, Stoddard PA (1995) Awake spinal anaesthesia for herniorrhaphy in ex-premature infants. (Editorial) Lancet 346:513-514
12. Oberlander TF, Berde CB, Lam KH et al (1995) Infants tolerate spinal anaesthesia with minimal overall autonomic changes: analysis of heart rate variability in former premature infants undergoing hernia repair. Anaesth Analg 80:20-27
13. Welborn LG, Rice JR, Hannallah RS et al (1990) Postoperative apnoea in former preterm infants: prospective comparison of spinal and general anaesthesia. Anaesthesiology 72:838-842

Chapter 9

Anaesthesia and postoperative care of children and neonates undergoing cardiac surgery, including transplantation

J. NEIDECKER

Despite prenatal diagnosis, the incidence, of congenital heart diseases remains between 5.5 to 8.6 per 1000 livebirths [1]. It is stable over the years. This overall rate encompasses a large combination of diseases which are not equally severe. Looking to critical congenital heart diseases requiring intervention in infancy, the reported number is rather constant: 3.5‰ [1].

In the last years, the new trend in surgical management is to operate on these infants very early in their lives, sometimes even within the first week. This has been made possible because of improvements and advances in early cardiological diagnosis, surgical techniques, anaesthetic management, and cardiopulmonary bypass technology. Nowadays the aim of any cardiac paediatric team is to provide the patient with the best care, i.e. to totally repair the diseased heart as far as possible. Thus, this lecture will be restricted to the management of paediatric patients undergoing total repair of the disease (procedure performed with the help of cardiopulmonary bypass) and will also approach a special way of treating some diseases: heart transplantation.

Pathophysiology

Due to the extreme complexity of congenital heart diseases, this short section on pathophysiology will focus on the main aspects of these abnomalitites and their possible consequences on the anaesthetic management.

Before birth, fetal and particularly pulmonary circulation are characterized by very high pulmonary pressure, virtually no pulmonary blood flow, and increased pulmonary vascular resistance [2]. At the time of birth, sudden modifications occur in normal newborns: pulmonary artery pressure and pulmonary resistance decrease while a pulmonary blood flow is generated. These modifications are different when congenital defects are present. In noncyanotic congenital heart disease at time of birth, pulmonary blood flow increases and remains high. This will have some effect on the pulmonary circulation: persistence of high pulmonary artery pressure and high pulmonary resistance. The "mid-term consequence" is the occurrence of insults of the pulmonary endothelium, leading to pulmonary vascular obstructive disease [2]. It has been shown that insults on the endothelium result in an increased release of endothelin, which is potentially vasoconstrictive, and in a decreased production of nitric oxide. All these phenomena induce pulmonary hypertension, which could be sudden or permanent and occur at any time during the surgical procedure and the postoperative course. These pathophysiological considerations must be taken into account when giving anaesthesia. Fluid intake should be carefully monitored because interstitial water and particularly extravascular lung water are increased. Any drug that can induce pulmonary hypertension directly or indirectly should be avoided [3].

Patients presenting with cardiomyopathy (primary myocardial dysfunction) are included in this group because their initial disease leads to increase pulmonary blood flow and pulmonary hypertension. During the perioperative period (operation is generally cardiac transplantation), the major problem is also pulmonary hypertension [4].

In cyanotic congenital heart diseases, pulmonary blood flow is usually reduced and, consequently, the pulmonary artery remains small. Pulmonary artery pressure is usually low because of the lack of flow while pulmonary resistance depends upon the complexity of the defect. Usually, the anaesthetic technique should avoid any systemic vasodilation (i.e. a drecrease in peripheral resistance) that would increase the right to left shunt and consequently increase the cyanosis.

Surgical repair increases the flow and sometimes the size of the pulmonary arteries. Nevertheless the occurrence of an increased postoperative blood flow will suddenly increase the right ventricular work, which is sometimes poorly tolerated and can lead to right ventricular failure. The latter will be very severe if, in addition, the pulmonary blood flow is reduced because of pulmonary stenosis.

When the anaesthesiologist is examining a newborn who is expected to undergo cardiac surgery, the same pathophysiology applies, of course, but the immaturity of several organs and particularly of the lung should be taken into account (surfactant deficiency).

The goal of anaesthetic management is to maintain the haemodynamics before surgical repair or transplantation and thereafter to adapt the heart and the circulation to the newly acquired circulation and sometimes physiological conditions.

Specific comment regarding heart transplantion [5]

Children scheduled for heart transplantation generally have end-stage congenital heart diseases; others present with acquired diseases which do not differ from those in adults. In addition to the pathophysiology described previously, there is global heart failure which is often treated by angiotensin-converting enzyme inhibitors (ACE inhibitors). The major problem concerning the indications for heart transplantation in children is correct assessment of pulmonary pulmonary pressure.

After transplantation, pathophysiological conditions change and move from a failing to a denervated heart. Denervation is complete and permanent; thus, the heart rate is the spontaneous resting rate, which is generally too slow. Just after reperfusion myocardial compliance is poor due to cold ischemic storage, which could explain a poor contractility and worsen the dysrhythmia.

Anaesthesia

Preoperative evaluation [3]

The preoperative evaluation of children undergoing cardiac procedures under cardiopulmonary bypass has several steps. The major one is the main diagnosis and is thus performed by the cardiologist: cardiac catheterization, echocardiography, etc. Anaesthesiologists are mainly interested in the biological data and the haemodynamic consequences of the disease. Appreciation of preoperative renal and hepatic functions allows better postoperative management, either by avoiding potentially toxic drugs (i.e., antibiotics) or by giving systemic treatment (i.e., diuretics). Coagulation tests are very important preoperatively because severe coagulation abnormalties are often associated with cyanotic diseases and sometimes require preoperative treatment. Otherwise, preoperative assessment is performed as in adult patients, with particular attention to reducing the blood sample volumes.

Generally, few adaptations of the preoperative treatment are necessary. Digoxin, if blood level is within therapeutic range, is usually continued until the day of surgery while β-blockers (mainly propranolol) are stopped 24 h before surgery when given to cyanotic patients. ACE inhibitors, anticoagulants, or aspirin are stopped according to the protocol used in the institution or for adult patients. When prostaglandin E1 is infused preoperatively in infants or neonates, some side effects of the drug can occur and thus should be known: mild fever (38°-38.5°C), hyperleukocytosis, and fluid retention. These side effects are not a contra-indication to cardiac surgery.

Premedication [3]

Children of any age should go into the operating room feeling confident and relaxed; therefore, premedication is required in the most cases. Premedication should be anxiolytic but not contain too much sedative, particularly in patients with cyanotic congenital heart diseases. In 1990, DeBock [6] and Levine [7] reported that premedication has an unpredictable effect regarding oxygen saturation in cyanotic children while there is only a mild decrease in oxygen saturation in noncyanotic patients. Light premedication is given usually 30 min to 1 h prior to surgery [6]. It can be administered intrarectally, intramuscularly, or sometimes orally. Various drugs, such as benzodiazepines, opioids, barbiturates or even ketamine, are routinely used. Together with premedication in older children in whom a direct peripheral venous puncture is expected, local anaesthesia of the site with EMLA cream may be useful.

Monitoring [8]

Routine monitoring of paediatric cardiac patients includes: ECG (at least four leads), invasive arterial blood pressure, pulse oximetry, capnography, urine output, temperatures (recorded at least in two different places: rectum, oesophagus, nasopharynx, ear, etc.). To assess central venous pressure, a double or triple lumen catheter is inserted. Swan-Ganz catheters are rarely used in paediatric cardiac patients because they are usually dificult to place correctly and sometimes may be dangerous. In addition, presence of indwelling catheters may hamper the surgeon. Usually, to complete the haemodynamic monitoring, the surgeon can insert various catheters at the end of cardiopulmonary bypass in the left atrium, in the pulmonary artery (in combination with a SVO^2 catheter or a probe to measure cardiac output by thermodilution) or in the right atrium. If transcutaneous vascular access is impossible at least one venous and one arterial line should be obtained by cutdown.

Transthoracic and transoesophageal echocardiography are, of course, part of noninvasive monitoring. Echocardiography is performed in the operating room or in the ICU. It assesses the myocardial contractility as well as pre- or afterload. After repair of any congenital heart disease, it allows also early diagnosis of any unsuspected residual defects.

All teams involved in the anaesthesia of patients with congenital heart defects must always bear in mind that intracardiac shunts may be present that have not been diagnosed preoperatively; therefore it is essential to ensure that there is no air (small bubbles) in any of the lines and syringes that could be transported to the brain because of an unknown intracardiac shunt or vessel abnormality. This will avoid neurological complications.

Induction of anaesthesia [3]

After a peripheral venous line has been inserted and the patient sedated with volatile anaesthetics (halothane or sevoflurane), induction of anaesthesia is performed intravenously. Barbiturates (thiopental) are the most commonly used hypnotic agents. They provide the necessary cerebral protection if a total circulatory arrest is required for the surgical procedure. Other hypnotics can be used. Etomidate is, like propofol, painful in children. In older children propofol can be safely used if early extubation is planned. All modern opiods (fentanyl, sufentanil, alfentanil) can be used and will correctly control catecholamine release [9-11]. Few data are available on paediatric use of remifentanil. All muscular relaxants can be chosen but pancuronium is often the preferred drug because it induces a mild tachycardia that inhibits bradycardia caused by the opioids, which is not desirable in children. The choice is very often made by the anaesthesiologist according to his personnal habits and to the cost.

Thereafter the nasotracheal intubation is undertaken; however, if early extubation is planned, the intubation can be performed orally.

During induction of anaesthesia, the anaesthesiologist must constantly bear in mind that vasodilation should be avoided in cyanotic patients while in non-cyanotic ones fluid intake should be carefully controlled.

After induction of anaesthesia and usually before skin incision, antiobiotic prophylaxis is initiated. The choice of antibiotics is adapted as usual to the microbiological environment and to the history of the patient. Further injections are performed according to the institution's protocols.

Maintenance of anaesthesia [3, 5, 9-11]

Further injections of hypnotics, opioids, and muscle relaxants are used to maintain anaesthesia. Volatile anaesthetics (isoflurane, sevoflurane or halothane) can be combined. Neonates have normal responses to surgical stress when as regards catecholamines release; therefore, systemic opioids should be given.

Transplant recipients do not receive different anaesthetic management than other paediatric cardiac patients do. The only particular point to focus on is that these children are receiving large doses of ACE inhibitors without any interruption. Intraoperatively, blood pressure may suddenly drop, which sometimes has to be corrected using very potent vasoconstrictors (norepinephrine, angiotensin, etc.).

Cardiopulmonary bypass [12, 13]

After administration of an average dose of 300 IU/kg of heparin (range from 200-500) cannulae are inserted into the vessels or into the right atrium.

The circuit and the volume of the oxygenator are generally adapted to the weight and size of the child. Thus, the prime volume of the circuit varies from 350 ml in neonates to 750 ml in "oversized" teenagers. As the dilution which is induced by such a prime volume is important regarding the child's volemia, red blood cells as well as fresh frozen plasma are added into the prime. Nevertheless, when a child's weight is close to 15 kg, total haemodilution can be attempted.

Cardiopulmonary bypass is conducted under deep hypothermia. In most of the cases 20°-25°C is required in combination with a low perfusion flow technique to reduce collateral circulation. When a total circulatory arrest is needed by the surgeon, the core temperature of the patient is lowered to 16°-20°C.

At the end of rewarming, haemofiltration is routinely used at some centres [14]. Intraoperative haemofiltration increases the mean blood pressure probably by several mechanisms which involve elimination of some vasoactive substances that have negative inotropic effects and water withdrawal inducing increased viscosity. Complement fragments and cytokines which are activated and released during paediatric cardiopulmonary bypass are also eliminated. Several techniques are proposed and at this point there is no agreement as to which one is the best.

Protamine is infused, like in adults, after termination of bypass and cannulae removal. The anaesthesiologist should infuse protamine cautiously in patients at risk of right ventricular failure or pulmonary hypertension because of protamine side effects.

Weaning from bypass: end of procedure

After total rewarming, the patients are progressively weaned from the cardiopulmonary bypass while keeping low filling pressures. Inotropics are progressively added if systemic pressure or contractility is poor. If preload is too high, vasodilators can be used. In pulmonary artery hypertension, vasodilators (sodium nitroprusside, nitroglycerine, prostaglandin E1) and, more specifically, nitric oxide are given.

Fluid can be infused as appropriate to maintain preload. In neonates and particularly after the arterial switch operation, it is important to stop the bypass with very low left atrial pressure.

Transplant recipients usually receive continuous infusion of isoproterenol before weaning from bypass because of the slow heart rate described above [5].

Sometimes at the end of the procedure, despite correct haemodynamic values, closure of the thorax is deleterious because of a dilated heart and/or myocardial edema the heart is compressed by the surrounding structures which limit the end-diastolic volume. Delayed chest closure is then advisable and final closure can be performed safely 48 h later [15]. This leads to a better outcome without any severe complications, such as mediastinitis.

Postoperative care

Standard postoperative care [3]

At the end of surgery children are transferred to the ICU where they stay until recovery. Postoperative monitoring is conducted as in adult patients but postoperative events are likely different because of the age, the initial disease, and the surgery.

Haemodynamic parameters – heart rate, systemic blood pressure, filling pressures (right and left atrial pressure), and pulmonary artery pressure – are recorded every hour. After some specific procedures, other data may be of interest: pressure in both vena cavae, mixed venous oxygen saturation (SvO_2), and cardiac output.

In children, peripheral perfusion and circulation are highly reflected by the temperature gradient (rectal or esophageal versus cutaneous) or urine output.

Mechanical ventilation is usually maintained for at least 3 h. Then patients with good haemodynamics who have undergone a simple procedure could benefit by early extubation (50%) [16]. Nevertheless, there is still a high reintubation rate (11%) and for the remaining patients Heinle [16] reports a mean duration of ventilation of 3.5 days.

Sedation is required when long-term mechanical ventilation is planned. Sedation is compulsory and often associated with muscular relaxants in cases of low cardiac output syndrome, pulmonary hypertension crisis, or delayed chest closure. It can be induced by continuous infusion of opioids (morphine, sufentanil)

[17]; benzodiazepines (midazolam) should be used cautiously because theis may accumulate if there is any evidence hepatic insufficiency [18]. They are of great interest in case of postoperative seizure. Nevertheless after 3 days if the haemodynamic values are correct, sedation must be interrupted to assess the neurogical status of the child, especially if a total circulatory arrest was used during surgery.

As soon as the patient is extubated, oral feeding can be started if there is no respiratory failure.

Specific complications are described below. Among the complications that are not described in detail, neurological ones have to be mentioned because of the severity, the unclear pathophysiological mechanism and the sometimes unpredictable development. They may ensue with simple seizures and progress to severe coma with stroke. Sometimes they are isolated or a consequence of a low cardiac output syndrome and part of multiple organ failure syndrome.

Biological examinations, chest radiographs, and echocardiography should be performed as often as required by the patient's condition.

Postoperative care of neonates

When they are in the ICU, neonates are managed like other children and the complications, if any, are the same. Nevertheless some particular points should be emphasized. First the use of incubators is compulsory to maintain correct temperature. Up to 50% of neonates enter the ICU with an open chest; therefore, mechanical ventilation is required for several days. In addition early extubation protocols are not suitable in neonates or are associated with a high reintubation rate [16]. During mechanical ventilation, high PaO_2 (over 120 mmHg for 6 h) should be avoided because it may cause, in conjunction with other factors due to immaturity, retrolental dysplasia leading to blindness [19]. In cases of persistent pulmonary hypertension associated with difficulty in performing mechanical ventilation, neonatal respiratory distress syndrome (surfactant deficiency) should be considered, which requires different management (oscillation ventilation and/or surfactant administration).

Management of specific aspects

Low cardiac output syndrome [3]

Low cardiac output syndrome occurring after paediatric cardiac surgery is different from that in adults: firstly, direct assessment of cardiac output is not common in children and sometimes not reliable; and secondly, initiation of the syndrome is generally concomitant with a right ventricular failure that will induce secondary global heart insufficiency.

Diagnosis will be established by several signs:
- clinical signs: pale face, peripheral cyanosis, hepatomegaly, and increased temperature gradient (increased central temperature and decreased cutaneous temperature);

– haemodynamics: decreased systemic pressure, and increased right or left atrial pressure, sudden (or permanent) increase in pulmonary artery pressure;
– low urine output (<0.5 ml/kg/per hour) together with biological signs of acute renal failure (hyperkalema and increased evels of urea and creatinine);
– biological signs of acute hepatic failure: hypoglycemia, and increased levels of enzymes or lactic acid;
– coagulation disorders (low fibrinogen and increased prothrombin time).

To correct the haemodynamics, treatment will mainly include inotropes (dopamine, dobutamine, epinephrine) to increase contractility and vasodilators (sodium nitroprusside, phentolamine, etc.) to decrease preload and afterload. Phosphodiesterase 3 inhibitors (milrinone, enoximone) combine inotropic and vasodilating effects and could be of interest because their mechanism of action is different [20, 21]. Phosphodiesterase inhibitors can be administered alone or in combination with other inotropics since the synergy is good. The dose of enoximone should be between 0.5 mg and 1 mg/kg every 6-8 h (own unpublished data) and should be adapted to haemodynamic response, renal function, and platelet count. When the patient is improving, reducing inotropics and/or vasodilators is generally difficult and the introduction of oral ACE inhibitors facilitates recovery and weaning from mechanical ventilation. While waiting for haemodynamic improvement, symptomatic treatment should be included: fresh frozen plasma, platelet, and high glucose intake.

Low cardiac output syndrome has still a high mortality rate despite improvements and advances in treatment. The initial disease and the surgical operation are some of the most important factors.

Pulmonary hypertension

Closure of congenital heart defects from left to right may result in postoperative pulmonary hypertension due to pulmonary obstructive vascular disease. It also occurs after heart transplantation. Clinically, in addition to the increase in pulmonary artery pressure, there is: a drop in blood pressure with cyanosis, bradycardia, and right ventricular failure. If present, SvO_2 will decrease. If it persists global heart failure occurs. Sometimes the increase in pulmonary artery pressure is sudden and will induce acute right ventricular dilatation that leads promptly to cardiac arrest.

Treatment is mainly based on prevention and avoidance of stimulation of the trachea (suction). Hyperventilation is basic to decreasing pulmonary pressure, generally associated with deep sedation. Pharmacological treatment consists of vasodilators given intravenously or sometimes directly into the pulmonary artery. A few years ago a more specific pulmonary vasodilator became available: nitric oxide. Nitric oxide is given by inhalation and doses commonly range between 5 and 20 ppm (but larger doses – up to 80 ppm – have been reported) [22]. When patients receive nitric oxide for a long period, methaemoglobin monitoring is mandatory to detect toxicity, which is rare but more frequent and dangerous in neonates [23]. This drug is rapidly efficient in controlling the pulmonary artery pressue and the patient will improve. Nevertheless, after normalization of pulmonary artery pressure, a deleterious rebound can be observed when nitric oxide is stopped. Such a rebound requires reintroduction of nitric oxide. Recently, the use of a nitric oxide donor drug (molsidomine or dipyridamole) has been reported to effectively prevent a rebound [24].

Renal failure

Postoperative renal failure is often the first organ dysfunction to develop. Initially, incremental dose of diuretics will effectively treat the oliguria. Usually, though, hyperkalemia, together with an increase in urea levels and fluid overload, will require a more active treatment – dialysis. In infants and neonates, peritoneal dialysis is preferable because it is easier to initiate and offers better haemodynamic stability [25]. It is effective in potassium and urea removal, but water removal is sometimes too slow. Conventional or continuous haemodialysis can be safely used in children [26] but in infants there is a problem of vascular access. Thus, it is chosen when weight is greater than 15-20 kg. The efficacy is greater (especially regarding water removal) but the haemodynamic stability is generally impaired at the initiation. Dialysis is progressively stopped in conjunction with renal improvement.

Management of the transplanted patients [5]

Management of children undergoing heart transplantation generally includes a combination of two protocols: 1) as in paediatric cardiac patients as described above; 2) according to the heart transplantation immunosuppressive protocol, which differs from one institution to another.

Regarding the haemodynamic status, the main complication is pulmonary hypertension, which has the same therapeutic scheme. Sometimes, bradycardia without a sinus rhythm requires a continuous infusion of isoproterenol for several days (sometimes before pacemaker implantation) to maintain an adequate heart rate for the age.

The basis of immunosupressive treatment is initially as in adults: Four-drug therapy during the first week (corticosteroids, azathioprine, cyclosporine A, and polyclonal anti-lymphocyte globulins, ALG) then triple-drug therapy (no ALG). Later treatment is adapted to acceptance and tolerance according to the age (especially for corticoids). Dosage and therapeutic levels of cyclosporine A are those currently accepted for adults. Careful monitoring of renal function is advisable and that requires often prolonged stay in the ICU.

To avoid the psychological trauma of repeated anaesthesia for endomyocardial biopsies in children and also to reduce the risk of repeated venous puncture, follow-up and detection of rejection are generally performed by transthoracic echocardiography. Endomyocardial biopsies which remain the primary and basic means of rejection detection, are undertaken only if the diagnosis is unclear [27].

Rejection is treated as in adults by corticosteroids (15 mg/kg), possibly associated with ALG; monoclonal anti-lymphocytes globulins (OKT3) are only used when conventional treatment is contraindicated or in case of renal failure, hepatic failure (which is not uncommon in end-stage congenital heart diseases, especially if a Fontan procedure was performed previously) or unresponsive rejection.

All other treatments are performed as in adults (i.e. prevention of infection).

Conclusions

The same basic concepts that regulate adult cardiac surgery apply to the perioperative management of children of any age undergoing cardiac surgery.

Factors specific to children are:
- the age and weight, which requires a constant adaptation of the technique and equipment;
- an extreme complexity of the disease, which requires a correct knowledge of the pathophysiology;
- complex surgical procedures that modify the preoperative pathophysiological conditions and move towards different ones.

Consequently, the perioperative management of these children should involve a team of cardiologists, radiologists, echocardiographers, anaesthesiologists, surgeons, and intensive care specialists.

References

1. Ferencz C, Neill CA (1992) Cardiovascular malformations: prevalence at livebirth. In: Freedom RM, Benson LN, Jeffrey F, Smallhorn JF (eds) Neonatal heart disease. Springer-Verlag, London, pp 19-29
2. Rudolph AM (ed) (1974) Congenital diseases of the heart. Yearbook Medical Publishers, Chicago
3. Hickey PR, Wessel DL (1987) Anaesthesia for treament of congenital heart disease. In: Kaplan JA (ed) Cardiac anaesthesia. Grune and Stratton, Orlando, pp 635-723
4. Meliones JN, Kern FH, Schulman SR, Ungerleider RM, Greeley WJ (1996) Pathophysiological directed approach to congenital heart disease: a perioperative perspective. In: Greeley WJ (ed) Perioperative management of the patient with congenital heart disease. Williams and Wilkins, Baltimore, pp 1-42
5. Dunn JM, Donner RM (eds)(1990) Heart transplantation in children. Futura, Mount Kisco
6. DeBock TL, Davis PJ, Tome J, Petrilli R, Siewers RD, Motoyama EK (1990) Effect of premedication on arterial saturation in children with congenital heart disease. J Cardiothorac Anaesth 4:423-424
7. Levine MF, Hartley EJ, Macpherson BA, Burrows FA, Lerman J (1993) Oral midazolam premedication for children with congenital cyanotic heart disease undergoing cardiac surgery: a comparative study. Can J Anaesth 40:934-938
8. Purday JP (1994) Monitoring during paediatric cardiac anaesthesia. Can J Anaesth 41:818-844

9. Hickey PR, Hansen DD (1984) Fentanyl- and sufentanil-oxygen-pancuronium anaesthesia for cardiac surgery in infants. Anaesth Analg 63:117-124

10. Moore RA, Yang SS, McNicholas KW, Gallagher JD, Clark DL (1985) Hemodynamic and anaesthetic effects of sufentanil as the sole anaesthetic for pediatric cardiovascular surgery. Anaesthesiology 62:725-731

11. Anand KJS, Hickey PR (1992) Halothane-morphine compared with high dose sufentanil for anaesthesia and postoperative analgesia in neonatal cardiac surgery. N Engl J Med 326:1-9

12. Kern FH, Schulman S, Greeley WJ (1996) Cardiopulmonary bypass: techniques and effects. In: Greeley WJ (ed) Perioperative management of the patient with congenital heart disease. Williams and Wilkins, Baltimore, pp 67-120

13. Gruenwald CE, Andrew M, Burrows FA, Williams WG (1993) Cardiopulmonary bypass in neonate. Adv Cardiac Surg 4:137-156

14. Pouard P, Journois D, Greeley WJ (1996) Hemofiltration and pediatric cardiac surgery. In: Greeley WJ (ed) Perioperative management of the patient with congenital heart disease. Williams and Wilkins, Baltimore, pp 121-132

15. Iyer RS, Jacobs JP, de Leval MR, Stark J, Elliott MJ (1997) Outcomes after delayed sternal closure in pediatric heart operations: a 10-year experience. Ann Thorac Surg 63:489-491

16. Heinle JS, Diaz LK, Fox LS (1997) Early extubation after cardiac operations in neonates and young infants. J Thorac Cardiovasc Surg 114:413-418

17. Pounder DR, Steward DJ (1992) Postoperative analgesia: opioids infusions in infant and children. Can J Anaesth 39:969-974

18. Lloyd-Thomas AR, Booker PD (1986) Infusion of midazolam in paediatric patients after cardiac surgery. Br J Anaesth 58:1109-1115

19. Obladen M (1981) Blood gas analysis. In: Wille L, Obladen M (eds) Neonatal intensive care. Springer-Verlag, Berlin Heidelberg New York, pp 55-72

20. Jayais P, Mauriat P, Pouard P, Journois D (1990) Enoximone et chirurgie cardiaque pédiatrique. Arch Mal Coeur 83:109-117

21. Hausdorf G (1993) Experience with phosphodiesterase inhibitors in paediatric cardiac surgery. Eur J Anaesth 10(Suppl 8):25-30

22. Selldén H, Winberg P, Gustafsson LE, Lundell B, Böök K, Frostell CG (1993) Inhalation of nitric oxide reduced pulmonary hypertension after cardiac surgery in 3.2 kg infant. Anaesthesiology 78:577-580

23. Aouifi A, Filley S, Neidecker J, Helal N, Bompard D, Vedrinne C, Blanc P, Laroux MC, Bouvier H, Girard C, Lehot JJ (1997) Methaemoglobin (MetHb) production during nitric oxide (NO) inhalation. Br J Anaesth 78(Suppl 2):47

24. Ivy DD, Kinsella JP, Ziegler JW, Abman SH (1998) Dipyridamole attenuates rebound pulmonary hypertension after inhaled nitric oxide withdrawal in postoperative congenital heart disease. 115:875-882

25. Giuffre RM, Tam KH, Williams WW, Freedom RM (1992) Acute renal failure complicating pediatric cardiac surgery. A comparison of survivors and non survivors following acute peritoneal dialysis. Pediatr Cardiol 13:208-213

26. Paret G, Cohen AJ, Bohn DJ, Edward H, Taylor R, Geary D, Williams WG (1992) Continuous arteriovenous hemofiltration after cardiac operations in infants and children. J Thorac Cardiovasc Surg 104:1225-1230

27. Balzer DT, Moorhead S, Saffitz JE, Huddleston CB, Spray TL, Canter CE (1995) Utility of surveillance biopsies in infant heart transplant recipients. J Heart Lung Transplant 14:1095-1101

Chapter 10

New modes of ventilation in paediatrics

G.A. MARRARO

Since its first extensive use during the polio epidemics of the 1950s, mechanical ventilation has proved to be of undoubted value in improving survival in many patients affected by severe respiratory failure of varying origin. In the last 25 years, artificial ventilation has tremendously improved the recovery of neonates, especially those born prematurely. However, mechanical ventilation can, in itself, result not only in pulmonary damage (interstitial emphysema, alveolar and bronchiolar damage, pneumothorax, and bronchopulmonary dysplasia) but also in damage to other organs, specifically when high FiO_2 has been used (i.e., retrolental fibroplasia) [1-4].

Side effects are connected with: a) inadequate ventilatory treatment due to incorrect correlation between the ventilatory strategy and lung pathology; b) delay in beginning artificial ventilation and subsequent treatment of a complicated and consolidated lung pathology and use of invasive and iatrogenic procedures; c) oxygen toxicity due to high FiO_2 [5-7]; d) large volume and high peak airway pressure [8-12]; and e) overinfection due to violation of the respiratory tract.

A new philosophy [13-17] is emerging in the application of mechanical ventilation:

1. to protect the ventilated lung (healthy or pathologic) using an *adequate* ventilatory support as soon as possible and for as short a time as necessary;
2. to prevent oxygen toxicity using the lowest FiO_2, applying complementary means of support which can lead to an improvement in PaO_2 (surfactant, nitric oxide, PEEP, etc.);
3. to recruit the infiltrated, atelectatic and consolidated lung using adequate PEEP level;
4. to maintain gas exchange, accepting a PaO_2 level between 50-70 mmHg and a moderate hypercapnia ($PaCO_2$ between 45-55 mmHg).

Complications of artificial ventilation are toxic effects due to high oxygen concentration used, alveolar injury barotrauma, reduction of cardiac output, laryngotracheal damage, pneumonia and bronchopneumonia.

Even though certain complications can be reduced by correct application of artificial ventilation, little can be done for others, given the necessity to guarantee gas exchanges and, therefore, survival.

In order to reduce side effects connected with artificial ventilation four principal areas are under investigation:

1. the use of ventilatory methods which allow the peak inspiratory pressure to be controlled or reduced, so as to reduce traumatic pulmonary lesions;
2. independent lung ventilation in order to ventilate only the more diseased lung, so as to reduce barotrauma in the healthier lung;
3. the use of mechanical support during spontaneous breathing in order to reduce work of breathing, oxygen consumption, and negative effects on haemodynamics connected with artificial ventilation and positive end-expiratory pressure (PEEP) application;
4. the use of perfluorocarbons instead of air for gas exchange.

Methods to reduce peak airway pressure

High frequency oscillatory ventilation

High-frequency ventilation (HFV) has been largely investigated over the past two decades. Despite its theoretical benefits it has not received unanimous consensus and has not been widely used, except for high frequency jet ventilation (HFJV) employed in tracheal and bronchial anaesthesia [18]. High frequency oscillatory ventilation (HFOV) is proving to be highly successful, however, mainly because adequate humidification of ventilated gases is now possible [19-21].

HFOV is recommended in order to reduce lung barotrauma and consequent lung injury in non homogeneous lung pathology and in the ventilation of premature babies. A number of mechanisms have been proposed to explain the gas exchange in HFOV: direct alveolar ventilation, asymmetric velocity profiles, Taylor dispersion, pandelluft, cardiogenic mixing, accelerated diffusion, and acoustic resonance, both individually and in combination [21].

The theoretical advantages of HFOV include:
1. maintaining open airways;
2. smaller phasic volume and pressure change;
3. gas exchange at significantly lower airway pressure;
4. less involvement of the cardiovascular system;
5. less depression of endogenous surfactant production.

Recent studies in premature babies with hyaline membrane disease and in term or near-term newborns affected with lung pathologies have demonstrated an important improvement in oxygenation and a reduced incidence of air leak with HFOV. HFOV has also proven to be a valuable ventilatory alternative in some newborns who meet criteria for extracorporeal membrane oxygenation (ECMO) [22]. There are limited published data on the use of HFOV in paediatric patients but its benefits, deriving from the reopening of alveoli and keeping them open, as well as the reduction of air leak, appear clear. The data available at present, which do not show haemodynamic compromise, increase in the incidence of barotrauma, or decline in oxygenation index require supplementary clinically controlled studies. The problems connected with permeability of the lung epithelium [23] and damage of trachea and bronchi [24, 25] have yet to be investigated.

Pressure-regulated volume control ventilation

A new mode of ventilation, pressure-regulated volume control (PRVC), is now available in newer ventilators [26-30]. This new mode delivers a controlled tidal and minute volume in a pressure-limited manner using the lowest possible pressure, which is constant during the inspiratory phase. The gas flow is decelerated, and pressure and flow constantly vary. Peak inspiratory pressure (PIP) is automatically reduced when compliance and airway resistance change.

Methodology

The ventilator tests the first breath at 5 cm H_2O above PEEP and calculates the pressure-volume ratio. The inspiratory pressure changes breath by breath until the set tidal volume is obtained with a maximum of 5 cm H_2O below the upper pressure limit set. At this stage the measured tidal volume corresponds to the preset value and the pressure level remains constant (Fig. 1). If the measured tidal volume increases above the preset level, inspiratory pressure will be adjusted until the set tidal volume is reached.

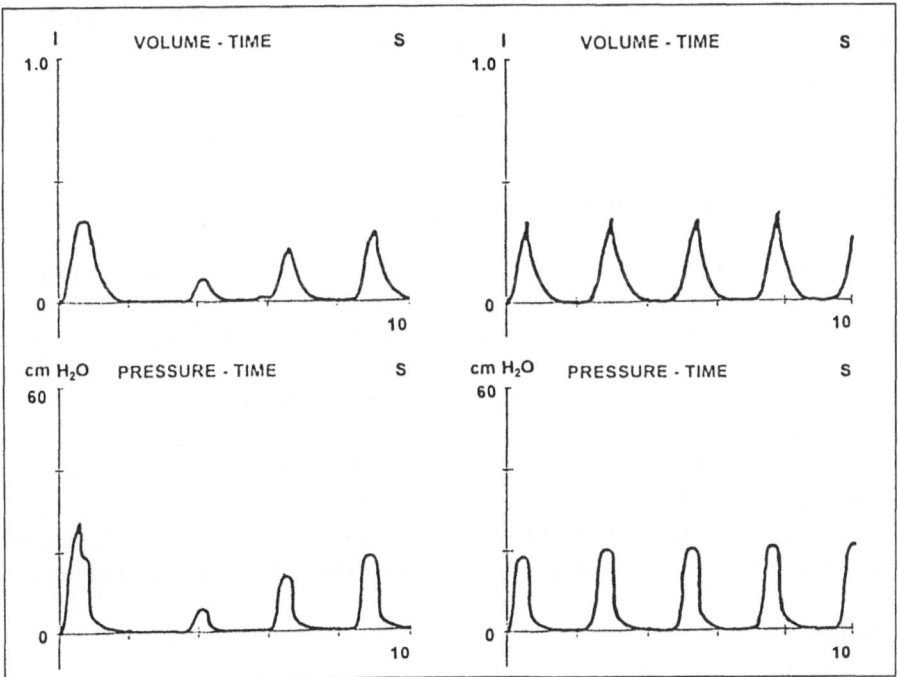

Fig. 1. The inspiratory pressure is tested, breath by breath, until preset tidal volume is reached. Subsequently, the inspiratory pressure is adapted according to the pressure volume ratio

Indications

This mode of ventilation appears to be indicated:
1. if within the lung compliance and resistance vary;
2. if there is an initial requirement of high flow in order to reopen closed pulmonary areas (i.e., atelectasis);
3. to reduce high ventilatory peak pressure (i.e., in premature infants, pneumothorax, interstitial emphysema, etc.);
4. to control ventilatory pressures from the moment nonventilated alveoli and bronchioles are reopened (i.e., surfactant, theophylline or nitric oxide administration, etc.);
5. in the presence of broncho- and bronchiole-spasms (i.e., asthma, bronchiolitis, etc.);
6. in all patients in whom PEEP levels must be reduced in order to avoid haemodynamic complications.

The method appears to be useful in improving respiratory mechanics and gas exchange, in reducing the barotrauma caused by PIP, in limiting oxygen toxicity due to the possibility of using reduced FiO_2 to maintain adequate gas exchange as compared with conventional mechanical ventilation [29-35]. It appears also beneficial when drugs such as surfactants, bronchodilators, nitric oxide, etc., which bring about a rapid change in compliance and airway resistance, are used [30, 32, 34].

Clinically controlled studies are required to evaluate its real benefits in the acute phase of the lung disease, in weaning from the ventilator, and in the ventilation of healthy lungs (i.e., neurosurgical patients).

Method to reduce monolateral lung overdistension

Independent lung ventilation

At present separate ventilation of the lungs of infants and children by means of selective bronchial intubation may be carried out using, for example, the Endobronchial Bilumen Tube (Portex® Ltd) [36]. It is available in different sizes and suitable for treating premature babies weighing more than 1500 g and children of up to 3 years [37-39]. Beyond this age selective intubation is possible only using a tube fitted with cuffs.

Left bronchial intubation is preferable to right because it reduces the possibility of exclusion of the upper right lobar bronchus and the resulting atelectasis. The correct positioning of the tube is checked by auscultation of the lungs and more reliably by X-ray examination of the chest after it has been put in place.

Ventilators

Independent lung ventilation (ILV) requires ventilators which permit different modes of ventilation to be applied to each lung (Fig. 2). Synchronization of the

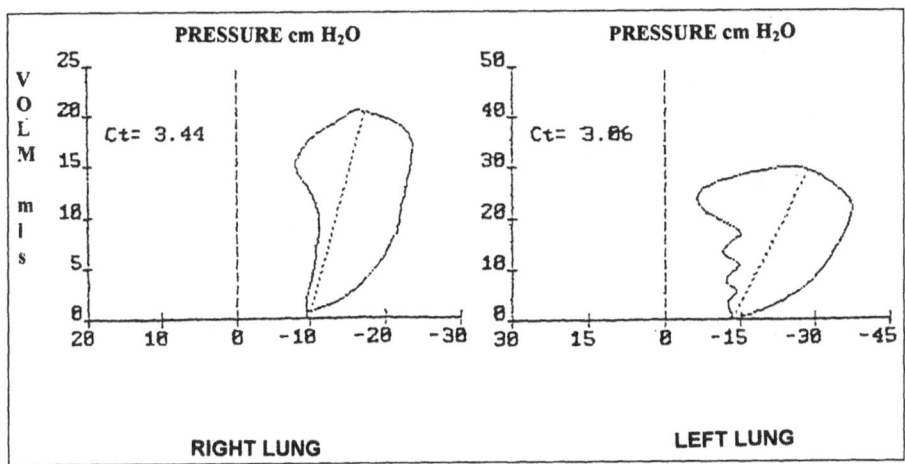

Fig. 2. Independent ventilation of the two lungs. Different levels of PEEP are applied to each lung

start of respiration ensures that there is no shifting of the mediastinum, which may create an obstacle to venous return to the heart and a resulting fall in cardiac output. Furthermore, the nonsynchronous insufflation of the lungs may produce severe ventilation disorders. These complications occur mostly at low respiratory frequencies (<30 times per minute) [38-42].

Application of ILV does not itself cause haemodynamic changes different from those which are encountered during intermittent positive pressure ventilation (IPPV) and continuous positive pressure ventilation (CPPV) with PEEP of 5 cm of H_2O. An increase in the central venous pressure and cardiac frequency and a reduction in arterial pressure are apparent when the levels of PEEP or tidal volumes are too high and interfere with intrathoracic pressure [38-40].

Less of CO_2 is eliminated from the more damaged lung than from the less damaged lung as long as the recruitment of the small airways and the alveoli has not normalized. Increasing the level of PEEP leads to an increase in the elimination of CO_2 since more areas are opened to ventilation. The improvement in the PaO_2 and the better elimination of CO_2 are rapid and constant. Excellent improvement in gas exchange takes place when selective ventilation and the best PEEP for each lung are applied (Fig. 3).

Advantages of independent ventilation are:
- increase in functional residual capacity and ventilation only in the more damaged lung;
- reduction in hyperventilation in the less damaged lung;
- possibility of using selective PEEP in the two lungs;
- isolation of secretions of the infected pulmonary areas and less risk of diffusion by contiguity of the infection from one to the other lung.

Several problems remain unsolved in the application of the methodology in infants:

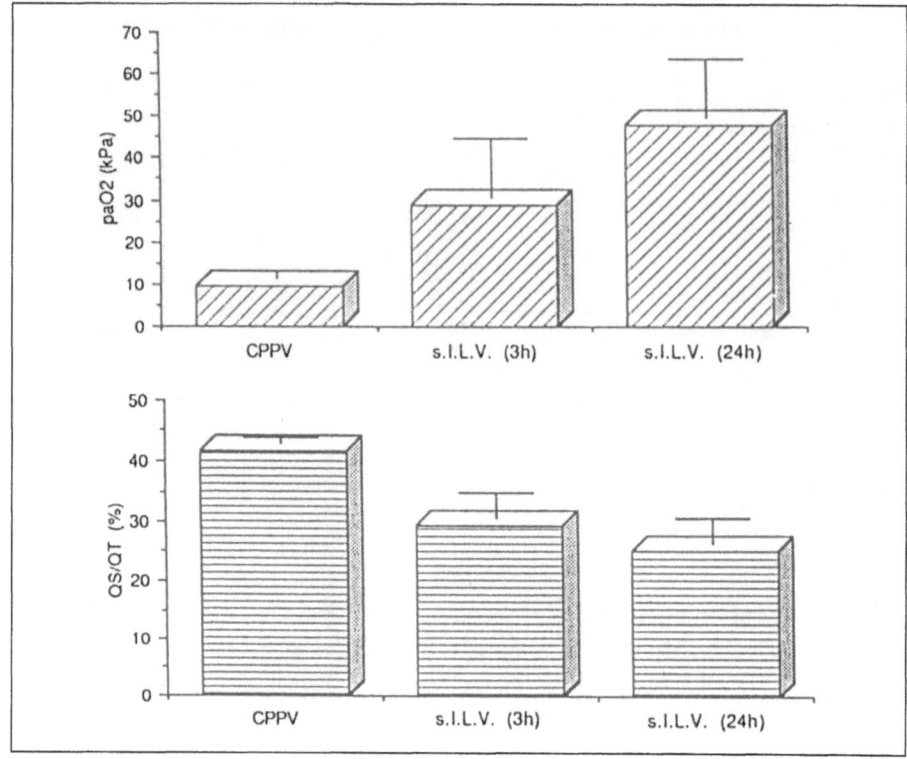

Fig. 3. PaO$_2$ and QS/QT improvement at different times of independent lung ventilation (*ILV*) of 15 infants affected by lung pathology with monolateral prevalence

– the absence of cuffs prevents the application of high PEEP levels because it is possible to detect gas losses;
– humidifying and heating the ventilated gases presents a considerable problem. The secretions must be kept fluid and easily suctionable so as to avoid obstruction of the lumina of the bilumen tube in view of the small gauge. This complication must be closely monitored [43]. The necessity of using two ventilators and the high operating cost should be reduced if the treatment is more intensive and its duration is shortened.

Methods to support spontaneous breathing

Pressure support ventilation

Pressure support ventilation (PSV) is designed to support spontaneous breathing during the inspiratory phase [26, 28, 30, 40-46]. Once the patient has triggered opening of the demand valve, a supplementary gas flow is delivered to the inspiratory circuit, thereby producing a positive inspiratory pressure at a preset

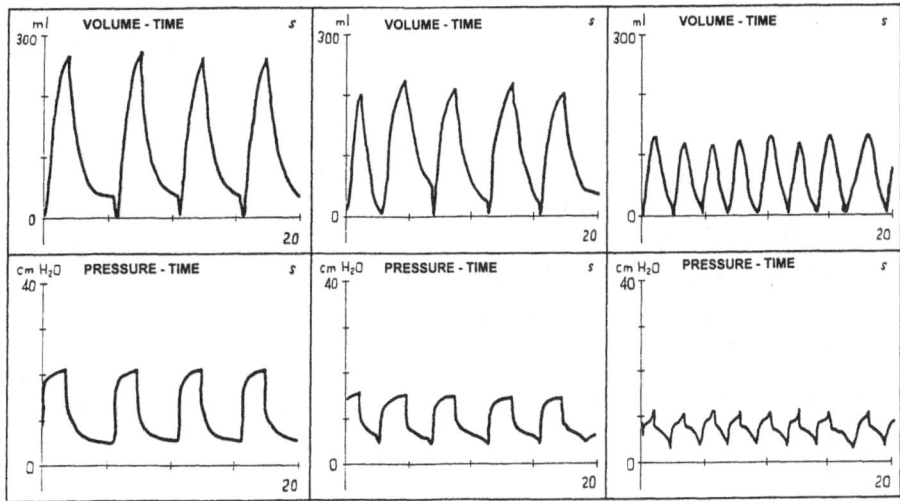

Fig. 4. Comparison of different levels of pressure support applied in a child. The correct pattern is in the middle. Increasing pressure support, a reduction in respiratory rate, and an increase in tidal volume were noted (left). Reducing pressure support, an increase in respiratory rate, and a decrease in tidal volume were obtained (right)

value. There is no preset tidal volume and cycles are pressure-limited. The ventilator assists each breath, regulated by the level of pressure preset. The patient triggers the assisted breathing and regulates the respiratory rate, inspiratory and expiratory time, and tidal volume [47-49].

Pressure support is regulated in order to supply tidal volumes and respiratory rates similar to the physiological values. If the pressure support is high, the patient tends to reduce respiratory rate and increase tidal volume. This could allow an increase in barotrauma and the humidifier would not be able to warm and humidify the ventilated gases sufficiently. In the case of low pressure support, the patient increases the respiratory rate and reduces the tidal volume, which leads to an increase in the work of breathing and oxygen consumption (Fig. 4).

In the presence of inhomogeneous ventilation, this model could expand the better ventilated areas without affecting the pathological areas. This method is best employed in weaning from ventilator when the lung condition has improved [50-53]. Beneficial effects are obtained in haemodynamics as far as ventilation control is concerned, because breathing begins spontaneously [53].

Volume support ventilation

Volume support ventilation (VSV) is another new means of assisting spontaneous breathing which avoids the disadvantages deriving from pressure support ventilation [29, 30]. The ventilator, breath by breath, adapts the inspiratory pressure support level to the changes in the mechanical properties of the lung and

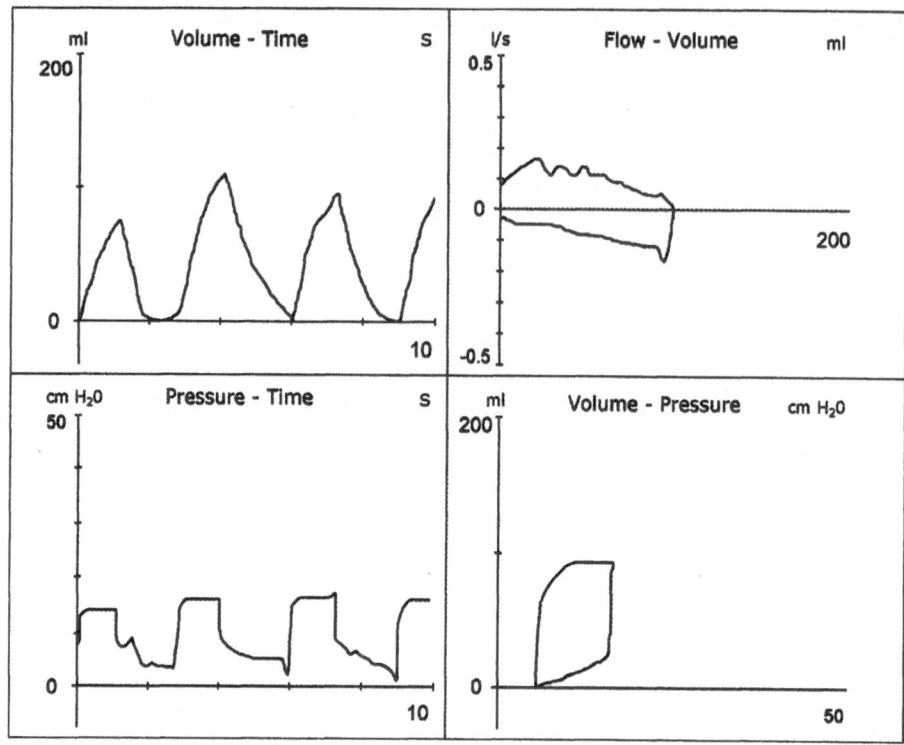

Fig. 5. Volume support ventilation, the same tidal volume is delivered, breath by breath, using the lowest possible inspiratory pressure level

the thorax in order to ensure that the lowest possible pressure is used to deliver the preset tidal and minute volume, which remain constant (Fig. 5). The inspiratory pressure is constant and the flow is decelerated. In cases of apnea the ventilator automatically switches to PRVC. The initial values for expected tidal and minute volume should be set, as should all parameters to be used in PRVC in the presence of apnea ventilation.

Indications for PSV and VSV

Intensive care:
- weaning from ventilation after improvement in lung pathology;
- weaning from long term ventilation [54];
- weaning of patients with chronic obstructive pulmonary disease, e.g., infants with severe bronchopulmonary dysplasia (BPD);
- to promote respiratory muscle training in critically ill patients;
- to compensate for the high resistance of endotracheal tubes during spontaneous respiration with continuous positive airway pressure (CPAP) [55].
Postoperative care:

- to preserve or reactivate spontaneous breathing;
- to reinflate areas of atelectasis after surgery.

Controindications to PSV and VSV

- Deep sedation and muscle relaxants;
- central neurological disorders;
- hypoventilation syndromes;
- small, premature infants who may be unable to trigger the demand valve.

Methods using liquid instead of air to effect gas exchange: liquid ventilation

The possibilities of using liquid instead of air in the exchange of gases has always fascinated researchers [56]. This possibility became a reality with the discovery of the properties of perfluorocarbon (PFC) liquids, when in 1963 Clark [57] demonstrated survival of mice and rats by immersing them in oxygenated PFC, thus opening the way to the clinical application of this concept.

Characteristics of perfluorocarbons

PFC can be derived from organic compounds, such as benzene. They are clear colorless and odorless and can be stored indefinitely at room temperature. They are resistant to autoclaving. They are insoluble in water or in lipids and water or lipids do not dissolve in them. However, oxygen, carbon dioxide, and many other gases are very easily dissolved in them. All PFCs have a low surface tension and rapidly evaporate at body temperature from the lung and the skin. The mechanisms for uptake, biodistribution, and elimination in the body are not clearly defined but are correlated to lipid tissue composition, organ perfusion, and the ventilation/perfusion ratio in the lung. The physiochemical characteristics of PFC, i.e. molecular structure and vapor pressure, and the lung pathophysiology play an important role. Small quantities of PFC can be absorbed in the blood and distributed to the tissues, with a preference for lipids and fats. The absorbed PFC can remain in the tissues for long periods but does not seem to exert any toxic effects. The persistence in the body and the predilection for fatty tissue warrants further investigation, particularly with respect to the developing central nervous system of neonates and premature babies.

Methods of administration

At present, there are two methods of administration of PFC. Total liquid ventilation (TLV) was developed by Moskowitz [58] and subsequently by Shaffer [59, 60]. Partial liquid ventilation (PLV) or perfluorocarbon-associated gas exchange (PAGE) was proposed by Fuhrman [61] and Lachmann [62].

Total Liquid Ventilation

TLV employs PFCs instead of gas for gas exchange. A volume of 30 ml/kg of warmed, oxygenated PFC is introduced in the lung and further quantities are administered until the lung has been completely filled. As soon as the air has been completely expelled, the patient is connected to a ventilator (similar to a dialysis pump). The tidal volume is subsequently set at 15-20 ml/kg of PFC. Respiratory rate is regulated to 4-5 breaths per minute. The maximum inspiratory peak pressure is 30 cm of H_2O but a pressure of between 15 and 20 cm H_2O is usually sufficient. The negative pressure required during the expiratory phase ranges from -15 to -30 cm of H_2O. At the end of the treatment conventional ventilation can be continued until the PFC has evaporated from the lung.

Partial Liquid Ventilation

PLV is a ventilatory technique employing PFCs to fill the functional residual capacity (FRC) of the lungs while gas tidal volumes are delivered by a conventional volume-regulated ventilator. A volume of 30 ml/kg of PFC is introduced in order to partially or fully replace the FRC. A further 10 m/kg of PFC is addeded every hour to replace redistribution or evaporative losses.

Problems in the use of PFC

A persistent problem noted in early use of PFC was a significant degree of lactic acidosis. A fall in cardiac output has been noted, possibly linked to an increase in pulmonary vascular resistence due to the compression of the pulmonary vessels by the heavier liquid.

CO$_2$ elimination is linked to the persistence of the PFC in the lung and to dead space. While PFC readily absorbs CO_2, it does not allow rapid diffusion of CO_2. PFC is highly viscous and dense and thus a very low frequency ventilatory rate is necessary. Unsuitable ventilatory rates can lead to an accumulation of CO_2 and, in turn, respiratory acidosis. At low frequencies CO_2, clearance is reduced because of inadequate diffusion time. Adjustment of tidal-volume during steady state ventilation can be made to keep $PaCO_2$ values within the normal physiological range, provided the frequency is low enough. In animals the most effective alveolar ventilation and CO_2 elimination occur at frequencies of 3-5 breaths per minute. Adequate oxygenation is achieved by manipulation of the FiO_2 of the inspired liquid and by maintaining an adequate FRC by altering inspiratory and expiratory volumes and PEEP level.

Advantages of TLV

Liquid ventilation is extremely effective in improving oxygenation [60, 63, 64]. Unlike the gas-filled lung, in which alveolar pressure are uniform and vascular pressures are subject to a hydrostatic gradient, the liquid-filled lung has trans-mural gradients that are relatively balanced. This results in uniformly distended pulmonary blood vessels and evenly distributed blood flow, thus improving ventilation/perfusion matching. The haemodynamic disturbances during PLV are less evident than during TLV. In areas of atelectasis, ventilation/perfusion matching and decreased pulmonary resistance through the lung leads to recruitment and unfolding of alveolar tissue and capillaries. The improvement in gas exchange and the increase in compliance indicate more effective oxygenation and ventilation, presumably because of a reduction in alveolar surface tension [59].

Any material present in the lung can be mobilized and eliminated and, therefore, these reventilated areas are recruited to ventilation [59, 65, 66]. Peak inspiratory pressure is lower during liquid ventilation than during conventional gas ventilation. The incidence of barotrauma and alteration of lung structure is thus reduced.

Advantages of partial liquid ventilation over total liquid ventilation

- Use of the same equipment as during conventional mechanical ventilation;
- does not require bulky, sophisticated equipment;
- better cardiovascular stability and fewer haemodynamic side effects and pH variations.

Indications for liquid ventilation

Liquid ventilation eliminates the air/liquid interface and reduces surface tension. It could be useful in lung pathologies such as respiratory distress syndrome (RDS) in premature babies and acute respiratory distress syndrome (ARDS) [67-69]. It may also be useful in meconium aspiration syndrome where it facilitates the removal of the meconium and eliminates inhomogeneous lung ventilation [59, 65, 66]. Future application could be in the treatment of inhalation syndrome, cystic fibrosis (mucoviscidosis), and proteinosis. In these cases PFC could remove the material present in the lungs, improve gas exchange, reduce the atelectactic tendency, and prevent the loss of surface activity. Liquid ventilation is also used in the study of the lung, for topical administration of drugs, heating pulmonary lobi to increase lobar or pulmonary blood flow, in the treatment of lung cancer, and as a ventilatory support for unusual types of treatment [60]. This is a fascinating and stimulating area requiring further studies. Some positive results have been reported in humans [66, 68-70].

Points remaining to be solved

- The safety of liquid ventilation over prolonged periods of time;
- the haemodynamic effects in the presence of pulmonary hypertension or patency of ductus arteriosus;

- the problems of returning to gas ventilation after a long period of liquid ventilation;
- the uptake and metabolism of PFC with regards to damage from long-term persistence in the tissues [64, 71, 72].

References

1. Northway WH, Rosan RC, Porter DY (1967) Pulmonary disease following respirator therapy of hyaline-membrane disease. Bronchopulmonary dysplasia. N Engl J Med 276:357-368
2. Goetzman BW (1986) Understanding bronchopulmonary dysplasia. Am J Dis Child 140:332-334
3. Chambers HM, van Velzen D (1989) Ventilator-related pathology in the extremely immature lung. Pathology 21:79-83
4. Wohl MEB (1990) Bronchopulmonary dysplasia in adulthood. N Engl J Med 323:1834-1836
5. Kafer ER (1971) Pulmonary oxygen toxicity. A review of the evidence for acute and chronic oxygen toxicity in man. Br J Anaesth 43:687-695
6. Holm BA, Matalon S, Finkelstein JH, Notter RH (1988) Type II pneumocyte changes during hyperoxic lung injury and recovery. J Appl Physiol 65:2672-2678
7. Saugstad OD (1985) Oxygen radicals and pulmonary damage. Pediatr Pulmonol 1:167-175
8. Nilsson R, Grossmann G, Robertson B (1980) Pathogenesis of neonatal lung lesions induced by artificial ventilation: evidence against the role of barotrauma. Respiration 40:218-225
9. Kolobow T, Moretti MP, Fumagalli R, Mascheroni D, Prato P, Chen V, Joris M (1987) Severe impairment in lung function induced by high peak airway pressure during mechanical ventilation. Am Rev Respir Dis 135:312-315
10. Dreyfuss D, Soler P, Basset G, Saumon G (1988) High inflation pressure pulmonary edema. Respective effects of high airway pressure, high tidal volume, and positive end-expiratory pressure. Am Rev Respir Dis 137:1159-1164
11. Tsuno K, Prato P, Kolobow T (1990) Acute lung injury from mechanical ventilation at moderately high airway pressures. J Appl Physiol 69:956-961
12. Dreyfuss D, Saumon G (1992) Barotrauma is volutrauma, but which volume is the one responsible? Intensive Care Med 18:139-141
13. Slutsky AS (1993) Mechanical ventilation. Chest 104:1833-1859
14. MacIntyre NR (1993) Clinically available new strategies for mechanical ventilatory support. Chest 104:560-565
15. Tobin MJ (1994) Mechanical ventilation. N Eng J Med 330:1056-1061
16. Slustsky AS (1994) Consensus conference on mechanical ventilation. Intensive Care Med 20:64-79
17. Stewart TE, Slutsky AS (1995) Mechanical ventilation: a shifting philosophy. Curr Opinion Crit Care 1:49-56
18. Smith BE (1990) High frequency ventilation: past, present and future? Brit J Anaesth 65:130-138
19. The HIFI Study Group (1989) High-frequency oscillatory ventilation compared with conventional mechanical ventilation in the treatment of respiratory failure in preterm infants. N Engl J Med 320:88-93

20. Kinsella JP, Clark RH (1993) High-frequency oscillatory ventilation in paediatric critical care. Crit Care Med 21:174-175
21. Arnold JH (1996) High frequency oscillatory ventilation: theory and practice in paediatric patients. Paediatr Anaesth 6:437-441
22. Carter MJM, Gerstmann DR, Clark MRH, Snider MG, Cornish JD, Null DM, deLemos RA (1990) High-frequency oscillatory ventilation and extracorporeal membrane oxygenation for the treatment of acute neonatal respiratory failure. Pediatrics 85:159-164
23. Man GCW, Ahmed IH, Logus JW, Man SFP (1987) High-frequency oscillatory ventilation increases canine pulmonary epithelial permeability. J Appl Physiol 63:1871-1876
24. Clark RH, Wiswell TE, Null DM, deLemos RA, Coalson JJ (1987) Tracheal and bronchial injury in high-frequency oscillatory ventilation compared with conventional positive pressure ventilation. J Pediatr 111:114-118
25. Mammel MC, Ophoven JP, Lewallen PK, Gordon MJ, Boros SJ (1991) Acute airway injury during high-frequency jet ventilation and high-frequency oscillatory ventilation. Crit Care Med 19:394-398.
26. Nielsen JB, Sjostrand UH, Edgren EL, Lichtwarck-Aschoff M, Svensson BA (1991) An experimental study of different ventilatory modes in piglets in severe respiratory distress induced by surfactant depletion. Intensive Care Med 17:225-233
27. Sjostrand UH, Lichtwarck-Aschoff M, Nielsen JB, Markstrom A, Larrson A, Svensson BA, Wagenius GA, Nordgren KA (1995) Different ventilatory approaches to keep the lung open. Intensive Care Med 21:310-318
28. Marraro G (1994) Pressure support ventilation (PSV) and pressure regulated volume control (PRVC): new methods of ventilation for newborns. In: Minoli I (ed) Neonatal Intensive Care. 16th Inter Symp, Sanremo, pp 33-34
29. Marraro G (1998) Intraoperative ventilation in paediatrics. Paediatric Anaesthesia 8:373-382
30. Marraro G (1997) New modes of pulmonary ventilation. In: Dalens B, Murat I, Bush G (eds) Advances in paediatric anaesthesia. FEAPA, Paris, pp 57-88
31. Hazelzet JA (1992) New ventilatory modes in severe respiratory failure. (Abstract). First World Congress of Pediatric Intensive Care, Baltimore
32. Marraro G (1994) Pressure regulated volume control ventilation and pressure support ventilation. CME Programme, Jaipur, pp 32-33
33. Marraro G, Mannucci F, Galbiati AM et al (1994) The advantages of a new mode of artificial ventilation: pressure regulated volume controlled (PRVC) ventilation. Pediatr Res 35(Suppl A344):2047
34. Marraro G, Casiraghi G, Galbiati AM (1995) A study of pressure regulated volume control ventilation in natural surfactant treated infants with RDS. Pediatr Res 4(Suppl A223):1321
35. Mori N, Suzuki M (1994) Trigger sensitivity of Servo 300 (Siemens Elema) for pressure support ventilation in an infant. Paediatr Anaesth 4:27-34
36. Marraro G (1994) Selective endobronchial intubation in paediatrics: the Marraro Paediatric Bilumen Tube. Paediatr Anaesth 4:255-258
37. Marraro G (1987) Synchronized independent lung ventilation in pediatric age. ACP Applied Cardiopulm Pathophys 2:283-288
38. Marraro G, Marinari M, Rataggi M (1987) The clinical application of SILV in pulmonary disease with unilateral prevalence in pediatrics. Int J Clin Mornit Comput 4:123-129
39. Marraro G (1990) Ventilation à poumons separés chez l'enfant au cours de la 1.ère année de vie. Cah Anaesthesiol 38:377-380

40. Marraro G (1992) Simultaneous independent lung ventilation in pediatric patients. Crit Care Clin 8:131-145
41. Versprille A, Hrachovina V, Jansen JRC (1995) Alternating versus synchronous ventilation of left and right lungs in piglets. Intensive Care Med 21:1009-1015
42. Frostell C, Hedenstierna G, Cronestrand R (1995) Asynchronous ventilation in the dogs: effects on lung blood flow and gas exchange. Clin Physiol 5(Suppl 3):59-64
43. Colombo A, Dell'Avo A, Nacci A, Personeni O, Spada P (1987) Hospital procedure and nursing for patients treated with synchronized independent lung ventilation (sILV). Intensive Care Nurs 3:117-124
44. Brochard L, Pluskwa F, Lemaire F (1987) Improved efficacy of spontaneous breathing with inspiratory pressure support. Am Rev Respir Dis 136:411-415
45. Mori N, Suzuki M (1994) Trigger sensitivity of Servo 300 (Siemens Elema) for pressure support ventilation in an infant. Paediatr Anaesth 4:27-34
46. Tokioka H, Kinjo M, Hirakawa M (1993) The effectiveness of pressure support ventilation for mechanical ventilatory support in children. Anaesthesiology 78:880-884
47. Bonmarchand G, Chevron V, Chopin C, Jusserand D, Girault C, Moritz F, Leroy J, Pasquis P (1996) Increased initial flow rate reduces inspiratory work of breathing during pressure support ventilation in patients with exacerbation of chronic obstructive pulmonary disease. Intensive Care Med 22:147-154
48. Brochard L, Harf A, Lorino H, Lemaire F (1989) Inspiratory pressure support prevents diaphragmatic fatigue during weaning from mechanical ventilation. Am Rev Respir Dis 139:513-521
49. Kacmarek RM(1988) The role of pressure support ventilation in reducing work of breathing. Respir Care 33:99-120
50. Esteban A, Frutos F, Tobin MJ (1995) A comparison of four methods of weaning from mechanical ventilation. N Engl J Med 332:345-350
51. Mancebo J, Amaro P, Mollo JL, Lorino H, Lemaire F, Brochard L (1995) Comparison of the effects of pressure support ventilation delivered by three different ventilators during weaning from mechanical ventilation. Intensive Care Med 21:913-919
52. Kanak R, Fahey PJ, Vanderward C (1985) Oxygen cost of breathing: changes dependent upon mode of mechanical ventilation. Chest 87:126-127
53. Gullberg N, Wimberg P, Selldèn H (1996) Pressure support ventilation increase cardiac output in neonates and infants. Paediatr Anaesth 6:311-315
54. Hird MF, Greenough A (1991) Patient triggered ventilation in chronically ventilator-dependent infants. Eur J Pediatr 150:732-734
55. Fiastro JF, Quan BF, Habib MP (1986) Pressure support compensation for inspiratory work due to endotracheal tubes and demand CPAP. Chest 89:441S
56. Kylstra JA, Tissing MO, Van der Maen A (1962) Of mice as fish. Trans Am Soc Artif Intern Organs 8:378-383
57. Clark LC, Gollan F (1966) Survival of mammals breathing organic liquids equilibrated with oxygen at atmophere pressure. Science 152:1755-1756
58. Moskowitz GD (1970) A mechanical respirator for control of liquid breathing. Fed Proc 29:1751-1752
59. Shaffer TH, Lowe CA, Bhutani VK, Douglas PR (1983) Liquid ventilation: effects on pulmonary function in meconium stained lambs. Pediatr Res 19:49-53
60. Shaffer TH, Wolfson MR, Clark LC (1992) Liquid ventilation. Pediatr Pulmunol 14:102-109
61. Fuhrman BP, Paczan PR, De Francisis M (1991) Perfluorocarbon-associated gas-exchange. Crit Care Med 19:712-722
62. Lachmann B, Tucuncu AS, Bos JA, Faithfull NS (1991) Intratracheal perfluorooctylbro-

mide (PFOB) in combination with mechanical ventilation. International Society for Oxygen Transport to Tissues, Willemstand, A24-A30

63. Fuhrman BP (1990) Perfluorocarbon liquid ventilation: the first human trial. J Pediatr 117:73-74

64. Marraro G (1997) La ventilation liquide partielle. Cah Anaesthesiol 45:383-388

65. Marraro G, Bonati M, Ferrari A, Barzaghi MM, Pagani C, Bortolotti A, Galbiati AM, Luchetti M, Croce A (1998) Perfluorocarbon bronchoalveolar lavage and liquid ventilation versus saline bronchoalveolar lavage in adult guinea pigs experimental model of meconium inhalation. Intensive Care Med 24:501-508

66. Foust R III, Tran NN, Cox C, Miller TF, Greenspan JS, Wolfson MR, Shaffer TH (1996) A liquid assisted ventilation: an alternative ventilation strategy for acute meconium aspiration injury. Pediatr Pulmonol 21:316-322

67. Shaffer TH, Wolfson MR (1996) Liquid ventilation an alternative ventilation strategy for management of neonatal respiratory distress. Eur J Pediatr 155(Suppl 2):30-34

68. Lowe Leach C, Greenspan JS, Rubenstein SD, Shaffer TH, Wolfson MR, Jackson JC, DeLemos R, Fuhrman BP, for the Liqui Vent Study Group (1996) Partial liquid ventilation with perflubron in premature infants with severe respiratory distress syndrome. N Engl J Med 335:761-767

69. Gauger PG, Prenikoff T, Schreiner RJ, Moler FW, Hirschl RB (1996) Initial experience with partial liquid ventilation in pediatric patients with the acute respiratory distress syndrome. Crit Care Med 24:16-22

70. Hirschl RB, Tooley R, Parent A, Johnson K, Bartelett RH (1996) Evaluation of gas exchange, pulmonary compliance, and lung injury during total and partial liquid ventilation in the acute respiratory distress syndrome. Crit Care Med 24:1001-1008

71. Modell JH, Tham MK, Calderwood HW, Ruiz BC (1973) Distribution and retention of fluorocarbon in mice and dogs after injection or liquid ventilation. Toxicol Appl Pharmacol 26:86-92

72. Shaffer TH, Wolfson MR, Greenspan JS, Hoffman RE, Davis SL, Clark Jr LC (1996) Liquid ventilation in premature lambs: uptake, biodistribution and elimination of perfluorodecalin liquid. Reprod Fertil Dev 8:409-416

Chapter 11

Weaning from artificial ventilation

A.J. Petros

When a child has recovered from the underlying disease which initially required intubation, the process of weaning from mechanical ventilation can begin, the endpoint being the removal of the endotracheal tube. Intensivists in the PICU, NICU, and CICU environment, on the whole tend to arrive at this end point by using "clinical judgement and years of experience". However, recent data from adult studies clearly show that specific weaning protocols decrease the duration of mechanical ventilation [1-3]. The criteria for determining whether the individual patient is capable of sustaining spontaneous respiration following withdrawal of respiratory support are becoming more clear. A number of specific variables have now been recommended to predict successful weaning in adults [4, 5]. Basing the decision of extubation upon clinical grounds alone can lead to problems, the incidence of reintubation and recommencing ventilation without weaning guidelines ranging between 17%-19% in adults [6] and 19%-28% in children [7] and neonates [8]. The imperative to extubate patients is determined by the higher incidence of nosocomial infection [9] and airway trauma and the associated risks of accidental extubation [10].

Pathophysiology of weaning

The ability to breathe depends upon three factors: central respiratory drive; the load placed upon the respiratory muscle pump, and the capacity of the muscles to sustain respiratory effort. When the balance among these three factors is lost, hypercapnic respiratory failure results. Capacity, load and drive can be influenced by many factors. In broad terms, a decrease in capacity is usually the result of a neuromuscular disease; an increase in workload is the result of airway obstruction; and a depression of central respiratory drive is due to a drug overdose [5, 11].

Capacity of respiratory muscles

The capacity of respiratory muscles to breathe spontaneously depends upon the ability of the muscles to generate adequate inspiratory pressure. This can be measured during a static effort against a closed airway. While a patient is ill and receiving intensive therapy there can be a 75% reduction in the capacity of his respiratory muscles. Systemic diseases, neuromuscular diseases or weakness of the muscles themselves account for this reduction. Metabolic abnormalities such as hypomagnesaemia, hypophosphataemia and hypocalcaemia can reduce respiratory muscle contractility. Infection and malnutrition can also affect respiratory muscles adversely.

Load

The work necessary to overcome the elastic forces of the lung and chest wall during inspiration and the minor forces of inertia and gravity all add to the load of breathing. The load may be further increase by any form of airway obstruction and the oxygen cost of breathing increases significantly in patients being weaned. If spontaneous respiration is to be successfully established and sustained the patient has to be able to accept and tolerate this load.

Central drive

The force generated by the respiratory muscles is also related to the output from the central nervous system. Any reduction of this central drive, for example in case of sedation, leads to a great reduction of the force generated. It is thus important to ascertain that patients are not oversedated and are sufficiently alert to maintain the central respiratory drive necessary to sustain breathing.

How to assess if sustained spontaneous breathing will be achieved

It is not entirely clear how useful these scoring systems are in practice. If a patient fails to meet the criteria and yet looks clinically well, should attempt at weaning be abandoned until the criteria are met? Do patients who easily satisfy the criteria need to be weaned or can they just be extubated? Do any of the quoted indexes have any relevance to the paediatric population?

Despite meeting the criteria for extubation, up to 20% adults can fail a weaning protocol [3, 12]. This is either because the criteria were not sufficently discerning or possibly because, though being capable of supporting spontaneous ventilation, the patients were actually impeded by the process of weaning. Up to 50% of accidental extubations do not require re-intubation [13, 14], indicating that we continue to ventilate some patients who simply do not need respiratory support.

Numerous indices have been used to quantify the adequacy of the ventilatory effort while receiving mechanical ventilation and to predict which patients are ready to resume sustained spontaneous respiration. Many univariate parameters have been studied in adult patients on mechanical ventilation to assess their readiness for extubation with different results. These include minute volume (MV), vital capacity (VC) maximal inspiratory pressure (MIP) and airway occlusion pressure (AOP). However, multiple factors can result in a patient's failure to wean and multivariate indices have to be considered when predicting ability to wean [7, 15]. By including a number of different measurements of respiratory muscle strength and assessments of respiratory mechanics it is assumed that an overall picture of success in weaning can be obtained. The most popular indices that have been used and studied in adults include: the ratio of inspiratory airway pressure to maximum inspiratory pressure; the inspiratory effort quotient; the weaning index; and more recently the rapid shallow breathing index (RSB) and the compliance, rate, oxygenation and pressure index (CROP).

Rapid shallow breathing index [4]

This index incorporates the rate of breathing and the result of the effort made.

$$\frac{\text{Respiratory frequency (bpm)}}{\text{Tidal Volume (ml)}} \quad \text{or} \quad \frac{f}{Vt}$$

It is claimed that values of ≤ 11 bpm^{-1}·ml^{-1} predict successful extubation in children [7].

Compliance, rate, oxygenation and pressure index

This index integrates the dynamic compliance (C_{dyn}) of the lungs; the maximal inspiratory effort (PImax); the respiratory rate (RR) and a measurement of gas exchange (PaO_2/PAO_2).

$$CROP = \frac{C_{dyn}\ PImax \cdot (PaO_2/PAO_2)}{RR}$$

Values of $\geq 0 \cdot 1ml^{-1} \cdot mmHg^{-1} \cdot bpm^{-1} \cdot kg^{-1}$ are claimed to be possible predictors of successful extubation [7].

Inspiratory drive

Inspiratory drive ($P_{0.1}$) is an important contributor to successful extubation and now available on many newer ventilators. The pressure during first 100 msec of an occluded breath is claimed to be an accurate measure of inspiratory drive in adults [6, 16]. The evidence in children is not so clear.

Value of these indexes in children

In the study reported by Yang and Tobin [4], minute ventilation was measured using a spirometer with the patient disconnected from the ventilator, and the frequency counted over 1 minute. Maximal inspiratory pressure was recorded over a 20-second period of airway occlusion with a unidirectional valve. Based on the results of this study, two indexes were proposed as having positive predictive value when extubating patients, and namely: the RSB index and the CROP index. Among adults 95% of patients with a f/Vt ratio or RSB index of ≥ 105 failed a weaning trial.

Baumeister et al. [7] evaluated the applicability of CROP and RSB indexes to intubated children. Of the 47 sets of patients studied 38 were successfully weaned and remained extubated for 24 h while 9 failed a trial of extubation. In this paediatric study a number of important modifications were made to obtain the measurements required to calculate the indexes. Vt was taken from the measurement made by the ventilator during spontaneous breathing. Continued attachment to the ventilatior was justified by the excess effort children have to make while breathing through narrower endotracheal tubes compared to adults. Therefore, to reduce this mechanical resistance Vt was measured while children were attached to the ventilator. Furthermore Vt was corrected for weight. Dynamic compliance was corrected for weight too. Weight correction was justified because of the wide age range of the paediatric population considered in practice and also in the reported study. No time limits were set to determine a MIP and airway occlusion continued only until MIP occurred. A 20 sec wait was considered too long for infants and airway occlusion was stopped when an MIP was obtained, usually within 12-15 seconds. Respiratory rate included spontaneous and mechanical breaths and percentile age correction for RR was also made. Measurements were time-averaged over 5-10 minutes. Baumeister at al. [7] concluded that the modified CROP and RSB indexes were useful predictors of successful extubation in the paediatric population. CROP more so than RSB. CROP cutoff values of $\geq 0.1 \ ml^{-1} \cdot mmHg^{-1} \cdot bpm^{-1} \cdot kg^{-1}$ would predict successful extubation with a specificity, sensitivity, positive and negative predictive value of 1.0 each. RSB cutoff values of $\leq 11 \ bpm^{-1} \cdot ml^{-1} \cdot kg^{-1}$ predicted successful extubation with a specificity of 0.779, a sensitivity of 0.789, a positive predictive value of 0.938 and a negative predictive value of 0.467. The opposite occurs in adults where RSB was found to be a more accurate predictor of successful extubation than CROP, once again emphasizing the importance of not extrapolating data from adult studies onto the paediatric population.

However, the validity of these indexes as a predictor of successful extubation is not universally accepted. Khan et al. found that neither CROP nor RSB predicted successful extubation [17]. However, this group determined the indexes as described for the adult study and not as modified by Baumeister at al. [7]. In contrast, Khan et al. [17] found that extubation failure rate increased significantly with decreasing Vt and increasing FiO_2, mean airway pressure, oxygenation index, fraction of total minute volume from the ventilator, and peak ventilator inspiratory pressure. Other indices which were supposed to predict outcome did not reach significance.

Once these indexes are set and accepted, how practical is to derive them and how frequently will they be used and, above all, are they really worth bothering about? Esteban et al. demonstrated that, despite numerous elaborate methods of weaning, the oldest and simplest one consisting in just using a T-piece for increasing periods was still a valid weaning method in adults [3].

Modes of weaning in children

Synchronized intermittent mandatory ventilation and pressure support

Patient-triggered modes such as synchronized intermittent mandatory ventilation (SIMV) and pressure support ventilation (PSV) have been widely used in adults to support ventilation while weaning. With many early ventilators, because of the time delay between triggering a breath and actually getting the volume, the WOB increases. Therefore, a continous flow system with a demand flow system was developed for most paediatric ventilators. However, in children over 15 kg, due to the relative large tidal volumes required, the Vt can exceed that delivered by the continuous flow through the circuit and thus a negative pressure can be generated during inspiration, which further increases the WOB. PSV reduces the WOB by shortening the response time for the delivery of the required tidal volume and provides the appropriate tidal volume at the predetermined pressure. Tokioka et al. demonstrated that PSV can effectively augment spontaneous breathing and reduce the work of breathing in children [18]. The use of SIMV plus PSV is thus increasing when weaning children. In many units it is now common practice to wean children from an SIMV rate of 5-10 bpm to PSV of 5-10 cmH_2O above a positive end expiratory pressure (PEEP) of 5 cmH_2O without a backup rate, to wean the peak inspiratory pressures (PIP) down to 5-10 cmH_2O and then extubate without going through a continuous positive airway pressure (CPAP) phase.

Patient-triggered ventilation

In a small group of neonates patient-triggered ventilation (PTV) with peak inspiratory pressures of 10 or 15 cmH_2O reduced the WOB of respiratory muscles by 40% compared to similar levels provided by intermittent mandatory ventilation (IMV) [19]. The authors conclude that PTV may be a possible way of weaning neonates from mechanical ventilation by reducing inspiratory pressures. PTV is a semantic definition and is in practice the same as PSV.

Continuous positive airway pressure

This mode of weaning is still popular when weaning children, infants and neonates. Levels of 5-8 cmH_2O are commonly used. The tendency to use continuous positive airway pressure (CPAP) for long periods is hard to resist to, but in our practice we limit to 4 h the duration of CPAP when used in a weaning mode.

If a decision cannot be made to extubate the child within this time then formal ventilation with a set rate is reinstitued.

Conclusions

Studies from the adult literature suggest that to optimize the weaning process all patients receiving mechanical ventilation should be assessed daily with the aim to identify those capable of breathing spontaneously. There are number of indexes which give a reliable prediction of success, CROP and RSB in particular. A short trial of spontaneous breathing should be undertaken and then, if the trial is successful, extubation should follow immediately. In adults Esteban et al. have demonstrated that trials of spontaneous breathing either through a T-tube or with pressure support of 7 cmH$_2$O are equally effective at determining successful extubation [20]. The implication being that all other newer and more sophisticated forms of wean are not better than a simple T-piece. The duration of the trial should be 30 min. The time has come to develop similar guidelines and protocols for weaning in the paediatric population.

References

1. Ely EW, Baker AM, Dunagan DP, Burke HL, Smith AC, Kelly PT, Johnson MM, Browder RW, Bowton DL, Haponik EF (1996) Effect on the duration of mechanical ventilation of identifying patients capable of breathing spontaneously. N Engl J Med 335:1864-1869
2. Saura P, Blanch L, Mestre J, Valles J, Artigas A, Fernandez R (1996) Clinical consequences of the implementation of a weaning protocol. Intensive Care Med 22:1052-1056
3. Esteban A, Frutos F, Tobin MJ, Alia I, Solsona JF, Valverdu I, Fernandez R, de la Cal M, Benito S, Tomas R, Carriedo D, Marcia S, Blanco J (1995) A comparison of four methods of weaning patients from mechanical ventilation. N Engl J Med 332:345-350
4. Yang KL, Tobin MJ (1991) A prospective study of indexes predicting the outcome of trials of weaning from mechanical ventilation. N Engl J Med 324:1445-1450
5. Goldstone J, Moxham J (1991) Assisted ventilation. Weaning from mechanical ventilation. Thorax 46:56-62
6. Tobin MJ, Perez W, Guenther SM, Semmes BJ, Mador MJ, Allen SJ, Lodato RF, Dantzker DR (1986) The pattern of breathing during successful and unsuccessful trials of weaning from mechanical ventilation. Am Rev Dis 134:1111-1118
7. Baumeister BL, el-Khatib M, Smith PG, Blumer JL (1997) Evaluation of predictors of weaning from mechanical ventilation in paediatric patients. Paediatr Pulm 24:344:352
8. Balsan MJ, Jones JG, Watchko JF, Guthrie RD (1990) Measurement of pulmonary mechanics prior to the elective extubation of neonates. Paediatr Pulm 9:238-243
9. Fagon JM, Chastre J, Domart Y, Trouillet JL, Pierre J, Darne C, Gibert C (1989) Nosocomial pneumonia in patients receiving continuous mechanical ventilation. Prospective analysis of 52 episodes with use of a protected specimen brush and quantitative culture techniques. Am Rev Respir Dis 139:877-884
10. Little LA, Koening JC, Newth CJL (1990) Factors affecting accidental extubation in neonatal and paediatric intensive care patients. Crit Care Med 18:163-165
11. Vassilakopoulos T, Zakynthinos S, Roussos C (1998) The pathophysiology of weaning

failure. In: Vincent J-L (ed) Yearbook of Intensive Care. Springer-Verlag, Berlin Heidelberg New York, pp 489-504

12. Esteban A, Alia I, Gordo F, Fernandez R, Solsona JF, Valverdu I, Macias S, Allegue JM, Blanco J, Carriedo D, Leon M, de la Cal MA, Taboada F, Gonzalez de Velasco J, Palazon E, Carrizosa F, Tomas R, Suarez J, Goldwasser RS (1997) Extubation outocome after spontaneous breathing trials with T-tube or pressure support ventilation. The Spanish Lung Failure Collaborative Group. Am Rev Respir Dis 156:459-465

13. Listello D, Sessler CN (1994) Unplanned extubation: clinical predictors for reintubation. Chest 105:1804-1807

14. Tindol GA Jr, DiBenedetto RJ, Kosciuk L (1994) Unplanned extubations. Chest 105:1804-1807

15. Stoller J (1991) Establishing clinical unweanability. Resp Care 36:186-198

16. Tobin MJ, Laghi F, Walsh JM (1994) Monitoring of respiratory neuromuscular function. In: Tobin MJ (ed) Principles and practice of mechanical ventilation. McGraw Hill, New York, pp 94-96

17. Khan N, Brown A, Venkataraman ST (1996) Predictors of extubation success and failure in mechanically ventilated infants and children. Crit Care Med 24:1568-1579

18. Tokioka H, Kinjo M Hirakawa (1993) The effectiveness of pressure support ventilation for mechanical ventilatory support in children. Anaesthesiology 78:880-884

19. Jarreau P-H, Moriette Mussat P, Mariette C, Mohanna A, Harf A, Lorino H (1996) Patient-triggered ventilation decreases the work of breathing in neonates. Am J Crit Care Med 1176-1181

20. Alia I, Esteban A, Gordo F (1998) What have we learned about weaning over the last five years. In: Vincent J-L (ed) Yearbook of Intensive Care. Springer-Verlag, Berlin Heidelberg New York, pp 505-516

MOTHER AND CHILD

Chapter 12

Fetal anaesthesia for surgery

J. Hamza, L. Simon, P. Sacquin

After extensive experimental study, fetal surgery has been undertaken in humans in a very few centers in the world [1, 2]. The purpose of this surgery is to correct a malformation before its effects have definitively compromised neonatal and fetal prognosis. Examples of this concept are the surgical correction of congenital diaphragmatic hernia [3-5] or bilateral hydronephrosis [6]; both of these conditions have been successfully treated before birth in some human fetuses.

Moreover, other diagnostic or therapeutic procedures can now be performed in the fetus and could generate fetal pain requiring adequate anaesthesia or analgesia of the fetus.

The implied roles of the anaesthetist in a fetal surgery program are the following [7, 8]: a) maternal safety; b) the need for adequate uterine relaxation which is essential for surgery; c) fetal anaesthesia as the fetus is the primary patient; d) intraoperative fetal monitoring, ensuring fetal well-being throughout surgery; and e) the need for adequate postoperative tocolysis to avoid preterm labor and fetal wastage.

Maternal safety

One of the major risks of general anaesthesia during late pregnancy is difficult intubation, which remains the primary cause of maternal death associated with general anaesthesia in obstetrics. It is therefore essential that the anaesthetist evaluate the risk of difficult intubation during a preoperative consultation.

The second potential risk is the inhalation of gastric contents. It is therefore necessary to prevent this complication with the administration of nonparticular antacids before the induction of general anaesthesia and with the use of a rapid-sequence anaesthetic induction with Sellick's maneuver, thus avoiding the risk of inhalation in case of gastroesophageal reflux.

The third risk is aortocaval compression syndrome, leading to a decreased venous return to the right ventricle and an increased risk of maternal arterial hypotension during anaesthesia. It can be associated to a certain degree of aortic compression, contributing to a decrease in uteroplacental flow and, therefore, to fetal asphyxia. It is therefore essential to prevent this aortocaval compression syndrome by the displacement to the left of the gravid uterus with a rolled blanket slipped under the right hip, or by tilting the operation table to the left.

Preoperative evaluation of these patients therefore has to be particularly careful: it should include the search for a previous cardiovascular problem completed by an ECG and maternal cardiac ultrasonography. Information about previous haemorrhage or blood transfusions and a complete blood typing and grouping with cross-match are mandatory as is immediate availability of blood products. In addition, information about previous thrombosis is particularly important because of the increased postoperative thromboembolic risk in pregnant women. Asymptomatic urinary tract infection is detected systematically before surgery and antibiotic prophylaxis is adapted to the bacterial flora found in vaginal smears.

Premedication with benzodiazepines is important to alleviate maternal anxiety, given the particular affective context of this type of surgery. This allows the patient to arrive relaxed in the operating room, which is useful to site the epidural catheter for postoperative analgesia under the best conditions.

After correct positioning of the patient, avoiding aortocaval syndrome and oxygenation by inhalation of 100% oxygen for 3 min, we use a rapid-sequence induction with thiopental (6 mg/kg) and succinylcholine (1.5 mg/kg) 2 min after a bolus intravenous dose of fentanyl (2 to 3 µg/kg). An endotracheal tube 6.5 or 7 mm in diameter is gently passed through the vocal cords, sometimes after local anaesthesia of the glottis to avoid a maternal stress response to endotracheal intubation which can compromise fetal oxygenation. We use controlled ventilation with 100% oxygen in order to optimize fetal oxygenation throughout surgery.

Maternal monitoring consists of continuous ECG, noninvasive arterial pressure, and pulse oximetry to continuously record the maternal oxygen arterial saturation. Capnography connected to the expiratory limb of the circuit allows to monitor end-tidal $°CO_2$ while the monitoring of end-tidal concentrations of halogenated agents allows rapid controlled variations in the administration of these agents to the mother. Finally, invasive, continuous monitoring of arterial pressure with a radial arterial catheter seemed necessary to rapidly assess the variations in maternal arterial pressure induced by frequent changes in the concentration of the halogenated agent used.

Fetal surgery

Hysterotomy and fetal extraction stimulate uterine contractility. It is essential to obtain an optimal relaxation of the uterine muscle just before fetal extraction [2]. The uterorelaxant effect of the halogenated agents is well known and there is a close relationship between the alveolar concentration of the halogenated agent and depression of uterine contractility [9, 10]. This goal necessitates high alveolar concentrations, substantially greater than the maternal MAC (minimum alveolar concentration) in the third trimester of pregnancy [11]. Later we will see the problems induced by the utilization of such high concentrations.

The unique problem posed by fetal surgery is that the fetus must be anaesthetized, in contrast to the classic situation of the Cesarean section where the objective is to avoid fetal depression. Considering this objective, several remarks have to be made. Thiopental rapidly crosses the placental barrier, but the peak plasma concentration in the umbilical artery is reached 3 min after injection, indicating an early redistribution to the maternal circulation. The association of thiopental with nitrous oxide is associated with fetal hypoxia, probably resulting from insufficient anaesthesia [12]. Fentanyl is highly liposoluble and easily crosses the placenta. However, the peak concentration, obtained in 1-2 min, decreases very rapidly to 10% of the peak value 15 min after maternal administration. Finally, the muscle relaxants used cannot induce fetal curarization because succinylcholine has a low liposolubility and therefore has difficulty crossing the placenta. This also applies to nondepolarizing agents such as vecuronium bromide whose transplacental passage is very low. In contrast, halogenated agents, having a high liposolubility and a low molecular mass, can easily cross the placenta. Fetal uptake is important [13], with an umbilical vein/umbilical artery ratio of 2.9 and a fetal cerebral concentration of halothane that increases rapidly. This probably explains why the arterial concentration of halothane sufficient to prevent the reaction of the fetus to a painful stimulus is much lower than the maternal arterial concentration. In an animal model (monkey), this resulted in a theoretical fetal MAC that is approximately 50% of the maternal MAC [14]. High concentrations of the halogenated agents used for uterine relaxation in fetal surgery are therefore sufficient to anaesthetize the fetus. It is probably why some medical teams do not use any other method of fetal anaesthesia than the halogenated agents administered to the mother.

Our attitude was, in contrast, to complete this anaesthesia by giving drugs directly through the umbilical vein. Indeed, in the animal experimentation, we observed several cases of imperfect fetal immobility with the use of halogenated agents alone [3]. Before fetal exteriorization, we injected vecuronium (0.1 mg/kg) in the umbilical vein, as we know from our experience of in utero fetal transfusions [15] that fetal paralysis can be obtained for 2 h, thus exceeding the duration of fetal surgery. We also decided to inject fentanyl (10 µg/kg of estimated fetal weight) in the umbilical vein at the same time. Indeed, it has been well demonstrated by the work of Anand that the premature neonate felt pain due to the surgical intervention [16] as judged by the stress reaction. In addition, the postoperative neonatal morbidity was less important in a group of premature babies who received sufficient analgesia by 10 µg/kg of fentanyl [17]. Therefore, we believe that the fetus submitted to fetal surgery had to undergo the same stress and would benefit from the same analgesic protocol.

Avoidance of perioperative fetal hypoxia

Fetal monitoring is essential during fetal surgery. It includes the monitoring of fetal heart rate throughout surgery, a pulse oximeter fixed to the fetal foot, a Doppler probe for monitoring the umbilical flow and a thermal probe to measure the rectal temperature of the fetus so as to avoid hypothermia. In addition, we measured blood gases and the hemoglobin concentration in the umbilical vein at the beginning and at the end of surgery. Some perioperative problems can affect the fetus, particularly maternal arterial hypotension, which can decrease uteroplacental blood flow. Indeed, the use of high concentrations of halogenated agents led to a dose-dependent decrease in the maternal arterial pressure and cardiac output [18, 19]. Beyond a certain threshold, these haemodynamic events can lead to a decrease in the uterine blood flow with the progressive development of fetal hypoxia, as detected by a decrease in the fetal oxygen saturation [19].

Animal studies of fetal haemodynamics during prolonged maternal administration of high concentrations of halogenated agents have shown a 30% decrease in the fetal arterial pressure [18, 20] without increase of the fetal heart rate, reflecting the abolition of the fetal baroreflex mechanism by the halogenated agents. However, a study by Biehl et al. [20] has shown that, despite arterial hypotension, fetal regional flows (myocardial, cerebral, placental) were preserved in the fetus, even after prolonged use of high concentrations of halogenated agents. In cases of maternal arterial hypotension, it is necessary to verify the absence of aortocaval compression, to decrease the concentration of halogenated agents, to increase maternal vascular expansion with crystalloids (Ringer Lactate), and to inject bolus doses (5-10 mg) of ephedrine.

The second most frequent problem is uterine hypertonia, especially during fetal extraction and the reinsertion of the fetus in the uterus. It is then necessary to rapidly increase the concentration of halogenated agents to obtain a rapid uterine relaxation.

Finally, if fetal bradycardia and/or hypoxia ensue, we rapidly search for a mechanical cause: umbilical cord compression, compression of the inferior vena cava by the fetus requiring immediate correction, or uterine hypertonia justifying the increase of concentrations of halogenated agents. Sometimes bradycardia is due to maternal hypotension or maternal hypoxia that would be immediately detected by the pulse oximeter, or to maternal hypocapnia due to excessive hyperventilation that can decrease the uteroplacental blood flow. Finally, fetal bradycardia due to overdosage of halogenated agents cannot be excluded, particularly in the presence of pre-existing fetal hypoxia: fetal haemodynamic adaptation to hypoxia, especially redistribution of cardiac output in favor of cerebral blood flow, could be altered in the presence of high concentrations of halogenated agents [21] although such a result was not reported in another study [22].

Ensuring postoperative maternal comfort and fetal safety

Maternal analgesia is an essential goal of the postoperative period, not only for maternal comfort, but also for fetal safety, as maternal stress due to untreated pain can decrease the uteroplacental blood flow [23]. It is for that reason that we think, with others [7], that epidural morphine (5 mg) administered postoperatively is important as it ensures a very good quality of analgesia.

Because of the thromboembolic risk in the postoperative period we prescribe subcutaneous low-molecular weight heparin while the patient is confined to bed so as to prevent a premature delivery.

Tocolysis presents the most difficult problem in the postoperative period. An i.v. infusion of salbutamol is generally used under cardiac monitoring (ECG, pulmonary auscultation) to detect complications, especially pulmonary oedema that can be prompted by excessive fluid administration during surgery [8]. Finally, indomethacin treatment, begun in the preoperative period, is continued for several days postoperatively and required fetal cardiac ultrasonographic examinations to detect premature closure of the ductus arteriosus as early as possible [24].

In conclusion, the role of the anaesthetist during fetal surgery is focused on three goals:

1. to ensure maternal security and optimal maternal comfort;
2. to remain vigilant during the entire perioperative period of all factors which might compromise fetal oxygenation, in order to correct them immediately;
3. to ensure jointly with the obstetrician an optimal tocolysis during surgery and the postoperative period, avoiding excessive dosages that could have a deleterious effect on maternal haemodynamics and, therefore, on fetal oxygenation.

References

1. Bargy F, Rouquet Y, Estève C, Toubas F, Gaudiche O, Meynaud L, Germain G (1987) Chirurgie in utero de la hernie diaphragmatique chez le singe Macaque. Chir Pediatr 28:108-111

2. Harrison MR, Anderson J, Rosen MA, Ross NA, Hendrickx AG (1982) Anaesthetic, surgical and tocolytic management to maximize fetal-neonatal survival. J Pediatr Surg 17:115-121

3. Estève C, Toubas F, Gaudiche O, Leveque C, Bargy F, Rouquet Y, Sapin E, Murat I, Saint-Maurice C (1992) Bilan de cinq années de chirurgie expérimentale in utero pour la réparation des hernies diaphragmatiques. Ann Fr Anaesth Reanim 11:193-200

4. Harrison MR, Adzick NS, Longaker MT, Goldberg JD, Rosen MA, Filly RA, Evans MI, Golbus MS (1990) Successful repair in utero of a fetal diaphragmatic hernia after removal of herniated viscera from the left thorax. N Engl J Med 322:1582-1584

5. Harrison MR, Langer JC, Adzick NS, Golbus MS, Filly RA, Anderson RL, Rosen MA, Callen PW, Goldstein RB, de Lorimier AA (1990) Correction of congenital diaphragmatic hernia in utero V. Initial clinical experience. J Pediatr Surg 25:47-57

6. Crombleholme TM, Harrison MR, Langer JC, Longaker MT, Anderson RL, Slotnik NS (1988) Early experience with open fetal surgery for congenital hydronephrosis. J Pediatr Surg 23:1114-1121

7. Johnson MD, Birnbach DJ, Burchman C, Greene MF, Datta S, Ostheimer GW (1989) Fetal surgery and general anaesthesia: a case report and review. J Clin Anaesth 1:363-367

8. Rosen MA (1992) Anaesthesia for fetal procedures and surgery. In: Shnider SM, Levinson G (eds) Anaesthesia for obstetrics. Williams and Wilkins, Baltimore, pp 281-295

9. Munson ES, Embro WJ (1977) Enflurane, isoflurane and halothane and isolated human uterine muscle. Anaesthesiology 46:11-14
10. Naftalin NJ, McKay DM, Phear WPC, Goldberg AH (1977) The effects of halothane on pregnant and nonpregnant human myometrium. Anaesthesiology 46:15-19
11. Palahniuk RJ, Shnider SM, Eger EI II (1974) Pregnancy decreases the requirement of inhaled anaesthetic agents. Anaesthesiology 41:82-83
12. Palahniuk RJ, Cumming M (1977) Foetal deterioration following thiopentone-nitrous oxide anaesthesia in the pregnant ewe. Can Anaesth Soc J 24:361-370
13. Biehl DR, Cote J, Wade JG, Gregory GA, Sitar D (1983) Uptake of halothane by the foetal lamb in utero. Can Anaesth Soc J 30:24-27
14. Gregory GA, Wade JG, Biehl DR, Ong BY, Sitar DS (1983) Fetal anaesthetic requirement (MAC) for halothane. Anaesth Analg 62:9-14
15. Lévêque C, Toubas F, Lepaul M, Poissonnier MH, Brossard Y, Saint-Maurice C (1989) Curarisation foetale au cours des exsanguinotransfusions réalisées in utero pour le traitement transfusionnel des iso-immunisations rhésus graves. Cah Anaesthesiol 37:479-482
16. Anand KJS, Hickey PR (1987) Pain and its effects in the human neonate and fetus. N Engl J Med 317:1321-1329
17. Anand KJS, Sippel WG, Ainsley-Green A (1987) Randomized trial of fentanyl anaesthesia in preterm neonates undergoing surgery: effects on stress response. Lancet 1:243-248
18. Eng M, Bonica JJ, Akamatsu TJ, Berges PU, Der Yuen D, Ueland K (1975) Maternal and fetal responses to halothane in pregnant monkeys. Acta Anaesth Scand 19:154-158
19. Palahniuk RJ, Shnider SM (1974) Maternal & fetal cardiovascular and acid-base changes during halothane and isoflurane anaesthesia in the pregnant ewe. Anaesthesiology 41:462-472
20. Biehl DR, Tweed WA, Cote J, Wade JG, Sitar D (1983) Effect of halothane on cardiac output and regional flow in the fetal lamb in utero. Anaesth Analg 62:489-492
21. Palahniuk RJ, Doig GA, Johnson GN, Pash MP (1980) Maternal halothane anaesthesia reduces cerebral blood flow in the acidotic sheep fetus. Anaesth Analg 59:35-39
22. Yarnell R, Biehl DR, Tweed WA, Gregory GA, Sitar D (1983) The effect of halothane anaesthesia on the asphyxiated foetal lamb in utero. Can Anaesth Soc J 30:474-479
23. Shnider SM, Wright RG, Levinson G, Roizen MF, Wallis KL, Rolbin SH, Craft JB (1979) Uterine blood flow and plasma norepinephrine changes during maternal stress in the pregnant ewe. Anaesthesiology 50:524-527
24. Eronen M, Pesonen E, Kurki T, Ylikorkala O, Hallman M (1991) The effects of indomethacin and a beta-sympathomimetic agent on the fetal ductus arteriosus during treatment of premature labor: a randomized double-blind study. Am J Obstet Gynecol 164:141-146

Chapter 13

Effects of anaesthesia/analgesia techniques in mother and child

M. Zakowski

Epidural analgesia produces many beneficial and a few potentially nonbeneficial effects in the mother or the fetus. Recently, possible nonbeneficial effects of epidural analgesia have received much attention in the scientific and lay press. We have examined the scientific validity of some of these concerns.

Epidural analgesia has been acknowledged by the American Society of Anaesthesiologists and the American College of Obstetricians and Gynecologists as providing the most effective method of pain relief during labor. Beneficial "side effects" of epidural analgesia include: decrease in maternal catecholamine levels [1], decrease in metabolic demands on the mother [2], improve in increase intervillous blood flow in pre-eclamptics [3], and decrease in maternal and fetal metabolic acidosis [4, 5]. Parturients with regional anaesthesia had a significantly reduced mortality rate from anaesthesia compared to general anaesthesia [6]. A parturient who had an emergency cesarean delivery for fetal distress with an epidural had a 1/16th chance of anaesthesia-related mortality compared to general anaesthesia.

The effect of epidural analgesia on maternal temperature during labor has recently received a lot of attention. Although epidural analgesia has been noted to increased maternal temperature slightly, the effect on the neonate has not been fully addressed. Unfortunately, no study examining temperature has randomized the type of maternal analgesia, and many studies do not even state what medications were administered via the epidural.

Camann et al. found that epidural analgesia increased maternal temperature after 5h of analgesia [7]. Parturients were free to choose type of analgesia (systemic narcotic, epidural). Women who chose epidural analgesia received 0.25% bupivacaine 8-12 ml to initiate analgesia and were randomized to receive 0.25% bupivacaine with or without fentanyl 2 µg/ml for continuous infusion at 10 ml/h. Oral temperature correlated with tympanic membrane temperature (r=0.61, $p<0.001$). There was a very weak, albeit statistically significant, correlation between fetal heart rate and maternal temperature (r=0.22, $p<0.005$). However, no patient had signs of infection, chorioamnionitis, or sepsis. In addition, the maximum degree of temperature elevation was <1°C, and patients remained below 38°C.

Fusi et al. found that maternal temperature started to rise after 6 h of epidural analgesia [8]. The maternal temperature rose 1°C in hour 6-13 of study. Again, parturients were not randomized, and more primigravidas chose epidural analgesia. Epidural analgesia was produced with 0.375% bupivacaine, intermittent dosing. Room temperatures were kept warm, on average at 25°C, with temperatures an average 0.5-0.7°C warmer in rooms where patients received epidural analgesia. Oral and vaginal temperature were well correlated (r=0.81, p<0.001). Higher vaginal temperature correlated with a higher fetal heart rate. The maximal mean vaginal temperature observed in the study, 37.6°C, was related to an average fetal heart rate of 160. Maternal fever was defined as oral temperature >37.5°C. It is interesting to note that the mean oral temperatures remained below 38°C in the 12 h of study. Further, no patient with fever developed bacteriological evidence of vaginal, uterine, or urinary tract infection. They postulated that the increased temperature was due to the result of vascular and thermoregulatory modifications induced by epidural analgesia.

Herbst et al. found that maternal fever was associated with nulliparity, a long duration of labor and epidural analgesia in a retrospective case control study [9]. In a matched-pair segment of their study, rupture of membranes longer than 24 h, latency phase longer than 8 h, admission temperature of 37.5-37.9°C, and epidural analgesia were independent risk factors for maternal fever. Although maternal fever was defined as a temperature of at least 38°C, all temperatures in this study had 0.5°C added to "correct" for oral measurements. Most fevers were for a short duration and occurred at a late stage of labor. The duration of fever was similar in the epidural and no-epidural groups (2.6 and 2.3 h, respectively) [9]. Importantly, none of the 250 parturients with fever during labor had a serious infectious complication. This occurred in spite of only 79/250 receiving antibiotics for fever. Is this marker, maternal fever of 37.5 °C, clinically significant?

In a retrospective analysis by Vinson et al., the duration of epidural analgesia correlated with maximum maternal temperature, increasing 0.07°C/h (0.05°C/h after adjustment for duration of labor) [10]. The authors also claim a trend was seen in the newborn's first temperature (≤30 min of life), although it was not statistically significant. In a prospective segment of their study, the maximum maternal (tympanic) temperature in the epidural and no-epidural groups were 37.5°C and 37.2°C, respectively. Parturients in the prospective group received bupivacaine for loading and a bupivacaine/sufentanil infusion for epidural analgesia. There was no difference in the incidence of epidural analgesia in mothers of infants who were febrile (51% vs 46%, respectively, p=0.6). When the authors controlled for the duration of labor, the duration of epidural analgesia was no longer a significant factors for newborn's first temperature. Parturients who received epidural analgesia tended to have lower parity and longer labor than those who did not. Antibiotics or diagnostic procedures performed in the neonate for fever (37.5°C, n=12) were equally distributed in the epidural and non-epidural groups. Only 4/600 infants were septic or presumed septic, two each in the epidural and non-epidural groups.

Lieberman et al. started a controversy over epidural analgesia, intrapartum fever, and neonatal sepsis evaluations [11]. Her group found a much greater incidence of fever in parturients receiving an epidural compared to parenteral narcotics alone (14.5% and 1%, respectively). The incidence of maternal fever increased with duration of labor in the epidural group, but not in the non-epidural group. Correspondingly, the rate of neonatal sepsis evaluations increased in the epidural group. The retrospective database used for this study was created prospectively to study the active management of labor [12]. Thus, many confounding variables were not controlled for. Epidural analgesia was not part of the original study protocol and was administered in the active and routine management of labor groups at the request of the patient. Women requesting epidural analgesia were more likely to have induced labor (28% vs 12% spontaneous labor), had labors about 6 h longer, and slightly greater but statistically significantly increased gestational age and mean birth weight. In addition, significantly more women in the nonepidural group received active management of labor, which shortened labor by almost 3 h in the original study, with a lower rate of fever (7% vs 11%) [12]. The association of fever and epidural use remained after logistic regression analysis controlled for these factors. However, statistical methods do not correct for any underlying bias introduced by a retrospective design. The duration of labor was increased in women who chose epidural for pain relief. In marked contrast, Bofill et al. found no difference in the length of first or second stages of labor between the epidural and parenteral narcotic groups [13]. This prospective study by Bofill et al. not only randomized the type of analgesia but also rigidly controlled the management of labor [13].

In the study by Lieberman et al., neonatal sepsis evaluations were more frequent in the epidural group than in the nonepidural group (34% vs 10%) and infants were more likely to receive antibiotics (15% vs 4%) [11]. However, maternal fever was the indication for only 33% of the neonatal evaluations for sepsis. The risk factors for evaluation of sepsis included rupture of membranes >12 h, maternal white blood count >15 000/mm^3, lower levels of intrapartum temperature elevations, and neonatal symptoms at the time of delivery. These criteria led to 25% of all infants at their institution being evaluated for sepsis. Even more importantly, only four of the 416 infants evaluated for sepsis actually had sepsis! Clearly, the clinical and diagnostic criteria of neonatal evaluation for sepsis need to be redefined. I can think of no place in medicine where a 1% specificity level is acceptable. Finally, the authors do state that "criteria for neonatal sepsis evaluation and antibiotic treatment should be re-examined, perhaps using a higher fever threshold for women with epidural". Other studies have included such diagnostic criteria as the presence of meconium and signs of infected amniotic fluid.

Mayer et al. found an increased antibiotic administration associated with epidural analgesia in labor [14]. In this retrospective review (n=300) of a computerized perinatal database, the incidence of intrapartum fever (oral temperature ≥37.8 °C) was 2%, 16%, and 24% in women who received parenteral narcotics, epidural analgesia (drugs not specified), or narcotics followed by epidural analgesia, respectively. Only ten patients had positive intrapartum cultures of placental pathology showing chorioamnionitis, although the criteria for performing cultures and pathologic examination were not defined. Indeed, based on information presented in their Table 2, significantly more patients in the epidural and narcotics-epidural group received an intrauterine pressure catheter. No parturient with proven chorioamnionitis had temperature elevation as an isolated finding! The implications of this study for clinical management is significant. The authors conclude: "Rather than treating all women with temperature elevations and epidurals for presumed chorioamnionitis, it is reasonable to target treatment to those with fetal tachycardia, meconium stained fluid, or abnormal amniotic fluid studies" [14].

The diagnostic criteria for intra-amniotic infection has been suggested as fever >37.8 °C, ruptured membranes, and two or more of the following: maternal pulse >100, fetal heart rate >160, uterine tenderness, malodorous amniotic fluid, white blood cell count >15 000, and no other site of infection [15]. Testing of amniotic fluid for glucose and gram staining and culture have also been suggested (see above).

There are many possible explanations for a temperature rise following several hours of epidural analgesia. Painful labor results in hyperventilation, which may lower oral temperature and increase heat loss. Sympathetic blockade of the lower extremities may block sweating, reducing heat loss. Shivering is fairly common after epidural drug administration and may be related to the temperature of the injectate [16]. The response of nursing staff may also be important. Sponging patients or covering them with layers of blankets in the presence of shivering, even though the patient does not feel cold may decrease heat loss and encourage pyrexia.

There are many problems inherent to a retrospective study design. Many factors are not controlled for, and multiple logistic regression cannot exclude all bias introduced with a retrospective study. Factors which may influence the measured outcome cannot be controlled for. Infection may cause painful but inefficient contractions [9]. The relationship between epidural analgesia and maternal fever may be confounded by labor dystocia, with the prolongation of labor resulting in more requests for epidural analgesia and an increased chance of fever and neonatal problems [17]. Epidural analgesia may be a risk marker rather than a risk factor for fever during labor [9].

In summary, epidural analgesia may increase maternal temperature to a small degree (0.5°C) in prospective, randomized trials. Whether women who request epidural analgesia have more painful labors because of a pre-existing uterine process (i.e., dystocia or infection) remains to be adequately studied. Epidural analgesia may be a risk marker for other processes during labor, including increased maternal temperature. Certainly, there is no increase in maternal infection or documented sepsis in infants of mothers who receive epidural analgesia, even for prolonged periods. The criteria for neonatal sepsis evaluation requires further investigation to yield a higher specificity and sensitivity rate.

References

1. Shnider SM, Abboud TK, Artal R et al (1983) Maternal catecholamines decrease during labor after lumbar epidural anaesthesia. Am J Obstet Gynecol 147:13-15

2. Sangoul F, Fox GS, Houle GL (1975) Effect of regional analgesia on maternal oxygen consumption during the first stage of labor. Am J Obstet Gynecol 121:1080-1083
3. Jouppila P, Jouppila R, Hollmen A et al (1982) Lumbar epidural analgesia to improve intervillous blood flow during labor in severe preeclampsia. Obstet Gynecol 59:158-161
4. Pearson JF, Davies P (1973) The effect of continuous lumbar epidural analgesia on the acid-base status of maternal arterial blood during the first stage of labour. J Obstet Gynaecol Br Commonwealth 80:218-224
5. Thalme B, Raabe N, Belfrage P (1974) Lumbar epidural analgesia in labour. II. Effects on glucose, lactate, sodium, chloride, total protein, haematocrit and haemoglobin in maternal, fetal and neonatal blood. Acta Obstet Gynecol Scand 53:113-119
6. Hawkins JL, Koonin LM, Palmer SK et al (1997) Anaesthesia-related deaths during obstetric delivery in the United States, 1979-1990. Anaesthesiology 86:277-284
7. Camann WR, Hortvet LA, Hughes N et al (1991) Maternal temperature regulation during extradural analgesia for labour. Br J Anaesth 67:565-568
8. Fusi L, Steer PJ, Maresh MJ et al (1989) Maternal pyrexia associated with the use of epidural analgesia in labour. Lancet 1:1250-1252
9. Herbst A, Wolner-Hanssen P, Ingemarsson I (1995) Risk factors for fever in labor. Obstet Gynecol 86:790-794
10. Vinson DC, Thomas R, Kiser T (1993) Association between epidural analgesia during labor and fever. J Fam Pract 36:617-622
11. Lieberman E, Lang JM, Frigoletto FJ et al (1997) Epidural analgesia, intrapartum fever, and neonatal sepsis evaluation. Pediatrics 99:415-419
12. Frigoletto FDJ, Lieberman E, Lang JM et al (1995) A clinical trial of active management of labor. N Engl J Med 333:745-750
13. Bofill JA, Vincent RD, Ross EL et al (1997) Nulliparous active labor, epidural analgesia, and cesarean delivery for dystocia. Am J Obstet Gynecol 177:1465-1470
14. Mayer DC, Chescheir NC, Spielman FJ (1997) Increased intrapartum antibiotic administration associated with epidural analgesia in labor. Am J Perinatol 14:83-86
15. Looff JD, Hager WD (1984) Management of chorioamnionitis. Surg Gynecol Obstet 158:161-166
16. Ponte J, Collett BJ, Walmsley A (1986) Anaesthetic temperature and shivering in epidural anaesthesia. Acta Anaesthesiol Scand 30:584-587
17. Douglas M, Shields SG (1997) Maternal fever after epidural analgesia. J Fam Pract 44:529-530

Chapter 14

Maternal complications

G. Zanconato, L. Fedele

Throughout the mean 40-week duration of a pregnancy, woman's life and that of her baby may be at stake. The threats to feto-maternal wellbeing may originate from the changes that pregnancy induces upon the maternal organism, may be facilitated by pre-existing maternal disease, or may be due to pathological processes of the fetoplacental unit. Whatever the reason, complications can be severe, at times developing rapidly.

Events that may complicate an otherwise normal pregnancy, as we all know, are also related to gestational age: ectopic pregnancy and trophoblastic disease are clearly an issue in the first half of pregnancy. Later on, in the second half of pregnancy, from 22 weeks on or so, just to name one of them, hemorrhage due to placental abruption with subsequent disseminated intravascular coagulation (DIC) may occur. At times, primarily the fetal life is in jeopardy: this is typically the case of a premature rupture of membranes or of a preterm delivery.

One could go on, and list the numerous pre-existing maternal diseases such as diabetes, hypertension, cardiovascular disease which coincidently complicate the pregnancy. All of these medical conditions, although well controlled, may undergo decompensation because of the important physical changes occurring in pregnancy.

Having said that, it is quite obvious that maternal complications represent a complex universe into which it is rather difficult to bring order, even if just for scholastic purposes.

An exhaustive list of such complications is bound to be a very long one. Therefore, it is worth focusing on some of them, starting from those that are most dangerous for the woman's life and that, because of this, can be found as leading causes of maternal death.

Maternal complications which can lead a pregnant woman to death are well known. They are responsible for a toll of 26 lives every 100 000 live births in the industrialized world [1]. Embolism, hypertensive problems with eclamptic crisis, and bleeding are the most common etiological factors. These are direct causes of maternal death, of obstetric nature in the true sense of the term.

Only in rare circumstances we have to deal with cases of septic abortion and infectious disease such as malaria, which instead claim hundreds of thousands of lives yearly in the developing world. Ectopic pregnancy, too, has become progressively less important as a maternal mortality cause in our countries, while being still a dramatic threat in developing countries.

As stated during the 1997 APICE Course [2], anaesthesia is not a major cause of maternal death anymore either, and it has been suggested that one should focus on hypertensive disorders, thromboembolism, and hemorrhage. In confirmation of this, among the figures concerning the admitting diagnosis at the intensive care unit (ICU) presented in 1997 [3], it has been emphasized that the most frequent obstetric causes for admission to the ICU were hypertensive disorders, with associated complications such as renal failure, placental abruption, and coagulopathies.

Deep vein thrombosis and pulmonary thromboembolism

The estimated incidence of deep vein thrombosis (DVT) in pregnancy is 0.05% to 1.8%, increasing to 2.2%-3% following cesarean section [4]. Thromboembolic (TE) complications occur antepartum (more in the first and second trimester) as often as postpartum, with known risk factors such as age over 35 years, as shown in the Table 1.

Table 1. Risk factors for thromboembolism

• Age >35 years
• Multiparity
• Obesity (>80 kg)
• Gross varicose veins
• Current infection and current major illness
• Pre-eclampsia
• Immobility prior to surgery
• Major pelvic or abdominal surgery
• Personal or family history of deep vein thrombosis, pulmonary embolism or thrombophilia
• Patients with antiphospholipid antibody

TE contributes substantially to mortality and morbidity in obstetric and gynecologic practice. The clinician must be aware of the risk factors for TE, as they are often present in patients who go on to develop deep vein thrombosis and pulmonary TE.

The diagnosis of deep vein thrombosis is crucial as pulmonary TE may occur in untreated DVT patients: it is noteworthy that many patients dying from pulmonary thromboembolism (PTE) do so without the preceding DVT being diagnosed [4].

The risk of DVT can be reduced by appropriate thromboprophylaxis with agents such as low-dose heparin and graduated elastic compression stockings employed in patients with risk factors.

Amniotic fluid embolism

Amniotic fluid embolism has an estimated prevalence of one out of 8 000 to one out of 80 000 births, with a maternal mortality rate of approximately 50%-60% and a high rate of long-term neurologic deficits among survivors [5].

It has recently been suggested that it should be considered as an anaphylactoid syndrome of pregnancy, to emphasize that the clinical findings are secondary to biochemical mediators rather than pulmonary embolic phenomenon.

The following five clinical signs often occur in sequence: respiratory distress, cyanosis, cardiovascular collapse, hemorrahge and coma.

Airway control and treatment of shock in the early phase need to be put into effect. There is a high likelihood that coagulopathy will develop and therefore supportive coagulation and volume therapy with blood and fresh frozen plasma should be administered as soon as possible.

Pre-eclampsia

Pre-eclapmsia is likely the result of a disturbance of placentation, that is, of uteroplacental arterial insufficiency.

In the clinical evolution of this pathological process an intermediate phase can be identified: the phase of maternal compensation to the placental ischemia with greater involvement of the cardiovascular, uropoietic, hepatic and coagulation systems [6]. When the compensation phase exceeds the systems' capacities, the critical situation of potentially fatal tertiary pre-eclampsia may develop in the woman (Table 2).

Cerebral hemorrhage, liver involvement, and disseminated intravascular coagulopathy are responsible for the maternal deaths related to hypertensive disorders in pregnancy.

Table 2. Tertiary pre-eclampsia manifestations

- Eclampsia
- Cerebral hemorrhage
- Cerebral oedema
- Retinal detachment
- Pulmonary oedema
- *DIC*
- *HELLP* syndrome
- Acute renal failure
- Subcapsular hematoma of the liver

DIC, denominated intravascular coagulopathy; *HEELP*, hemolysis, elevated liver enzymes, low platelets

Hemorrhage

Hemorrhage in obstetric patients represents an acute and dramatic problem. Risk factors for an obstetric hemorrhage greater than 1000 cc are placental abruption, placenta previa, multiple pregnancy, and retained placenta. The situation can be worsened by DIC, which is the activation of the coagulation cascade in response to the presence of large amounts of tissue phospholipids (Table 3). Such conditions also include retained dead fetus and amniotic fluid embolism.

Table 3. Stimuli for DIC in obstetrics

Condition	Mediated by
• Pre-eclampsia • Hypovolemia • Sepsis	Endothelial damage
• Placental abruption • Amniotic fluid embolism • Retained abortion • Intrauterine sepsis • Throphoblastic disease • Placenta accreta	Thromboplastin
• Intravascular hemolysis • Fetomaternal hemorrhage • Sepsis • Incompatible blood transfusion	Phospholipids

The conditio sine qua non of successful management of DIC is treatment of the initiating event. Once the cause has been identified and treated, the process can be solved with replacement of essential factors contained in fresh frozen plama.

Other maternal complications exist whose implications for the mother's health are more benign than those mentioned above, but which are still very serious in terms of fetal prognosis.

Such is preterm labor, and undoubtedly, the preterm premature rupture of membranes.

The birth of a premature baby is still the principal cause of perinatal mortality and morbidity. Despite abundant new knowledge about the factors that underlie preterm birth, 8%-9% of births still occur before 37 weeks' gestation, and 1%-2% of births that occur before 32 weeks account for half the perinatal deaths [7]. Risk factors have been identified with genital infection, abnormal cervical function, physical exertion, sexual activity, uterine volume and contractility, and even vaginal bleeding.

Obstetricians have treated the incompetent cervix and have administered drugs to inhibit labor, antibiotics to avoid infection, and corticosteroids to reduce the neonatal consequences of prematurity. This has reduced the neonatal morbidity and mortality, but not the rate of preterm birth.

When amniotic fluid leakage begins before 37 weeks' gestation, the clinical condition is defined preterm premature reapture of membranes (PROM).

As for preterm labor, several similar risk factors have been associated with a higher risk of preterm PROM: genital tract infection, coitus, low socioeconomic status, poor nutrition, smoking and bleeding in pregnancy have all been linked to an increased chance of preterm PROM (premature rupture of membranes).

Intrauterine infection is a potentially serious complication to the mother, and, in fact, a clinical diagnosis of chorioamnionitis accompanies preterm PROM in approximately 10% of cases.

Although amnionitis usually responds well to antibiotic administration and delivery, maternal deaths from sepsis do occur.

Amnionitis is more common when PROM occurs before 30-32 weeks than later in pregnancy.

As for the mother, infection is a major potential complication for the fetus and the neonate, too. Other serious complications include frank or occult cord prolapse, placental abruption occurs in 4%-6% of cases; and overall cesarean delivery is more common for fetal distress in labor and failed induction.

When women present with preterm PROM very early in pregnancy, as for example around 26-28 weeks, it is possible to apply expectant management in an attempt to delay delivery and reduce the risk of fetal prematurity. This can be done by reducing the risk of infection with antibiotic treatment, administering steroids to accelerate fetal lung maturation, and treatment with tocolytic drugs.

It should be noted that β-mimetic drugs are still the tocolytics of first choice since there is no clearly superior agent to suppress uterine contractions. However, it is important to know that they carry severe risks to the mother, such as pulmonary oedema, and that they have absolute (maternal cardiac disease; severe pre-eclampsia or other hypertensive disorders; uncontrolled diabetes mellitus; maternal hyperthyroidism) and relative (febrile patient; diabetes, diet or insuline controlled; history of severe migraine, headaches) contraindications [8].

Among the subjects which deserve special attention because of the implications they carry for fetomaternal wellbeing, one must not neglect the multiple gestations, namely, triplet gestations. Without getting into the dramatic problems that are associated with higher-order (four or more) multiple gestations, such as the need for selective reduction, it is a fact that the advent of ovulation inducing agents and reproductive technologies has led to a tenfold increase in the prevalence of triplet pregnancies [9].

As a result of both the physiologic changes seen with triplet gestations, such as uterine sovradistension, and the treatments used, such as prolonged bedrest and tocolytic use, numerous maternal complications may develop.

Since the chances of preterm labor are estimated to be very high – in some studies as high as 86% – treatment for this complication is often necessary: this may mean increased hospitalization and increased maternal complications. Among the others, various authors have reported gastrointestinal bleeding after indomethacin therapy, pulmonary edema due to i.v. magnesium sulfate, DVT with pulmonary embolism because of the prolonged bedrest. Also, postpartum uterine atony and consequent hemorrhage caused by uterine overdistension. This complication has been frequently seen in some series, often making blood transfusion necessary and, in rarer instances, Caesarean hysterectomy.

Other maternal complications include higher rates of pre-eclampsia and gestational diabetes.

In conclusion, a triplet pregnancy, like all higher-order multifetal gestations, requires intensified surveillance, in order to avoid the more frequently associated maternal complications. The pregnancy, in this case, may exaggerate its effects upon the cardiovascular, hepatic and renal functions, just to name some of them. Modern obstetricians, while waiting for the embryo transfer and superovulation effects to subside, should be aware that maternal complications may have also less familiar etiologies, borne within the daring progress of their own profession.

References

1. World Health Organization (WHO) (1991) Weekly epidemiological record. Geneva 47:2
2. Lyons G (1998) Risk factors and maternal mortality. In: Gullo A (ed) Critical care medicine. Springer-Verlag, Milano, pp 523-527
3. Capogna G et al (1998) High risk patients and ICU management. In: Gullo A (ed) APICE. Springer-Verlag, Milano, pp 543-548
4. Greer IA (1997) Epidemiology, risk factors and prophylaxis of venous thromboembolism in obstetrics and gynaecology. Clin Obstet Gynaecol 11:403-430
5. Clark S et al (1995) Amniotic fluid embolism: analysis of the national registry. Am J Obstet Gynecol 1158:1167
6. Redman CWG (1995) Ipertensione in gravidanza. In: Chamberlain G (ed) Turnbull's obstetrics. Churchill Livingstone, New York, pp 345-367
7. Iams J (1998) Prevention of preterm birth. N Engl J Med 338:54-55
8. Iams J (1996) Preterm birth. In: Gabbe SG et al (eds) Obstetrics. Normal and problem pregnancies. Churchill Livingstone, New York, pp 743-820
9. Albrecht JL (1996) The maternal and neonatal outcome of triplet gestations. Am J Obstet Gynecol 174:1551-1556

Chapter 15

Asphyxia and hypoxic-ischemic encephalopathy in neonates: postnatal interventions

G. Motta, L. Gagliardi, P. Introvini

The birth of an asphyxiated neonate is a dramatic event that can affect both the probability of survival and the quality of life of the neonate. About 6/1 000 newborn infants develop asphyxia [1], with a mortality rate of 15%-20% (due to a multiorgan failure syndrome and respiratory complications) and a further 25% probability of later neurodevelopmental sequelae due to hypoxic-ischemic encephalopathy (HIE) [2]. Even when electronically monitoring fetal heart rate, asphyxia is not detected before birth in about 50% of severe cases [3].

Therefore, in recent years research has focused on the mechanisms of brain damage after asphyxia, in search of an effective treatment for HIE, but this new information has not translated into clinical practice yet, and some of the promising therapies have not proven effective in the clinical arena [4-6].

Several excellent reviews are available, describing recent developments in the field of understanding the mechanisms of HIE and the possible new therapies [7-13]; this article will briefly summarize some of the more promising findings that could translate into clinical practice in the next future, with particular interest for clinical references.

Clinical presentation

Birth asphyxia is often not preventable [3], and so every hospital must be able to guarantee immediate and adequate resuscitation and care of the asphyxiated newborn. Symptoms of asphyxia at birth are well known and include hypotonia, bradycardia, apnea, pallor, and absence of reflexes. They are classically estimated using the Apgar score. All these derangements can be effectively reverted with a proper resuscitation; however, prognosis can be poor in spite of an effective and rapid resuscitation.

Neither the Apgar score, which is influenced also by resuscitation maneuvers, nor the degree of acidosis are reliable indicators of the severity of asphyxia and of the probability of later development of neurologic sequelae [14]. There is no good way of rapidly recognizing (in the first days of life) which neonates will later develop such sequelae [14] that are associated with depletion of energy substrates in the hours to days after the hypoxic-ischemic (HI) insult, as demonstrated by nuclear magnetic spectroscopy [15] (see below).

Table 1. Sarnat and Sarnat stages of hypoxic-ischemic encephalopathy. (Modified from [16])

	Stage 1 (mild)	Stage 2 (moderate)	Stage 3 (severe)
• Level of consciousness	Hyperalert; irritable	Lethargic or obtunded	Stuporous, comatose
• Neuromuscular control	Uninhibited, overreactive	Diminished spontaneus	Diminished or absent spontaneous movement
- Muscle tone	Normal	Mild hypotonia	Flaccid
- Posture	Mild distal flexion	Strong distal flexion	Intermittent decerebration
- Stretch reflexes	Overactive	Overactive, disinhibited	Decreased or absent
- Segmental myoclonus	Present or absent	Present	Absent
• Complex reflexes	Normal	Suppressed	Absent
- Suck	Weak	Weak or absent	Absent
- Moro	Strong, low threshold	Weak, incomplete high threshold	Absent
- Oculovestibular	Normal	Overactive	Weak or absent
- Tonic neck	Slight	Strong	Absent
• Autonomic function	Generalized sympathetic	Generalized parasympathetic	Both systems depressed
- Pupils	Mydriasis	Miosis	Midposition, often unequal; poor reflex
- Respirations	Spontaneous	Spontaneous; occasional apnea	Periodic; apnea
- Heart rate	Tachycardia	Bradycardia	Variable
- Bronchial and salivary secretion	Sparse	Profuse	Variable
- Gastrointestinal motility	Normal or decreased	Increased diarrhea	Variable
• Seizures	None	Common focal or multifocal (6 to 24 h of age)	Uncommon (excluding decerebration)
• Electroencephalographic findings	Normal (awake)	Early: generalized low-voltage, slowing (continuous delta and theta) Later: periodic pattern (awake); seizures focal or multifocal; 1.0 to 1.5 Hz spike and wave	Early: periodic pattern with isopotential phases Later: totally isopotential
• Durations of symptoms	<24 h	2 to 14 days	Hours to weeks
• Outcome	About 100% normal	80% normal; abnormal if symptoms last more than 5-7 days	About 50% die; remainder with severe sequelae

Clinically, the severity of HIE during the acute phase can be quantified in term neonates with the Sarnat and Sarnat classification [16] (Table 1). This classification is widely used, but requires prolonged observation and cannot be applied in the first days of life.

Recent data indicate that the evaluation of the so-called "general movements" (spontaneous global body movements) is particularly reliable in identifying infants who will be neurodevelopmentally handicapped. This mode of assessment calls for prolonged, planned, qualitative observation of the pattern of spontaneous movements of the infant that become altered in perinatal brain injury. The results published so far indicate that this elegant technique is simple, totally noninvasive, and compares favorably with "classical" neurologic examination and neuroimaging data in identifying infants that need other examinations or early intervention for brain damage, both in term and preterm infants [17, 18].

Pathophysiology

Asphyxiated infants initially increase their cardiac output, heart rate and arterial pressure, with an increase in central venous pressure (CVP) and pulmonary flow. The systemic blood flow is preferentially diverted towards the brain, heart (coronary arteries), and adrenals. With continuing hypoxia, pH and CVP fall, causing a fall in cardiac output and in perfusion, with HI damage. The limited ability of the cerebral circulation to autoregulate in neonates (maintain blood flow in the face of a falling systemic flow) renders them particularly susceptible to hypotension; especially in distal territories, ischemia rapidly ensues.

The clinical picture is that of a multiple organ failure, and the therapeutic interventions tend to break the vicious circle, by restoring oxygenation and perfusion.

After the HI event is treated and resolved, however, a delayed secondary injury develops. Recent observations indicate a possible "therapeutic window" of about 2-3 h after birth for the drugs to be effective in reducing the severity of the HIE [13].

From a biochemical point of view, this secondary phase is not completely understood, but probably involves cellular injury mediated by excitatory neurotransmitters, free radical formation and lipid peroxidation, activation of immune mechanisms and removal of trophic factors that normally support cell survival [9-13].

Cells undergo a shift from aerobic to anaerobic metabolism, with impaired oxidative phosphorylation and depletion of energy substrates, and formation of lactic acid, with subsequent alteration of the Na/K pump. At the cerebral level, the release of glutamate and excitotoxic amino acids and their accumulation in the synaptic cleft produce entry of excess sodium and water into the cell (leading to cytotoxic edema), and hyperstimulation of N-methyl-d-aspartate (NMDA) receptors (which open calcium channels). The high Ca concentration in the postsynaptic cells stimulates oxidative substances, production of nitric oxide, and the activation of proteases and lipases that further damage the cell [7-10].

Reperfusion of previously ischemic tissue may also cause the activation of the hypoxanthine-xanthine oxidase system and promote the formation of excess oxygen free radicals (i.e., superoxide ion, hydrogen peroxide, hydroxyl radicals, singlet oxygen) that, when they overwhelm endogenous scavenger mechanisms, may damage cellular lipids, proteins, and cell membranes [11, 12].

Therapies for birth asphyxia

Although birth asphyxia is such a common problem, effective therapies are lacking. The decrease in mortality and morbidity attributable to asphyxia is due to an improvement in general pre- and postnatal care, with a better ability to treat cardiac, renal, respiratory, and other organs complications, rather than to an improvement in treating HIE per s. In Table 2, commonly used therapeutic interventions for severe birth asphyxia are reported.

Most therapeutic interventions are based on common sense, and some – though widely used – are not supported by evidence of efficacy. Recently the editor of Paediatrics (the official journal of the American Academy of Paediatrics) in an article on neuroprotection and perinatal brain care has recalled that "present therapies to prevent or treat perinatal brain damage are ineffective" [19]. Research is very active in this area, but there are several causes of difficulty in translating experimental research into clinical research and practice.

Table 2. Summary of management of severe birth asphyxia

Immediate management
- Establish effective ventilation
- Assist circulation if necessary

Early management
- Restrict fluids to 20% less than the normal values for the postnatal age of the baby
- Monitor blood pressure and treat hypotension vigorously
- Assess respiratory effort and
  - ventilate if baby is breathing spontaneously with arterial carbon dioxide tension >52.5 torr (7 kPa)
  - If baby is ventilated, maintain arterial carbon dioxide tension at 30-45 torr (4-6 kPa)
- if clinical signs of raised intracranial pressure are present, mannitol may be given; corticosteroids are probably useless
- Phenobarbital at high doses (40 mg/kg) may be useful
- Avoid hypo- or hyperglycemia

Anticonvulsants if
- frequent convulsions >3 per hour
- prolonged convulsions lasting ≥3 min

First, the results of experimental studies (in animals) are often contradictory, and it is often difficult to understand the clinical relevance of such studies. The causes lie in the difficulty of standardizing experimental models; confounding variables include the species studied, the time-course of the insult and treatment, the preexisting chemical environment of the subject and the effects of temperature variations. Adult animal models may not apply to neonates, as asphyxia in adult animals can exert effects that are different from those in the fetus or newborn.

Moreover, in translating to the human being, beyond ethical concerns, further difficulties are encountered. Differences between subjects are greater than in animal studies; most of the variables are outside the control of the researcher, and all interventions can only be given after the insult, at variable time.

Moreover, in animal studies the rate of cerebral damage in control animals can be as high as 100%; in practice in human studies it is particularly difficult to select cotrol groups with such high rates of cerebral injury, making the demonstration of effect more difficult.

Another problem is the lack of interest of the pharmaceutical industry. HIE seems to be a "therapeutic orphan": in 1997 there were 146 new medicines in development for children in the USA; only eight of these are for neurologic disorders of children, and all are for epilepsy. No therapies for HIE in children are being developed [19].

Nonetheless, some interventions (Table 3) [7-13, 20] have attracted some interest.

Some therapies have been tried also in human neonates, but so far with disappointing results [4-6], and others are a refinement of old therapies [20]. Two interventions, however – namely, the resuscitation of asphyxiated infants with room air and the use of moderate hypothermia – are now the focus of particular interest in clinical journals, because of their simplicity and apparent ease of use. Because their clinical application is under way, they will be reviewed more in depth.

Table 3. New therapies for hypoxic-ischemic encephalopathy

- Resuscitation with room air instead of 100% oxygen
- Moderate hypothermia, whole body or brain only
- High-dose phenobarbital
- $MgSO_4$
- Oxygen-free radical inhibitors, allopurinol
- Calcium channel blockers
- Inhibitors of nitric oxide production
- Monoganglioside GM
- NMDA receptor antagonists (MK801)
- Nerve growth factor (IGF)
- CO_2 control
- SNO S-nitrosohemoglobin
- Combination of above

Resuscitation with room air

The Apgar score is a well known and universally used scale to rate the degree of "viability" of the newborn. Although its usefulness as a marker of perinatal distress is disputed [14], especially in preterm infants [21], it is useful for guiding resuscitation.

Obviously some items (heart rate, respiratory efforts) are more important than others (skin color, reflexes), and if a neonate does not have a good heart rate or does not breathe spontaneously, resuscitation maneuvers are immediately begun, without waiting for the first minute to pass.

The resuscitation maneuvers in the delivery room are well standardized and are based on classical "ABCD" (airway management, breathing, circulation, drugs) of basic life support. The aim is that of trying to "normalize" the disorders as soon as possible. The American Heart Association and the American Academy of Paediatrics have jointly produced guidelines [22] and a manual [23] to be used for field courses of resuscitation that report these standards. An Italian translation of the manual has been published and is currently used by the Italian Society of Neonatology for field courses aimed at paediatricians and other personnel that work in delivery rooms.

In particular, manual ventilation with 100% oxygen, with mask and bag or after endotracheal intubation is the standard, in order to obtain a rapid normalization of heart rate, color, and other Apgar items. However, no data are available to support this long-standing practice.

In recent years a growing body of knowledge has accumulated concerning the possible toxic effect of oxygen administration, because of the formation of unstable oxygen radicals, especially after a HI insult [11, 12]. In other words, oxygen could be detrimental to asphyxiated infants, adding free-radical damage to that caused directly by HI. This has led to the suggestion of using room air, instead of oxygen, in the resuscitation maneuvers in the delivery room [24].

Several studies [25-28] both in animals and in term and preterm human neonates have been carried out, including two randomized controlled trials [27, 28]. Though there are differences in the methodology of the studies, a consensus seems to emerge that air is at least as good as 100% oxygen to resuscitate an asphyxiated neonate.

Recent studies in the experimental animal (newborn piglets) suggest that biochemical markers of intracellular hypoxia and energy depletion such as hypoxantine levels are greater in the cerebral cortex of the animals treated with oxygen than in the group treated with air, while the levels are the same in the muscle and in plasma [26]. One possible mechanism for this paradoxical response to oxygen could be the reduction of cerebral blood flow and of the level of vasodilating substances as prostacyclin produced by oxygen inhalation [2, 29, 30].

The studies carried out in human neonates are, however, only short-term studies, focusing on the immediate effect of resuscitation maneuvers such as the time to first spontaneous breath or the length of manual ventilation in the delivery room etc., without any long-term (prognostic) study reported to date.

These studies are necessary to change a long-standing practice such as using 100% oxygen in resuscitation, but the data available so far suggest that the possibility could be real.

Moderate hypothermia

There is a growing consensus that not only do some cells die during a HI insult, but that late damage occurs, and many more cells die in the hours to days after the insult has ceased [31-33]. In the 1980s it was shown with magnetic resonance spectroscopy studies that asphyxiated newborns have a normal cerebral metabolism immediately after resuscitation, but that severe energy depletion (impaired oxidative phosphorylation) develops 9-24 h later, even without continuing hypoxia and with a normal acid-base status. The magnitude of this late energy depletion correlated well with the severity of neurological impairment and reduced brain growth at follow-up [15, 32, 33]. Recent data have confirmed these findings and have shown that cerebral metabolism is disturbed for a long period of time (weeks to months) after an HI episode [34, 35].

This biphasic sequence that occurs in asphyxiated neonates has been well studied and characterized in animals. This late damage is associated with delayed cell death; the mechanisms underlying this phenomenon are not completely clear, but apoptosis (or programmed cell death) is surely an important part of it [31, 34]. Histological studies have shown that the death of cerebral cells during the late phase of HIE presents the features of apoptosis (the cell shrinks and the nucleus becomes small and dense, the plasma membrane invaginates with vacuolization, and eventually the cell separates into multiple small apoptotic bodies that are phagocytosed by healthy neighboring cells, without inflammation). These are clearly different from what happens in the immediate phase where cell death presents with the features of necrosis (the cell swells after an overwhelming insult, organelles become disrupted until the cell bursts, spilling the cytoplasmic content in the extracellular space, where phagocytes migrate to remove the debris with classical signs of inflammation) [31].

This has led to the hypothesis that inappropriate activation of the apoptotic program contributes (at least in part) to the delayed cell death and has arisen some hope in the possibility to break the circle and prevent the late phase of cerebral damage.

In animals, some interventions applied after a HI insult, including the infusion of insulin-like growth factor 1 (IGF-1) [36] and the moderate cooling of the brain [37, 38], have resulted in amelioration of the cerebral injury.

Of particular interest, given its simplicity, is the application of moderate hypothermia (32°-33°C) to the brain. The idea is not new. As Edwards et al. note, "to many people, especially writers of science fiction interested in preserving brains for narrative purposes, it seems self-evident that cooling the brain protects it against hypoxic-ischemic damage" [34]. Indeed, reducing cerebral temperature during HI is a standard procedure during cardiac and neurosurgery.

Observational data supporting the use of hypothermia in asphyxiated neonates were collected by Swedish researchers some 40 years ago [39]. However, animal studies using drastic temperature reductions failed to show any benefit [40, 41]. Moreover, during the 1950s seminal investigations on the effect of environment on the survival of preterm neonates were produced, and randomized clinical trials showed that failing to maintain a neutral thermal environment increased mortality in preterm neonates [42]. This led to the widespread notion, permeating the culture of the subsequent generations of neonatologists, that hypothermia is bad and must be avoided.

The resurgence of the idea of moderate cooling is based on the demonstration that hypothermia reduces, sometimes dramatically, the degree of late cerebral injury without (apparent) serious adverse effects, in term neonates, whereas hyperthermia increases it [43]. Re-examination of earlier research in humans has shown that the benefit of maintaining high environmental temperatures is only apparent in (tiny) preterm neonates, whereas term neonates tolerate moderate cooling wery well. Some authors have even suggested that perhaps neonates are meant to become a little cold after birth, and that moderate hypothermia is an adaptive mechanism of our species, as shown by the large surface of the usually bald head of the newborn whose abundant blood vessels do not vasoconstrict in response to cold [38]. This hypothesis needs to be proven, before it is accepted [44].

How hypothermia works is still unclear; presumably it reduces cerebral energy demands so that, during HI, high-energy phosphate reserves are maintained at relatively normal levels [13]. This may prolong the "therapeutic window" after HI and exert a synergistic action with other rescue therapies [38].

It must be stressed that profound hypothermia has deleterious effects not only on preterm infants but also on term ones [34, 37, 38]. It decreases perfusion and oxygenation by impairing myocardial function, shifting the oxygen dissociation curve to the left and causing peripheral vasoconstriction and ventilation-perfusion mismatch, increasing blood viscosity, and thus leading to renal failure, metabolic acidosis, and decreased cerebral blood flow. Other adverse effects of severe hypothermia are coagulation disturbances, pulmonary hemorrhage, impairment of the immune system, hypoglycemia, and disturbances in potassium and acid-base balance etc. Obviously, profound hypothermia must be avoided. Less severe hypothermia does not seem to cause severe adverse effects, but more studies are necessary, especially if moderate hypothermia has to be maintained for longer periods of time to offer greater neuroprotection after an episode of asphyxia.

The duration of brain cooling, its degree, and the way of producing it, are other areas that need further research.

As stated above, great differences exist between experimental settings, where the investigator regulates the degree and duration of the HI insult and can control for many other important variables that can influence the outcome, and the case of asphyxia in human neonates, where most of the variables are outside the control of the investigator. From animal studies, however, it seems that the duration of cooling must be of at least 12h for maximal protection to occur [34, 45].

As far as how to provide brain cooling, research is hampered by the lack of precise and handy ways to measure deep brain temperature. Most animal studies have been carried out by cooling the whole animal, but it is likely that if head-only cooling can be obtained, this should result in a similar neuroprotection with fewer side effects. A "cooling cap" has been succesfully used in some animal species and is not technically difficult to build.

To date, only animal studies have been published, but two preliminary studies of moderate hypothermia in asphyxiated neonates are under way in New Zealand and in England. No published results are available, but a comment states that so far there are no data to suggest that moderate hypothermia is unsafe, and that the results suggest a beneficial effect sufficient to justify further trials [45].

However, simple as it may seem, organizing a clinical trial on this subject is not easy, and the difficulties are well summarized by the recent review by Edwards and Azzopardi [45].

Conclusions

At least two promising and potentially useful therapeutic interventions for neurologic rescue after asphyxia have passed the phase of animal study and are now being tested in randomized controlled trials. Together with the continuing improvement in critical care of the sick newborn, and with advances in basic research and understanding of HIE, it is possible that in the near future the neonatologist will not be left without effective therapies for HIE, as is still the case today.

References

1. Levene MI, Kornberg J, Williams THC (1985) The incidence of and severity of postasphyxial encephalopathy in full-term infants. Early Hum Devel 11:21-28
2. Levene MI (1995) Management and outcome of birth asphyxia. In: Levene MI, Bennett MJ, Punt J (eds) Fetal and neonatal neurology and neurosurgery. Churchill Livingstone, Edinburgh, pp 427-442
3. Spencer JAD (1998) Deaths related to intrapartum asphyxia. Br Med J 316:640
4. Levene MI, Gibson NA, Fenton AC et al (1990) The use of a calcium-channel blocker, nicardipine, for severely asphyxiated newborn infants. Dev Med Child Neurol 32:567-574
5. Russell GA, Cooke RW (1995) Randomised controlled trial of allopurinol prophylaxis in very preterm infants. Arch Dis Child 73:F27-F31
6. Bennet P, Edwards AD (1997) Use of magnesium sulphate in obstetrics. Lancet 350:1491
7. Levene MI (1993) Management of the asphyxiated full-term infant. Arch Dis Child 68:612-616
8. Shankaran S (1993) Perinatal asphyxia. Clin Perinatol 20(2)

9. Edwards AD (1993) Protection against hypoxic-ischaemic cerebral injury in the developing brain. Perfusion 8:97-100
10. Bowen FW (1996) Management issues for the neonatal patient. Clin Perinatol 23:1-30
11. Saugstad OD (1996) Role of xantine oxidase and its inhibitor in hypoxia: reoxygenation injury. Pediatrics 98:103-107
12. Saugstad OD (1996) Mechanisms of tissue injury by oxygen radicals: implication for neonatal disease. Acta Paediatr 85:1-4
13. Vannucci RC, Perlman JM (1997) Intervention for perinatal hypoxic-ischemic encephalopathy. Pediatrics 100:1004-1014
14. Patel J, Edwards AD (1997) Prediction of neurological outcome after perinatal asphyxia. Curr Opin Pediatr 9:128-132
15. Azzopardi D, Wyatt JS, Cady EB et al (1989) Prognosis of newborn infants with hypoxic-ischemic brain injury assessed by phosphorus magnetic resonance spectroscopy. Pediatr Res 25:445-451
16. Sarnat HB, Sarnat MS (1976) Neonatal encephalopathy following fetal distress. A clinical and electroencephalographic study. Arch Neurol 33:696-705
17. Prechtl HFR, Ferrari F, Cioni G (1993) Predictive value of general movements in asphyxiated fullterm infants. Early Hum Devel 35:91-120
18. Cioni G, Ferrari F, Einspieler C et al (1997) Neurological assessment of preterm infants: comparison between observation of spontaneous movements and neurological examination. J Pediatr 130:704-711
19. Lucey JF (1997) Neuroprotection and perinatal brain care: the field of the future, currently going nowhere. Pediatrics 100:1030-1031
20. Hall RT, Hall FK, Daily DK (1998) High-dose phenobarbital therapy in term newborn infants with severe perinatal asphyxia: a randomized, prospective study with three-year follow-up. J Pediatr 132:345-348
21. Catlin EA, Carpenter MW, Brann BS et al (1986) The Apgar score revisited: influence of gestational age. J Pediatr 109:865-868
22. American Heart Association, Emergency Cardiac Care Committee and Subcommittees (1992) Guidelines for cardiopulmonary resuscitation and emergency cardiac care. VII. Neonatal resuscitation. JAMA 268:2276-2281
23. Bloom RS, Cropley C (1987) Textbook of neonatal resuscitation. AHA and AAP, Dallas
24. Saugstad OD (1996) Resuscitation of newborn infants; do we need new guidelines? Prenatal Neonatal Med 1:26-28
25. Lundstrom KE, Pryds O, Greisen G (1995) Oxygen at birth and prolonged cerebral vasoconstriction in preterm infants. Arch Dis Child 73:F81-F86
26. Feet BA, Yu X-Q, Rootwelt T et al (1997) Effects of hypoxemia and reoxygenation with 21% or 100% oxygen in newborn piglets: extracellular hypoxanthine in cerebral cortex and femoral muscle. Crit Care Med 25:1384-1391
27. Ramji S, Ahuja S, Thirupuram S et al (1993) Resuscitation of asphyxic newborn infants with room air or 100% oxygen. Pediatr Res 34:809-812
28. Saugstad OD, Rootwelt T, Aalen O (1998) Resuscitation of asphyxiated newborn infants with room air or oxygen: an international controlled trial. The RESAIR 2 study. Pediatrics 102:E1
29. Leahy FAN, Cates D, MacCallum M, Rigatto H (1980) Effects of CO_2 and 100% O_2 on cerebral blood flow in preterm infants. J Appl Physiol 48:468-472
30. Rahilly PM (1980) Effects of 2% CO_2, 0.5% CO_2 and 100% oxygen on cranial blood flow of the human neonate. Pediatrics 66:685-689
31. Mehmet H, Edwards AD (1996) Hypoxia, ischaemia, and apoptosis. Arch Dis Child 75:F73-F75

32. Roth SC, Edwards AD, Cady EB et al (1992) Relation between cerebral oxidative metabolism following birth asphyxia and neurodevelopmental outcome and brain growth at one year. Dev Med Child Neurol 34:285-295

33. Lorek A, Takei Y, Cady EB et al (1994) Delayed ("secondary") cerebral energy failure following acute hypoxia-ischaemia in the newborn piglet: continuous 48-hour studies by 31P magnetic resonance spectroscopy. Pediatr Res 36:699-706

34. Edwards AD, Wyatt JS, Thoresen M (1998) Treatment of hypoxic-ischaemic brain damage by moderate hypothermia. Arch Dis Child 78:F85-F91

35. Du C, Hu R, Csernansky CA et al (1996) Very delayed infarction after mild focal cerebral ischemia: a role for apoptosis? J Cereb Blood Flow Metab 16:195-201

36. Gluckman PD, Klempt N, Guan J et al (1992) A role for IGF-1 in the rescue of CNS neurons following hypoxic-ischemic injury. Biochem Biophys Res Commun 182:593-599

37. Thoresen M, Wyatt JS (1997) Keeping a cool head, post-hypoxic hypothermia-an old idea revisited. Acta Paediatr 86:1029-1033

38. Wyatt JS, Thoresen M (1997) Hypothermia treatment and the newborn. Pediatrics 100:1028-1030

39. Westin B, Miller JA, Nyberg R et al (1959) Neonatal asphyxia pallida treated with hypothermia alone or with hypothermia and exchange transfusion of oxygenated blood. Surgery 45:868-879

40. Oates RK, Harvey D (1976) Failure of hypothermia as treatment of asphyxiated newborn rabbits. Arch Dis Child 51:512-516

41. Sirimanne E, Blumberg RM, Bossano B et al (1996) The effect of prolonged modification of cerebral temperature on outcome following hypoxic-ischemic brain injury in the infant rat. Pediatr Res 39:591-597

42. Silverman WA, Fertig JW, Berger AP (1958) The influence of the thermal environment upon the survival of newly born premature infants. Pediatrics 22:876-886

43. Grether JK, Nelson KB (1997) Maternal infection and cerebral palsy in infants of normal birth weight. JAMA 278:207-211

44. Silverman WA (1998) Cooling the asphyxiated newborn-responsibly. Pediatrics 101:697-698

45. Edwards AD, Azzopardi D (1998) Hypothermic neural rescue treatment: from laboratory to cotside? Arch Dis Child 78:F88-F91

Chapter 16

The parents in neonatal intensive care units and the kangaroo-mother method

U. DE VONDERWEID

As early as 1907, Pierre Budin, the father of neonatology, noted in his book "The Nursling" that some mothers may find it very difficult to cope with the experience of having a low-birth-weight newborn and that encouraging mothers to participate in the care of their offspring and to breastfeed could help them to overcome the crisis and establish a healthier relationship with the infant.

Unfortunately, this aspect of care did not find its way into nurseries being established in the United States and Europe: with rare exceptions, most hospitals were concerned with preventing infections and excluded parents completely both from well-baby nurseries and special care units. Klaus and Kennel [1], in a survey of hospital nurseries in the 1970s found that only 30% of mothers were allowed into the nurseries in the first days of life.

The fear of parent-infant transmission of infections was not based on any scientific evidence at that time. Actually, there are only limited data associating the transmission of bacterial colonization or infectious diseases with either family visitation or physical contact. But several reports in the 1980s stated there are no significant differences in bacterial colonization or the number of infants with infections comparing infants with visitation or contact to those who are isolated [2-4]. Furthermore, some trials on the effect of family visitation in nurseries on the isolation of pathogens from the umbilicus actually show a decrease in isolated pathogens [5-7].

So, there is no bacteriological reason for restricting parental access to neonatal nurseries and special/intensive care units.

The question now is to what extent the presence of parents in neonatal intensive care units (NICUs) may be beneficial for the parents and the infants themselves. In order to answer this question it is first necessary to understand the feelings of the parents of preterm/low-birth-weight infants in the context of the theory of parent/infant bonding.

Klaus and Kennell defined mother/infant attachment or bonding as "perhaps the strongest bond in the human and the wellspring for all the infant's subsequent attachments. Throughout his lifetime, the strength and character of this attachment will influence the quality of all future bonds to other individuals" [1]. The foundations of this attachment are laid long before conception: entering parenthood represents the completion of human generation cycle. Multiple factors are at work, going back to the care each parent received from his/her own parents: especially for mothers, the quality of the interaction with their own mothers in the first months of life is particularly important. Parental attitudes are further shaped by lifelong experiences of caring and by cultural and social values and situations.

Once pregnancy is confirmed, multiple factors in the mother's life and relationships influence her acceptance of the pregnancy and the fetus growing inside her. Quickening generally marks the beginning of a mother's perceptions of the fetus as a separate individual. Hopes and plans, fears and phantasies intermingle as pregnancy progresses. A picture of the hoped-for, normal baby forms in the mother's mind as she prepares for labor and delivery. Most pregnant women, however, also have conscious or unconscious fears of producing a dead or malformed child.

After birth, parents face the task of resolving the discrepancy between features of the real baby and the phantasized ideal: time spent together in the first days of life allows this task to be accomplished. Much has been written about a "sensitive period" in the mother (and father) in the hours or days immediately after birth and its importance in the establishment of a bond from parent to infant. Despite some methodological limitations, most studies indicate that prolonged early contact of mother and newborn has significant effects and benefits [8-11].

When the pregnancy is prematurely interrupted by a preterm delivery and especially when the infant is of very low birth weight (VLBW) and/or needs intensive care procedures, many psychoaffective problems arise to complicate the process of mother(father)/infant attachment [12, 13].

Quite often, a preterm delivery is the product of a pathological pregnancy and delivery is preceded by a period of suffering related to obstetrical problems. The suffering is then accentuated by the grief for the premature interruption of the pregnancy and the difficulty of elaborating the untimely physical and psychological separation from the infant. Many mothers experience a sense of irreality of the child, since the interval between the beginning of the perception of the fetus as an individual growing inside her and the interruption of this intrauterine relationship is too short. A premature birth implies many "losses" for the woman: the loss of the pregnant woman status without fully achieving the status of mother, the loss of the physical and psychological processes of pregnancy (especially that of "making" a baby inside her), the loss of the dream of a normal pregnancy (with personal, familial, and social realization), and of a perfect child (narcissistic wound).

The crisis is then aggravated by a complex of guilt feelings, related to the suffering of the infant, his/her possible (or actual) death, or long-term handicap. These guilt feelings produce a sense of worrying, extraneousness, defeat, and refusal of the child, which manifest themselves in the fear of seeing and touching a child so small, fragile, strange, frightening, etc.

All these relational problems are aggravated by the environment of the NICU with all its strange machinery: Winnicott's "primary maternal preoccupation" is substituted by a sort of "primary medical preoccupation" and the mother feels she is useless to the child in the face of all the life-sustaining equipment around him/her.

Coping with such a psychological crisis is not easy for the majority of parents of a very premature and/or VLBW infant, and it is a very delicate task for the staff of the NICU to help parents in this process. For some parents, "coping through distance", that is avoiding contact with the child for some time, may be the only way to preserve their psychological equilibrium, but for all parents, sooner or later (and very soon for most), "coping through commitment", that is, seeing, talking to, touching, handling the child, and being involved in his/her care is the only way to heal the psychological wound and to start creating a healthy relationship with the child [13].

It is thus very important that no restriction is posed to the entering of parents in the NICU at any time: visitations to the infant must be encouraged and the staff must be prepared to help parents with information and reassurance.

Among the many ways for enhancing parent/infant relationships in the NICU a very special place is held by the kangaroo-mother care (KMC) method. The procedure is very simple: it only implies putting the tiny infant, naked except for a diaper, at direct skin-to-skin contact with the mother's body, and covering him/her with a blanket. The method was originally adopted in developing countries with the aim of improving survival and growth of preterm/low-birth-weight infants where the availability of technological resources is limited [14-16]. Mothers are encouraged to breastfeed their infants early and frequently and provide heath and protection from infections with their body. Early discharge from the hospital and follow-up at home or in outpatient clinics is an essential part of the program [17].

In the developed world KMC does not represent an alternative to technological intensive neonatal care for VLBW infants, especially for those who need respiratory support, but has been successfully integrated in modern care with the main objective of supporting mother-infant relationships and the infant's well-being and development.

When it was first applied to VLBW infants in the developed world, the main concern was for its safety, which was tested in a number of observational before/after studies. Acolet first demonstrated in 1989 that body temperature and oxygen saturation of VLBW infants placed on KMC were not different from incubator nursing: furthermore, some infants with chronic lung disease actually had better oxygen saturation [18]. Ludington in 1990 observed a reduction of restlessness and improvement of quiet sleep during KMC, again without modifications of heart and respiratory rates [19]. De Leeuw studied eight VLBW infants treated with nasal continuous positive airway pressure and reported no modifications of respiration, oxygen saturation, apneas, and bradycardyias during 1 h of KMC as compared to standard incubator care [20]. Similar results come from Bosque's study of spontaneously breathing VLBW who were offered longer periods (4 h/day) of KMC [21].

In two very elegant studies, Bauer and Bauer demonstrated a slight increase in body temperature during KMC as compared to incubator care, without any modifications of oxygen consumption and CO_2 production, and concluded that KMC is not accompanied by any metabolic stress for the infant [22, 23].

A randomized, controlled trial of KMC vs standard incubator care was performed by Ludington in a North American NICU. She studied 24 moderately preterm infants (≥34 weeks gestational age) aged 18 days and demonstrated a positive effect on body temperature and respiration, a reduction of uncoordinated motor activity, and an increase in quiet sleep [24]. In another randomized controlled trial of KMC vs incubator care for VLBW infants, Blaymore Bier demonstrated better oxygenation during KMC with no differences in heart and respiratory rate and body temperature [25].

It is now possible to conclude that KMC is safe for stable, spontaneously breathing VLBW infants and possibly also for those on long-term respiratory support.

The effect of KMC on mothers has only been studied on limited samples so far.

In an observational study, Affonso reported that KMC is effective in favoring the process of mother/infant reconciliation and healing of the psychological wound of the preterm birth, but no standard care controls were included in her study [26].

Whitelaw published in 1988 a randomized controlled trial of KMC in UK [27]. He concluded that, in a context where psychorelational support for mothers of VLBW infants was largely available, KMC did not improve total visitation and handling time, but had a positive effect on the duration of breastfeeding. Similar observations were made by Blaymore Bier [25].

Further studies are necessary to understand the limits of KMC (how early can it be applied? how long? in babies on mechanical ventilation?...) and the benefits for the infant (well-being, neurophysiological development) and the mother (recreation of the physical and psychological relationship with the child), but there is sufficient evidence to support its widespread use for promoting the preterm infant's wellbeing in NICUs.

References

1. Klaus MH, Kennell J (1976) Maternal-infant bonding. Mosby, St. Louis
2. Sosa R, Kennell J, Klaus M, Urrutia J (1976) The effect of early mother-infant contact on breast feeding, infection and growth. Ciba Found Symp 45:179-187
3. Trause MA, Voos D, Klaus M, Kennell J, Boslett M (1981) Separation for childbirth: the effect on the sibling. Child Psychiatry Hum Dev 12:32-39
4. Maloney M, Ballard J, Hollister L, Shank M (1983) A prospective controlled study of scheduled sibling visits to a newborn intensive care unit. J Am Acad Child Adolesc Psychiatry 6:565-570
5. Barnett CR, Liederman PH, Grobstein R, Klaus M (1970) Neonatal separation: the maternal side of interactional deprivation. Paediatrics 45:197-205
6. Umphenour JH (1980) Bacterial colonisation in neonates with sibling visitation. J Obstet Gynecol Neonat Nurs 9:73-75
7. Kowba MD, Schwirian PM (1985) Direct sibling contact and bacterial colonisation in newborns. J Obstet Gynecol Neonat Nurs 14:412-417

8. Klaus MH, Jerauld R, Kreger NC, McAlpine W, Steffa M, Kennell JH (1972) Maternal attachment: importance of the first post partum days. N Engl J Med 286:460-463
9. O'Connor S, Vietze PM, Sherrod KB, Sandler HM, Altmeier WA (1980) Reduced incidence of parental inadequacy following rooming-in. Paediatrics 66:176-182
10. Seashore MJ, Leifer AD, Barnett CR, Leiderman PH (1973) The effects of denial of early mother-infant interaction on maternal self-confidence. J Pers Soc Psychol 26:369-378
11. Leiderman PH, Seashore MJ (1975) Mother-infant neonatal separation: some delayed consequences. Parent-infant interaction. Ciba Found Symp 33:213-239
12. Druon C (1996) A l'écoute du bébé prématuré. Une vie aux portes de la vie. Aubier, Paris
13. Klaus MH, Kennell JH (1986) Care of the parents. In: Klaus MH, Fanaroff AA (eds) Care of the high risk neonate, 3rd ed. WB Saunders, Philadelphia, pp 147-170
14. Rey ES, Martinez HG (1983) Manejo racional del niño prematuro. I Curso de Medicina Fetal y Neonatal. University of Bogotà, Bogotà, pp 137-151
15. Sloan Nl, Leon Camacho LW, Rojas EP, Stern C, Maternidad Isidro Ayora Study Team (1994) Kangaroo mother method: randomized controlled trial of an alternative method of care for stabilized low birthweight infants. Lancet 344:782-785
16. Vaivre-Douret L, Papiernik E, Relier JP (1996) Méthode et soins kangourou. Arch Pediatr 3:1262-1269
17. Cattaneo A, Davanzo R, Uxa F, Tanburlini G (1998) Recommendations for the implementation of Kangaroo Mother care for low birthweight infants. Acta Paediatr 87:440-445
18. Acolet D, Sleath K, Whitelaw A (1989) Oxygenation, heart rate and temperature in very low birthweight infants during skin-to-skin contact with their mothers. Acta Paediatr Scand 78:189-193
19. Ludington SM (1990) Energy conservation during skin-to-skin contact between premature infants and their mothers. Heart Lung 19:445-451
20. De Leeuw R, Colin EM, Dunnebier EA, Mirmiran M (1991) Physiological effects of kangaroo care in very small preterm infants. Biol Neonate 59:149-155
21. Bosque EM, Brady JP, Affonso DD, Wahlberg V (1995) Physiological measures of kangaroo versus incubator care in a tertiary-level nursery. J Obset Gynecol Neonat Nurs 24:219-226
22. Bauer J, Sontheimer D, Fischer C, Linderkamp O (1996) Metabolic rate and energy balance in very low birth weight infants during kangaroo holding by their mothers and fathers. J Pediatr 129:608-611
23. Bauer K, Uhrig C, Sperling P, Pasel K, Wieland C, Versmold H (1997) Body temperatures and oxygen consumption during skin-to-skin (kangaroo) care in stable preterm infants weighing less than 1500 grams. J Pediatr 130:240-244
24. Ludington SM, Thompson C, Swinth J, Hadeed AJ, Anderson GC (1994) Kangaroo care: research results and practice implications and guidelines. Neonatal Network 13:1-9
25. Blaymore Bier JA, Ferguson AE, Morales Y, Liebling JA, Archer D, Oh W, Vohr BR (1996) Comparison of skin-to-skin contact with standard contact in low-birth-weight infants who are breast-fed. Arch Pediatr Adolesc Med 150:1265-1269
26. Affonso D, Bosque E, Wahlberg V, Brady JP (1993) Reconciliation and healing for mothers through skin-to-skin contact provided in an American tertiary level intensive care nursery. Neonatal Network 12:25-32
27. Whitelaw A, Heisterkamp G, Sleath K, Acolet D, Richards M (1988) Skin to skin contact for very low birthweight infants and their mothers. Arch Dis Child 63:1377-1381

PERIOPERATIVE SEDATION
AND ANALGESIA

Chapter 17

Models of pharmacokinetics in the treatment of acute postoperative pain in paediatrics

M. Calamandrei, P. Busoni

The development of new, sensitive techniques for assaying drugs and drug metabolites together with progress in computer technology have made possible remarkable advances in pharmacokinetics studies. Pharmacokinetics is the mathematical description of drug disposition over time. In other words, it is what the body does to the drug over time. Pharmacokinetics deals with the fate of the drugs in the body, including the mechanisms and kinetics of drug absorption, distribution, elimination (excretion and metabolism), and transport to the site of action (biophase). The latter process can be considered as a link between pharmacokinetics and pharmacodynamics; fundamentally, however, it is a pharmacokinetic process. The volume of pharmacokinetic drug evaluations in children falls considerably behind that performed in the adult population, with the exception of a few limited areas. There are some appropriate reasons for the limited availability of pharmacokinetics data in children. The thalidomide tragedy led to more stringent regulations. Consequently, manufacturers began omitting drug studies in infants and children, creating a population of "therapeutic orphans". Performing research in children is not only problematic for ethical reasons but also due to logistic difficulties. Patient and parent cooperation may be poor and phlebotomy is typically more difficult to perform in children. Limited patient populations present a problem even in large centers. The use of meta-analysis, although controversial, has tremendous potential for overcoming some of the problems with small sample size.

The constant intravenous infusion of a drug has been demonstrated to provide better postoperative pain relief than that provided by intermittent intramuscolar doses. This also avoids the necessity for unpleasant i.m. injections. The total dose which is given may be higher than that of traditional methods, but this is considered an index of the inadequacy of those previous methods. Pharmacokinetics data can be used to calculate the rate of infusion for the desired steady-state plasma concentration, the time to achieve a steady-state, and the size of a loading dose. During intravenous infusion, the concentration of drug in the plasma increases until the rate of elimination is equal to the rate of infusion. The time required to reach the steady-state drug concentration in the plasma is dependent on the elimination half-life of the drug. For practical purposes, plateau is said to be reached when the concentration is 90% of the concentration of the drug at the steady state. An increase in the rate of infusion will not shorten the time to reach the steady-state drug concentration. If the drug is given at a higher infusion rate, a higher steady state will be obtained. In order to maintain instant steady-state level, the loading dose should be equal to the ratio R/k, where R is the infusion rate (zero order) and k is the elimination rate constant (first order). Because of distribution kinetics, the time to reach the plateau differs between plasma and tissue.

Opioid analgesics are the mainstay of pain management in paediatric patients postoperatively. Opioids have similar pharmacodynamic properties but have widely different kinetics properties. The most important of these is the delay between the blood concentrations of an opioid and its analgesic effects, which probably relate to the delay required for blood and brain and spinal cord equilibrium. The half-lives of these delays range from 34 min for morphine to 1 min for alfentanyl [1]. The clearance of morphine varies with age [2]. In infants, clearance approaches the adult levels at 2-3 months of age. Pharmacokinetics studies of premature neonates in the first 24 h of life [3] and between 1 day and 10 weeks of age in infants born after 36-41 week's gestation [4] demonstrated a longer elimination half-life and a lower plasma clearance than in adults. (Tables 1, 2).

Epidural administration of narcotic analgesic drugs via lumbar or caudal route has been shown to be effective in the management of postoperative pain in infants and children. Following an extradural injection of 50 µg/kg of morphine, Attia et al. [7] found the plasma C_{max} to be 29 µg/ml at the T_{max} of 10.3 min, which could be compatible with clinical analgesia. However, at 1 h the C_{max} had fallen to less than 10 µg/ml, which could not account for the good degree of analgesia which was noted at that time. They found pharmacokinetic parameters in children between the age of 2 and 15 years similar to those observed in adults.

The effect of the pharmacokinetics of local anaesthetic agents is different than for most other drugs, as these agents are applied directly to the site of their action rather than being transported in the blood stream to this site. Following an epidural injection, the classic biphasic absorption curve is not seen in chil-

Table 1. Intravenous morphine pharmacokinetics

Age	Gestational age	Vd (l/kg)	t 1/2 (h)	Cl (ml/kg/min)	Reference
1 day	26-34 weeks	1.8	8.75	2.4	[3]
1-4 days	36-41 weeks	3.4	6.8	6.3	[4]
11-182 days		2.0	1.15	21.5	[5]
Infants and children		2.8	2.0	23.6	[2]

Table 2. Recommended dosage for morphine infusion [6]

	Dosage (µg/kg/h)
Preterm neonates	2
Term neonates	7
Infants and children	20

dren and, thus, the absorption is much more rapid than in adults. Total plasma concentrations of bupivacaine in neonates are similar to those of older children after a single caudal bolus dose [8]. Due to the relationship $t1/2=(Vd \cdot \ln 2)/C$, any increase in Vd will raise the $t1/2$. Despite an augmented clearance, neonates have an increase in Vd due to their total body water and consequently a longer $t1/2$. This has implications for continuous infusions in small children as there is a change in the local anaesthetic accumulation. The total plasma concentrations of bupivacaine 0.3 mg/kg/h measured during an infusion at 180 min and 300 min were higher in neonates than in children [9]. On the basis of these and other data, Berde [12] has recommended that neonates receive a bolus dose of bupivacaine of no more than 2-2.5 mg/kg and no more than 0.2 mg/kg/h by infusion (Table 3). These empirically derived rates in neonates result in steady-state concentrations of about 1 mg/l and follow age-related total clearance changes.

In conclusion pharmacokinetics data are the theoretical basis of postoperative pain management in children but despite extensive clinical experience knowledge is, again, fragmentary.

Table 3. Pharmacokinetics of epidural bupivacaine [8, 10, 11]

Age	Cl (ml/min/kg)	Vd ss	t1/2 (h)
1-6 months	7.1	3.9	7.7
5-10 years	10	2.7	4.6
Adults	6.3	1	2.7

References

1. Upton RN, Semple TJ, Macintyre PE (1997) Pharmacokinetic optimisation of opioid treatment in acute pain therapy. Clin Pharmacokinet 33:225-244
2. Kart T, Christrup LL, Rasmussen M (1997) Recommended use of morphine in neonates, infants and children based on a literature review. Part 1: Pharmacokinetics. Paediatr Anaesth 7:5-11
3. Hartley R, Green M, Quinn M, Levene MI (1993) Pharmakokinetics of morphine infusion in premature neonates. Arch Dis Child 69:55-58
4. Lynn AM, Slattery JT (1987) Morphine pharmacokinetics in early infancy. Anaesthesiology 66:136-139
5. Olkkola KT, Munuksela EL, Korpela R, Rosemberg PH (1988) Kinetics and dynamics of postoperative intravenous morphine in children. Clin Pharmacol Ther 44:128-136
6. Kart T, Christrup LL, Rasmussen M (1997) Recommended use of morphine in neonates, infants and children based on a literature review. Part 2: Clinical use. Paediatr Anaesth 7:93-101
7. Attia J, Ecoffey C, Sandouk P, Gross JB, Samii K (1986) Epidural morphine in children: pharmacokinetics and CO^2 sensivity. Anaesthesiology 65:590-594
8. Mazoit JX, Denson DO, Samii K (1988) Pharmacokinetics of bupivacaine following caudal anaesthesia in infants. Anaesthesiology 68:387-391
9. Luz G, Innerhofer P, Fishhut B et al (1996) Bupivacaine plasma concentrations during

continuous infusion epidural anaesthesia in infants and children. Anaesth Analg 82:231-234

10. Ecoffey C, Desparmet AM, Maury M et al (1985) Bupivacaine in children: pharmacokinetics following caudal anaesthesia. Anaesthesiology 63:447-448
11. Tucker GT (1986) Pharmacokinetics of local anaesthetics. Br J Anaesth 58:717-731
12. Berde CB (1992) Convulsions associated with pediatric regional anesthesia. Anesth Analg 75:164-166

Chapter 18

Techniques of continuous or intermittent analgesia

G. Ivani, P. De Negri

The International Association for the Study of Pain defined pain as "an unpleasant and emotional experience associated with actual or potential tissue damage, or described in terms of such damage... pain is always subjective. Each individual learns the application of the word through experiences related to injury in early life" [1]. In this form the definiton of pain cannot be applied to living organisms (newborn, infants, small children) incapable of self-report. Consequences of this definition are evident in the clinical care given to neonates and small children: in fact the distress experienced by infants undergoing injuries as a part of medical care is often neglected and undertreated if compared to older children or adults. The hypothesis that the later in gestation the neonate is born the more pain they experience contrasts with neurophysiological evidence, indicating that the ability to experience pain comes early in fetal development [2]. As facial responses and body movements seem to provide the best information about pain sensations [3], what appears to be deficient are the motor mechanisms needed to communicate distress to observers. Moreover, as only recently are preterm babies more likely to survive, the capacity to communicate distress has not yet completely evolved. During the course of a hospital stay, children may experience pain from a variety of sources; pain is often severe in the postoperative period. Some authors studied the incidence of postoperative pain based on child ratings and studied prescription of analgesics and administration: approximately 40% of patients studied reported moderate to severe pain during the operative and first postoperative day even with pain medications and 16% did not receive any analgesics [4]. Children often receive less pain-killing medication than adults undergoing similar surgery [5]; Johnston observed that 57% of patients rated their pain as moderate or severe and half of these patients did not receive any analgesics [6]. These findings indicate that pain in children is often unrecognized and undertreated; children with acute illness are at a greater risk for significant pain than children with chronic illness. Children in pain received less medication than prescribed (often on a pro-re-nata, PRN, basis); lack of medication can occurr because pain has not been assessed,because children may refuse medication or may deny pain for fear of needles, because staff prefer not to administer medications due to disagreement with route or fear of side effects. Sometimes children still feel pain because the prescribed dosage of analgesics is inadequate. Objectives of adequate postoperative analgesia must include pain relief with as few unwanted and undesired side effects as possible, a

satisfactory restoring of vital function, and a reduction of surgical and anaesthetic trauma. Pain management needs to be tailored to location, extent, inva-
siveness of surgical procedure and to expected severity of postoperative pain.
Postoperative pain management is essential and must be approached as an inte-
gral part of perioperative care; it has to be viewed as a process which starts before the surgical incision and continues during anaesthesia until the complete
recovery of the child from the surgical procedure. In choosing a method, various
factors must be considered, including the physician's skill, knowledge of analgesics and routes of administration, patient-related and clinical circumstances,
the availability of an environment supportive of effective pain management, and
the knowledge and skill of staff to assess and monitor patients.

In this paper we will examine postoperative analgesia induced by opioids and
antinflammatory agents not administered by the spinal route.

Opioid analgesia

Opioids are the mainstay of pain management postoperatively in the paediatric
patient; no matter what opioid is used, careful titration and adjustment is usually needed as the patient progresses through the postoperative course.

Inter- and intrapatient variations in the pharmacokinetic and pharmacodynamic behavior of opioids, as well as psychological differences make it impossible to obtain consistent analgesia with intermittent intramuscular injections.
Intravenous administration of opioids can be managed as continuous or intermittent infusion. Intermittent i.v. administration requires accurate titration in
order to achieve an analgesic blood level; boluses infused in a short period of
time have the advantage of frequent observation and assessment of pain.The
major disadvantage of this technique is the need to use relatively large dose of
opioids in order to avoid the necessity of frequent boluses: the blood levels of
drug will be relatively high after the dose and relatively low immediately before
the successive dose, exposing the patient to side effects of high opioid concentration and pain associated with low level of drug. Constant infusion of opioid
prevents the ups and downs of intermittent dosing; when used in conjunction
with intermittent doses or rescue doses, constant infusions produce relatively
stable blood analgesic levels.

In 1983, Bray studied 20 children undergoing major surgery and observed
that the group that received i.v. bolus of morphine 200 µg kg^{-1} followed by a
continuous infusion of 20 µg kg^{-1} h^{-1} showed lower pain scores than the group
receiving i.m. morphine 200 µg kg^{-1} q 4 h PRN [7]. Hendrickson compared 26
children receiveing i.v. morphine infusions 10-40 µg kg^{-1} h^{-1} with 20 children
receiving i.m. morphine 100 µg kg^{-1} q 3 h; pain scores were higher in the i.m.
group [8]. Koren gave morphine infusion to newborns, observing a large interpatient variability in plasma concentrations, elimination half-life and clearance;
he recommended a maximum infusion rate of 15 µg kg^{-1} h^{-1}[9]. Olkkola felt
that the pharmacokinetic profile of morphine reached that of on older child or

adult by 1 or 2 months of age [10]. Kupferberger, studying newborn rats, suggested that an incompletely developed blood-brain barrier allowed greater penetration of morphine to the infant brain: the findings may not be applicable to human neonates because the blood-brain barrier in the newborn rat is relatively incompleted if compared with higher mammals [11]. Lynn found that infants with a normal cardiovascular system undergoing surgery clear morphine more efficiently than infants of the same age undergoing cardiac surgery; morphine clearance from the body is slow in newborns but increases to reach adult values in the first months of life. This maturation occurs more quickly in infants undergoing noncardiac surgery (by 1-3 months of age) than in those receiving morphine after cardiac surgery (by 6-12 months of age) [12]. Wolf suggested in children under 4 years undergoing major abdominal surgery, after a loading dose of 0.15 mg kg^{-1}, a continuous i.v. infusion of morphine 5 µg kg^{-1} h^{-1} for patients <10 kg and 10 µg kg^{-1} h^{-1} for patients >10 kg [13]. It would seem safe to use continuous opioid infusions in children over 6 months of age on paediatric wards, with hourly monitoring of vital signs, level of consciousness and pain scores.

Another interesting way to administer opiods is representd by the use of patient-controlled analgesia (PCA); the first report of PCA use in a paediatric patient was in 1987 [14]. PCA is now used in children as young as 5 years for the treatment of postoperative pain; a typical program uses a bolus of morphine of 10-20 µg kg^{-1} h^{-1} with a lockout period of 10 min. PCA has been used with or without a continuous background infusion. Some authors found in adults that background infusions did not improve pain scores or the number of demands by the patients, nor decrease the number of patients who had difficulty in sleeping due to pain [15, 16]. One study in children found an improvement in analgesia without an increase in side effects with a background infusion of morphine 15 µg kg^{-1} h^{-1} [17]; another study found that a background infusion of morphine did not improve pain scores but was associated with a better sleep pattern [18]. Doyle found that the use of background infusion of morphine 4 µg kg^{-1} h^{-1} in a PCA regimen for children after lower abdominal surgery caused no increase in side effects if compared with no background infusion and was associated with less hypoxemia and a better sleep pattern. The reason why a background infusion of 4 µg kg^{-1} h^{-1} of morphine gave less hypoxemia may be that the infusion produces better analgesia and improves ventilation [19]. It is useful to monitor arterial oxygen saturation in children receiving PCA; studies revealed that children normally have periods of saturation between 90% and 95% during sleep. An SpO$_2$ of 94% indicates mild hypoxemia; some authors reported that a more common reason for hypoxemia is pain and not opioid overdosage [19]. In another study, Doyle found that the use of a background infusion of morphine 20 µg kg^{-1} h^{-1} in a PCA regimen for children who have abdominal surgery caused a significant increase in morphine consumption without improving pain relief and a significant increase of respiratory depression, oversedation and nausea and vomiting; however, there was no increase of side effects with the duration of PCA use as the severity of postoperative pain declined. The author observed in

15% of cases an SpO_2 <94% but he stated that there is no information on the incidence of hypoxemia detected by pulse oximetry in children breathing air and given i.m. opioids [20]. Broadmann found that children using PCA received twice as much narcotic as those undergoing similar operations and receiving intermittent i.m. injections, underscoring the inadequacy of the tradtional management of postoperative pain in children [21]. McNeely found that the use of a nightime infusion of morphine in a group of 36 school-age children, whose oxygen saturation has been recorded continuously for the duration of PCA use, did not appear to offer any advantage over the use of PCA alone [22]. Considerable preparation is needed in order to establish a PCA program; candidates for PCA are children at least 5 years of age undegoing major surgical procedures.

It is stated frequently that the major reason for avoiding i.m. administration of opioids is the associated pain of injection; the use of a rectal route of administration had a fatal outcome as a result of inappropriate alternative prescription [23]. Rectal route is questionable because of the unpredictable blood levels achieved as a result of the variable absorption through the systemic and biliary venous system.

An interesting alternative route for morphine infusion is represented by subcutaneous (s.c.) route. A cannula can be placed s.c. at the time of anaesthesia, covered with a sterile dressing and flushed with heparinized saline in the postoperative period [24]; the cannula can be used for administration of morphine or a different drug as the sole method of providing analgesia or to supplement other techniques. Moreover, the s.c. route is particularly useful in patients whose veins are at a premium, such as those with burns or chronic and terminal pain. Lloyd Thomas suggested that the dosage of morphine administered by a continuous s.c. infusion should not differ much from on i.v. regimen [25]. Continuous infusion of morphine would appear to be superior to intermittent injections because a small volume of morphine is injected over a short period of time and breakthrough pain, the main drawback of "à la demande" analgesia, is avoided. Lloyd Thomas suggested that a dosage of s.c. morphine 20 $\mu g \ kg^{-1} \ h^{-1}$ is sufficient to prevent pain caused by major surgery [23]. McNicol underlined the safe use of continuous s.c. infusion of morphine, observing a reduction in consumption in the first 24 h if compared with other authors using PCA systems and suggested that s.c. delivery may also be possible if pulse oximetry is not available [26, 27]. The same PCA can be used by s.c. cannula.

Doyle used a PCA device through a 22-gauge catheter sited over the deltoid muscle. Patients received bolus doses of 20 $\mu g \ kg^{-1}$ with a lockout interval of 5 min and a background infusion of 5 $\mu g \ kg^{-1} \ h^{-1}$. PCA s.c. seemed to be as effective and safe for acute postoperative pain as PCA i.v.; there was a lower consumption of morphine with reduced hypoxic episodes if compared with PCA i.v. It may be that the reduced consumption of opioids determines ventilatory depression; as an alternative, the s.c. route should be safer because delivery of morphine is slower and can cause lower peak concentrations in case of morphine boluses. The delay for patients in receiving analgesia by the s.c. route was on the order of a few minutes [28]. Semple used a continuous s.c. infusion of diamorphine 20 μg kg^{-1} h^{-1}; he underlined the benefit of a continuous s.c. infusion over intermittent s.c. administration because, in the latter case, periods of unrelieved pain alternating with episodes of sedation or nausea due to high plasma concentration of opioid after bolus can occur [29].

Nonopioid analgesia

Nonopioid analgesics have an increasing role in the management of postoperative pain. Of particular importance are the nonsteroidal anti-inflammatory drugs (NSAIDs). With a direct action on the local mediators of inflammation and a possible role in the reduction of the systemic response to surgery, NSAIDs appear to be an useful addition in the treatment of postoperative pain. The same analgesics used in adults can be safely used in children after the newborn period; for successful treatment in paediatrics it is mandatory to pay attention to drug administration, correct dose and timing and the choice of drug. The oral route is preferable whenever possible but in the immediate postoperative period of major surgery, gastric stasis has been commonly observed, making oral administration ineffective. Moreover, the onset of analgesia after oral administration is too slow to obtain adequate and rapid pain relief. So, oral administration is better used for mild to moderate postoperative pain (minor surgery) when gastric stasis is no longer a problem. Rectal administration is widely used, particularly for young children, because it is considered a better choice than injection even if this route, as discussed above, is questionable. Oral or rectal drugs must be administered well in advance because the analgesic effects of NSAIDs are reached slowly, also if the drug is given by i.v. route. The intramuscular route does not offer particular advantages regarding bioavailability, nor a better or faster analgesic effect. The margin of safety of NSAIDs is wide and the individual variations as with opioid analgesics have not been observed. Except during the neonatal period, the pharmacokinetic and pharmacodynamics of NSAIDs in children do not seem to differ markedly from those in adults.

Analgesia based on regular oral/rectal administration or continuous i.v. infusions improves the postoperative period in children if compared with the ups and downs of PRN medication. Use of NSAIDs in conjunction with an opioid allows a reduction of dosage and of side effects of the latter.

NSAIDs have to be considered as first-line agents in the treatment of paediatric pain. In children undergoing adenotonsillectomy, the largest group studied for postoperative pain, NSAIDs are able to reduce pain without having any particular effect on bleeding [30]. Ketoprophen 0.5 mg kg^{-1} i.v. provided good analgesia with fewer adverse effects in a group of 107 children between 1-7 years after adenoidectomy [31]. Diclofenac sodium was effective when administered prophylactically via the oral or rectal route for pain treatment after tonsillectomy [30, 32]. Continuous infusion of indomethacin (bolus 0.35 mg+1.7 mg kg^{-1} day^{-1}) or rectal ibuprofen (40 mg kg^{-1} day^{-1}) resulted in adequate analgesia, reducing the need for additional opioid [33]. Acetaminophen (paracetamol) with codeine administered in the preoperative period demonstrated a superior efficacy if compared with acetaminophen alone after bilateral myringotomy with placement of PE tubes [34].

In the same procedure preoperative administration of oral acetaminophen is more effective [35]. Bennie suggested that neither preoperative oral acetaminophen 15 mg kg^{-1} nor ibuprofen 10 mg kg^{-1} is effective in providing analgesia in children undergoing myringotomy [36]. Romsig said that recommended doses of acetaminophen (60 mg kg^{-1} day^{-1} orally or 90 mg kg^{-1} day^{-1} rectally) do not provide sufficient pain relief in children following tonsillectomy [37]. Anderson found that a plasma acetaminophen concentration of 25 mg/l^{-1}, corresponding to a satisfactory analgesia for 65% of patients after tonsillectomy, can be achieved after a loading dose of 70 µg kg^{-1} and a maintenance dose of 50 mg kg^{-1} every 8 h; doses over 150 mg kg^{-1} day^{-1} must be avoided due to liver toxicity [38]. Maunuksela administered ibuprofen 40 mg kg^{-1} divided in three or four doses rectally; he found that scheduled administration of ibuprofen decreases the need of opioid analgesic, improving pain relief during recovery, and did not cause additional side effects such as bleeding [39].

The recommended i.v. dosage of ketorolac in children is 0.5 mg/kg, followed either by bolus injections of 1.0 mg/kg every 6 h or an i.v. infusion of 0.17 mg kg^{-1} h^{-1}. The maximum daily dosage is 90 mg, and the maximum duration of treatment is 48 h. The recommended oral dosage is 0.25 mg/kg to a maximum of 1.0 mg/kg/day, with a maximum duration of 7 days. Older children may require somewhat lower dosages, while infants and young children may require slightly higher dosages to achieve the same level of pain relief. Ketorolac is not recommended for use in infants aged <1 year.

Ketorolac demonstrated efficacy when used for postoperative pain management; the i.v. route is preferred during the immediate postoperative period (particularly when additional respiratory depression or sedation is not desired), until the patient can tolerate oral medication.

Intramuscular injections are not recommended in children, unless the intravenous route is unavailable. There are pharmacokinetic differences, but the dosage interval is similar in children and adults. Pharmacokinetics studies in children indicate that, because of the greater volume of distribution and the plasma clearance of drug, a higher relative dosage per weight may be required in children [40]. The recommended i.v. dosage of ketorolac in children is 0.5 mg/kg, followed either by bolus injections of 1.0 mg/kg every 6 h or an i.v. infusion of 0.17 mg kg^{-1} h^{-1}. The maximum daily dosage is 90 mg, and the maximum duration of treatment is 48 h. The recommended oral dosage is 0.25 mg/kg to a maximum of 1.0 mg/kg/day, with a maximum duration of 7 days. Older children may require somewhat lower dosages, while infants and young children may require slightly higher dosages to achieve the same level of pain relief. Ketorolac is not recommended for use in infants aged <1 year [41]. Watcha demonstrated, in children undergoing elective surgery, that an intraoperative dose of ketorolac 0.9 mg kg^{-1} i.v. provided postoperative analgesia similar to that of morphine 0.1 mg kg^{-1} and that ketorlac was associated with less emesis.

He suggested that ketorolac may have a "ceiling" effect and that doses between 0.5 and 0.9 mg kg^{-1} may produce a similar degree of pain relief [42]. Munro showed that ketorolac 0.75 mg kg^{-1} provides analgesia comparable with that of morphine 0.1 mg kg^{-1} [43].

In summary, ketorolac in children undergoing myringotomy, hernia repair, tonsillectomy, or other surgery associated with mild or moderate pain provides comparable analgesia to morphine, pethidine or acetaminophen. Combined therapy with ketorolac and an opiod results in reduction of opioid requirements and, in some patients, this is accompanied by a concomitant decrease in opioid-induced adverse effects, a more rapid return of gastrointestinal function and a shorter stay in hospital [44]. Bleeding time is usually slightly increased, but in most patients it remains within normal values. There is conflicting evidence of the potential for increased surgical-site bleeding after tonsillectomy but, for other types of paediatric surgery, numerous clinical studies have confirmed that ketorolac is not associated with increased bleeding.

Propacetamol hydrochloride, a water-soluble formulation of paracetamol attached to a molecule of dietylglycine, is in fact a prodrug of paracetamol. When it reaches the plasma it is cleaved either spontaneously or by nonspecific plasma esterases. One gram of propacetamol releases 0.5 g of paracetamol. Propacetamol is a useful analgesic that can be administered after surgery with a faster onset and a better analgesic efficacy than oral administration. Pharmacokinetics of paracetamol in infants and children after infusion of propacetamol (15 mg kg^{-1} in single or repeated doses or 30 mg kg^{-1} in single doses) is similar to that described for adults; it is different in neonates where a lower clearance level has been observed due to both hepatic immaturity and slow renal excretion [45, 46]. For these reasons the dose of propacetamol should be adapted only on a weight basis. Granry demonstrated the analgesic efficacy of proparacetamol 30 mg kg^{-1} i.v. in children 6-12 years old undergoing orthopedic surgery [47].

In conclusion, we have now the key to control pain in children. There are drugs, devices and techniques sufficiently safe to work with and it is up to us to make pain therapy in paediatrics real and effective.

References

1. Merskey H (1991) The definition of pain. Eur J Psychiatry, 6:153-159
2. Anand KJS, Hickey PR (1987) Pain and its effects in the human neonate and fetus. New Engl J Med 317:1321-1329
3. Craig KD (1997) The facial display of pain in infants and children. In GA Finley and PJ McGrath (eds), Measurements of pain in infants and children. IASPPress, Seattle
4. Mather L, Mackie J (1983) The incidence of postoperative pain in children. Pain 15:271-282
5. Beyer JE, de Good DE et al (1982) Patterns of postoperative analgesia use with adults and children following cardiac surgery. Pain 17:71-81
6. Johnston CC, Abbott FV et al (1992) A survey of pain in hospitalised patients aged 4-14 years. Clin J Pain 8:54-163

7. Bray RJ (1983) Postoperative analgesia provided by morphine infusion in children. Anaesthesia 38:1075-1078
8. Hendrickson M, Myre L et al (1987) Postoperative analgesia in children: a prospective study of intermittent intramuscular injection vs continuous intravenous infusion of morphine. J Pediatr Surg 22:264-266
9. Koren G, Butt W et al (1985) Postoperative morphine infusion in newborn infants :assessment of disposition characteristics and safety. J Pediatrics 107:963-967
10. Olkkola KT, Maunuksela EL et al (1988) Kintics and dynamics of postoperative morphine in children. Clin Pharmacol Ther 44:128-136
11. Kupferberger HJ, Way EL (1963) Pharmacologic basis for the increased sensitivity of the newborn rat to morphine. J Pharmacol Exp Ther 141:105-112
12. Lynn A, Nespeca MK et al (1998) Clearance of morphine in postoperative infants during intravenous infusion: the influence of age and surgery. Anesth Analg 86:958-963
13. Wolf AR, Hughes D (1993) Pain relief for infants undergoing abdominal surgery: comparison of infusions of iv morphine and extradural bupivacaine. BJA 70:10-16
14. Brown RE, Broadmann LM (1987) Patient controlled analgesia for postoperative pain control in adolescents. Anesth Analg 66:S22
15. Owen H, Szekely SM et al (1989) Variables of PCA Concurrent infusion Anaesthesia 44:11-13
16. Wu MYC, Purcell GJ (1990) PCA - the value of a background infusion. Anaesth Int Care 18:575-576
17. Berde CB, Lehn BM et al (1991) PCA in children and adolescents: a randomised prospective comparison with intramuscular administration of morphine for postoperative analgesia. J Pediatrics 118:460-466
18. Skues MA, Watson DM et al (1993) PCA in children. A comparison of two infusion techniques. Ped Anesth 3:223-228
19. Doyle E, Harper I et al (1993) PCA with low dose background infusions after lower abdominal surgery in children. BJA 71:818-822
20. Doyle E, Robinson D et al (1993) Comparison of PCA with and without a background infusion after lower abdominal surgery in children. BJA 71:670-673
21. Broadmann L, Vaughan M et al (1989) PCA provides more effective pain control following pectus excavatuum repair in children than does conventional narcotic therapy. Can J Anesth 36:S96
22. McNeely JK, Trentadue NC (1997) Comparison of PCA with and without nighttime morphine infusion following lower extremity surgery in children. J Pain Sympton Manage 13:268-273
23. Gourlay GK, Boas RA (1992) Fatal outcome with use of rectal morphine for postoperative pain control in infant. BMJ 304:766-767
24. Lavies NG, Wandless JG (1989) Subcutaneous morphine in children: taking the sting out of postoperative analgesia. Anaesth 44:1000-1001
25. Lloyd Thomas AR (1990) Pain management in pediatric patients. BJA 64:85-104
26. McNicol R (1993) Postoperative analgesia in children using contnuous sc morphine. BJA 71:752-756
27. Irwin M, Gillespie JA et al (1992) Evaluation of a disposable PCA device in children. BJA 68:411-413
28. Doyle E, Morton NS et al (1994) Comparison of PCA in children by iv and sc routes of administration. BJA 72:533-536
29. Semple D, Alridge LA et al (1996) Comparison of iv and sc diamorphine infusion for the treatment of acute pain in children. BJA 76:310-312

30.   Walters CH, Patterson CC et al (1988) Diclofenac sodium for the post tonsillectomy pain in children. Anaesthesia 43:641-643, 1988
31.   Nikanne E, Kokki H et al (1997) Comparison of perioperative ketoprofen 2.0 mg kg-1 with 0.5 mg kg-1 iv in small children during adenoidectomy. BJA 79:606-608
32.   Bone ME, Fell D (1988) A comparison of rectal diclofenac with im papaveretum or placebo for pain relief after tonsillectomy. Anaesthesia 43:277-280
33.   Maunuksela EL, Okkola KT et al (1988) Does prophylactic intravenous infusion of indomethacin improve the management of postoperative pain in children? Can J Anaesth 35:123-127
34.   Tobias J, Lowe S et al (1995) Analgesia after bilateral myringotomy and placement of PE tubes in children: acetaminophen vs. acetaminophen with codeine. Anesth Analg 81:496-500
35.   Verghese S, Davis R et al Acetaminophen treatment for pain relief in pediatricpatients undergoing myringotomy and tube placement: oral vs. rectal. Anesthesiology 81:A1363
36.   Bennie R , Dierdorf S et al (1995) Prophylactic oral acetaminophen or ibuprofen are not effective for postoperative pain relief in children undergoing myringotomy. Anesth Analg 80:S40
37.   Romsig J, Hertel S, et al (1998) Examination of acetaminophen for outpatients management of postoperative pain in children. Paediatr Anaesth 8:235-239
38.   Anderson BJ, Holford NH (1997) Rectal paracetamol dosing regimens: determination by computer simulation. Paediatr Anaesth 7:451-455
39.   Maunuksela EL, Ryhanen P et al (1992) Efficay of rectal ibuprofen in controlling postoperative pain in children. Can J Anaesth 39:226-230
40.   Olkkola KT, Maunuksela EL (1991) The pharamcokinetics of postoperative intravenous ketorolac tromethamine in children. Br J Clin Pharmacol 31:182-184
41.   Forrest JB, Heitlinger EL et al (1997) Ketorolac for postoperative pain management in children Drug Saf 16:309-329
42.   Watcha MF, Jones MB et al (1992) Comparison of ketorolac and morphine as adjuvants during pediatric surgery. Anesthesiology 76:368-372
43.   Munro HM, Riegger LQ et al (1994) Comparison of the analgesic and emetic properties of ketorlac and morphine for pediatric outpatient strabism surgery. BJA 72:624-628
44.   Gillis JC, Brodgen RN (1997) Ketorolac, a reppraisal of its pharmacodynamic and pharmacokinetic properties and therapeutic use in pain management. Drugs 53:139-188
45.   Granry JC, Rod B et al (1992) Pharmacokinetics and antipyretics effects of an injectable prodrug of paracetamol in childre. Paed. Anaesth. 2:291-295
46.   Autret E, Dutertre JP et al (1993) Pharmacokinetics of paracetamol in the neonate and infant after administration of propacetamol chlorydrate. Dev Pharmacol Ther 20:129-134
47.   Granry JC, Monrigal JP et al (1997) The analgesic efficacy of an injectable prodrug of acetaminophen in children after orthopaedic surgery. Paediatr Anaesth 7:445-449.

Chapter 19

Sedation and acute pain management: association/combinations of drugs

A.R. WOLF

In recent years there has been an increasing understanding that combinations of drugs, acting at different effector sites, can provide higher-quality analgesia or sedation than single drugs acting alone. This concept of co-analgesia has become routine practice in paediatric postoperative analgesia, and has proved to be highly effective. The combined action of the different drugs allows individual drug dosing to be reduced, thereby minimising side effects while maintaining adequate analgesia. Analgesic agents can also be combined in mixtures (such as in the epidural space) which can alter efficacy and duration of the technique, and this, too, has been a recent development in paediatric anaesthetic practice. However, all drugs have side effects, and each time a new drug is added, it brings with it an increasing possibility of drug interactions. Therefore, while drug combinations are undoubtedly beneficial, the clinician must have detailed knowledge of the pharmacology and interactions of the drugs used.

At the outset it should be made clear that analgesia and analgesic techniques pertain to pain relief, while sedation and sedative techniques are directed at lowering conscious levels or reducing responses to discomfort. These two techniques should be regarded as independent, although in appropriate clinical situations both analgesia and sedation may be required together. Clear distinctions between different types of pain or discomfort are therefore needed for the clinician to make an informed and rational approach to therapy. The four main areas of pain to be treated are described as follows.

1. Point pain: the pain associated with a brief procedure which may be painful, such as heel prick drip or drain insertion or dressing change.
2. Postoperative pain: this may vary from minor somatic pain from procedures such as hernia repair to major somatic and visceral pain associated with major thoracic or abdominal surgery. The pain from major surgery may continue for several days or longer.
3. Discomfort: patients on the intensive care unit that are confined to bed often with endotracheal tubes, drains etc. These patients initially may have postoperative pain from surgery but with time pain becomes less of a feature compared to chronic discomfort. In addition, critically ill children often do not understand their situation and may struggle in attempt to remove the causes of their discomfort (drips drains, nasogastric tubes, etc.). These children may require sedation rather than analgesia, together with complementary non-pharmacological coping strategies.

4. Chronic pain syndromes: true chronic pain in children is rare but well recognised in practice. Discussion of combined treatment for this highly specialised area is outside the scope of this text.

These broad definitions of pain and discomfort are influenced by age, and therapy must be chosen accordingly. For example postoperative pain in the newborn infant after abdominal surgery can be managed by a pure, nonsedative technique such as that provided by epidural local analgesia combined with oral or rectal paracetamol [1], avoiding complications associated with systemic opioid analgesia such as oversedation, ventilatory depression and gastrointestinal disturbance [2]. In contrast, a 3-year-old having similar surgery rarely manages well with this approach, even when the analgesia is complete. This is due to the additional emotional component of the child's situation (fear, anger, and unhappiness), which results in the child becoming agitated, restless and often unmanageable in the postoperative period unless additional sedation is given.

Clearly, specific individual approaches are needed for pain management and sedation, using knowledge of both the therapeutic effects and side effects of the drugs and situation age and environment in which they are to be used. Pharmacokinetic and pharmacodynamic properties change considerably with age and this needs to be taken into account. This article will review the properties and uses of the available drugs and discuss a rational approach to the use of particular combinations of drugs in both postoperative pain management and in the paediatric intensive care unit (PICU).

Drugs and techniques available for analgesia and sedation

Drug options can be broadly divided into five areas (Table 1).

The requirements and the end points for adequate sedation or analgesia are very different. Clearly, great care is therefore needed in selection of the appropriate group of drugs for the task required. Before discussing combinations of drug groups, it is useful to point out specific features of some of the drugs (from Table 1).

Group 1: analgesic drugs

This group contains analgesic drugs varying from high efficacy (opioids) to relatively low efficacy (paracetamol). Opioids provide dose-dependent analgesia but higher doses of opioids are associated with an increasing risk of serious side effects. In contrast, local anaesthetic drugs offer the potential for absolute analgesia without dose-dependent side effects.

Opioids

Morphine is a water-soluble opioid with useful sedative properties. Neonates are highly sensitive to morphine due to an overall sensitivity to all CNS depres-

Table 1. Drugs and techniques available for analgesia and sedation

Systemic analgesic drugs	Opioids: morphine, fentanyl, alfentanil, remifentanil, ketamine Paracetamol, propacetamol NSAIDS: ketorolac, diclofenac α-2 agonists- clonidine, dexmetatomidine tramadol
Hypnotic/anaesthestic drugs	Benzodiazepines: midazolam, diazepam, lorazepam Chloral hydrate, trichlofos Propofol Barbiturates: phenobarbitone, pentobarbitone
Other sedative agents	Neuroleptics: phenothiazines, butyrophenones Antihistamines: trimeprazine, promethazine Anticholinergics: hyoscine
Local techniques	Local anaesthesia: topical, regional, epidural, spinal Central local anaesthesia block with admixtures: adrenaline/opioids/clonidine/ketamine
Nonpharmacological strategies	Massage, sucrose pacifiers, complementary medicine

sant drugs and their increased blood brain barrier permeability. Elimination half-lives in the neonate are over 12 h compared to 3 h or less in the older child [3]. Elimination of the drug in the neonatal period is initially poor due to limitations of liver conjugation. The kidney's limited ability to excrete the active morphine 6-glucuronide may also prolong analgesic action [4].

Fentanyl has a rapid and profound onset in the infant due to the drug's high fat solubility and its distribution kinetics in this age group [5]. After short-term infusion, this drug has a rapid offset due to its favourable context-sensitive half-life. Longer-term infusions are associated with slow offset once the peripheral compartments have been saturated. The elimination half-life is about 3 h in the older child but it can be greater than 17 h in the preterm infant [6]. Tolerance to the drug increases rapidly when given as an infusion due to both pharmacokinetic and pharmacodynamic effects [7, 8].

Remifentanil is a relatively new drug with predictable and rapid offset that is independent of duration of infusion. In the limited studies in children so far it appears to be a very promising drug that may allow profound analgesia with haemodynamic stability during surgery, and rapid offset without ventilatory depression after surgery. This drug is potentially ideal for neonatal use provided local analgesia has been instituted before the end of surgery to ensure continuity of analgesia.

Ketamine

Ketamine is a phencyclidine derivative with NMDA antagonist properties. It is one of the few analgesic drugs that can increase blood pressure and has therefore

found use as an analgesic/induction agent in patients with circulatory insufficiency. Ketamine inhibits re-uptake of catecholamines at the nerve terminal,
thereby increasing levels of catecholamines. While it is grouped with the analgesic drugs, it can be regarded as an anaesthetic agent in that bolus doses or high
levels of infusion can produce unconsciousness as well as analgesia. It has become popular as an analgesic/anaesthetic agent in the PICU for treatment of severely asthmatic patients because of its bronchodilating properties. Side effects
include raised intracranial/ocular pressure and hallucinations.

Clonidine

Clonidine is a centrally acting α-2 agonist acting presynaptically at noradrener-
gic sites in the locus coeruleus and dorsal horn neurones. It can provide analgesia and, like morphine, has a sedative profile. It can reduce haemodynamic hor-
monal and metabolic responses to surgery and has been used as a sedative in the
critically ill neurologic patient [9]. Its use to date in paediatrics has been as an
adjunct in caudal anaesthesia and to ease the withdrawal from morphine in the
intensive care unit.

Group 2: hypnotic/anaesthetic drugs

Drugs in this group comprise agents used for premedication or those used for
intravenous anaesthesia. They have the common property of lowering levels of
consciousness and this can be useful both in the agitated child after surgery or as
a sedative agent in the intensive care unit. The heterogeneous nature of this
group results in the drug's having useful additional properties. For example, the
memory loss associated with benzodiazepines or the reduction in cerebral metabolism associated with high dose thiopentone and propofol.

Benzodiazepines

These drugs do not provide analgesia but are useful for single-dose administration in the agitated child. The use of midazolam as a single-agent infusion at
doses of up to 300 µg/kg/per hour for sedation of the critically ill infant has been
associated with tolerance and a prolonged and sometimes severe withdrawal reaction. It is the view of the author that midazolam should only be used for sedation in combination with other agents and should rarely be used at doses exceeding 100 µg/kg/per hour. Lorazepam has particularly powerful amnestic
properties with a long duration of action. It has proved to be a useful drug for
short-term intermittent use in the PICU.

Propofol

Propofol has returned as a popular drug for short-term sedation or anaesthesia
in the PICU. Initial reports of deaths from this agent appear to be associated

with the excessive dosage [10]. Resistance to the drug after long-term infusion can make it impossible to use as a single agent and prolonged recovery and withdrawal phenomena can be problematic. Its use on intensive care units as part of a cohesive sedation protocol is discussed below.

Barbiturates

Thiopentone infusions are used in combination with anti-epileptics to treat status epilepticus or to render the EEG isoelectric after head injury or during cardiac surgery. The long elimination half-life of the drug can result in delayed return of consciousness, which can take many days, and may mask the underlying neurological damage. Unfortunately, thiopentone also has significant major effects on immune function. Children receiving high-dose infusions of thiopentone are at major risk of sepsis.

Group 3: other sedative agents

Unlike the group 2 drugs, these agents do not provide anaesthesia and unconsciousness. Their main role is as additional drugs to be used in combination with group1 or group 2 agents. Phenothiazines such as chlorpromazine can be an invaluable agent in the long-term PICU patient that has become tolerant to a variety of analgesic and sedative drugs. Butyrophenones such as droperidol can produce severe dysphoric states unless combined with a benzodiazepine. There are particularly likely to produce dystonic reactions (orofacial dyskinesia, akathesia) in children

Group 4: local anaesthesia

The major advantage in choosing local anaesthesia is its potential to provide complete analgesia without CNS depression. This makes it valuable for children in whom reduction in consciousness is likely to be associated with adverse events (apnoea, ventilatory depression). Appropriate local blocks or epidural techniques are therefore useful in neonates and children with head injuries. Specific examples include the use of spinal anaesthesia for hernia repair in the ex-premature neonate prone to ventilatory depression or the use of femoral nerve blockade in children with reduced consciousness and fractured femoral shaft. The other advantages of local techniques for analgesia include improved pulmonary function, reductions in intraoperative blood loss, postoperative catabolism, and the incidence of postoperative venous thrombosis.

While bupivacaine and lignocaine have provided the mainstay of local anaesthetic agents, new drugs such as ropivacaine and l-bupivacaine with improved therapeutic ratios and analgesic profiles are now becoming available. The use of drug combinations with local anaesthetics is discussed below.

Group 5: nonpharmacological strategies

This group contains techniques that are often dismissed, ignored or taken for granted. However, they have a major place as an adjunct to pain relief and sedation. Simple examples include parental presence, which can be effective in calming an otherwise inconsolable child. Massage has been shown to reduce haemodynamic and stress responses in the ventilated preterm neonate [11] and may even improve outcome [12].

Studies in the human neonate have shown a dose-dependent effect of sucrose in reducing behavioural and heart rate responses to pain [13], although other work has shown that the cardiovascular and stress responses are not reduced [14]. Comforting procedures alter behavioural responses to pain but cannot be regarded as analgesic drugs. They should be viewed as coping strategies which can modulate "pain experience" rather than true analgesics.

Drug combinations in postoperative analgesia

The underlying principles in drug combinations are to maximise analgesia, reduce individual side effects and to select agents that deliver adequate duration of analgesia. The choice of drug combination is dependent on the operation, the age of the patient and the environment (i.e., day care surgery, general hospital ward, high dependency unit). Below are examples of how drug combinations can be selected in this fashion.

Neonate

Neonates are highly susceptible to CNS depressant drugs. A better understanding of opioid pharmacokinetics and pharmacodynamics has made the use of these drugs far safer in the postoperative period in recent years [15]. Opioids delivered by continuous intravenous infusion or nurse-controlled analgesia in this age group can be used in the spontaneously breathing neonate in an appropriate environment (intensive care unit or high dependency unit). Local techniques such as caudal, epidural or spinal analgesia are highly effective in this age group. Complete analgesia is obtainable with pure local anaesthetic agents for central blocks. The use of combinations of local anaesthesia with admixtures such as fentanyl are not necessary and are relatively contraindicated. Paracetamol is an invaluable adjunct to neonatal analgesia and should be given on a regular rather than on an as required basis to obtain the maximum value.

Tonsillectomy

With the advent of day case tonsillectomy it has been necessary to re-evaluate analgesia strategies for tonsillectomy. Morphine reduces pain and provides sedation but results in a high incidence of nausea and vomiting after surgery. The potency of nonsteroid anti-inflammatory drugs (NSAIDs) such as ketorolac and diclofenac are not enough to provide adequate analgesia in the immediate post-operative period. However, the combination of regular paracetamol before and after surgery, a single dose of fentanyl during surgery and regular intraoperative and postoperative diclofenac has allowed analgesia to be maintained without major sedation or vomiting. NSAIDs potentially can increase the risk of bleeding but this does not appear to be significant in clinical practice. A large proportion of children coming for tonsillectomy have asthma, and the use of these drugs in true asthmatics remains controversial.

Orchidopexy

Caudal analgesia with local anaesthetic agents alone do not provide adequate analgesia. The height of the block may be insufficient, given that failure of the immediate block and the pain from this surgery usually outlasts the duration of a single shot caudal block (6-8 h). Combinations of a single intravenous dose morphine at the time of surgery and regular paracetamol and diclofenac afterwards can greatly improve analgesia but at the expense of a high incidence of nausea and vomiting. This can result in overnight hospital admission. The use of admixture of clonidine or ketamine can increase efficacy and duration of analgesia for this procedure (Fig. 1) [16].

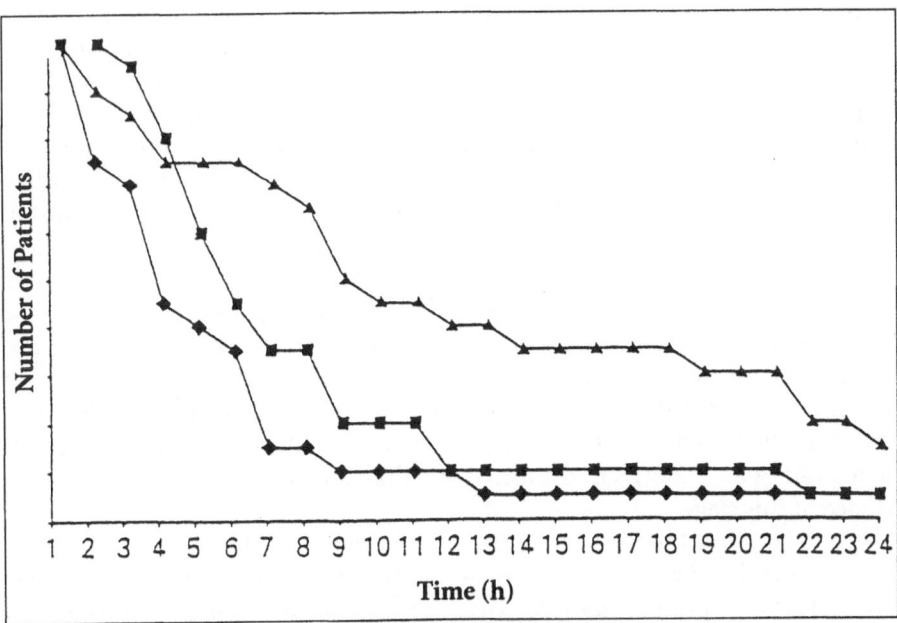

Fig. 1. Duration of caudal analgesia after orchidopexy using: bupivacaine and adrenaline (◆), bupivacaine and clonidine (■), bupivacaine and ketamine (▲)

Agent choices for epidural techniques

The choice of which opioid to add to a local anaesthetic agent depends on whether a single-shot technique or a continuous infusion are to be used. Morphine is a water-soluble agent that has a long half-life in the CSF. These properties result in its long duration of action (up to 24 h) after single injection and therefore makes it a useful drug in this context [17]. Because of its solubility in CSF it spreads to provide analgesia in a non-segmental fashion and therefore caudal administration can provide analgesia even after thoracic surgery. However this same property allows the drug to migrate rostrally to give sudden ventilatory depression. Fat-soluble opioids such as fentanyl are not rational choices for single-dose epidurals. These drugs are rapidly absorbed from the epidural space, making their duration of action short. Combinations of local analgesia and fat-soluble opioids such as fentanyl provide excellent analgesia when given by continuous infusion. Drug is delivered continually to the epidural space, where it can diffuse across the dura mater and CSF into the substantia gelatinosa. While fentanyl does produce specific spinal analgesia, most of the drug eventually becomes systemically absorbed to produce general analgesia and sedation.

Drug combinations in intensive care sedation

Sedation and analgesia in the intensive care unit require a clear understanding of the goals required (the patients'optimum level of sedation), the tools available (which drugs) and a technique for evaluating levels of sedation/comfort (pain/sedation scores). Oversedation delays extubation, promotes lung atelectasia after extubation (increasing the risks of reintubation), promotes tolerance and withdrawal, and results in increased side effects from the ever-increasing doses of drugs. In contrast, undersedation allows discomfort and pain, increases haemodymamic and stress responses and may, in the post-operative cardiac patient, result in pulmonary hypertensive crises. For a patient arriving in the PICU after surgery, high levels of analgesia are required initially for postoperative pain relief or reduction of stress responses to surgery. Immediately after surgery a neonate will not require more than 20 µg/kg/per hour morphine for analgesia and a child will not require more than 40 µg/kg/per hour. These are doses based on observational behavioural data in the awake, spontaneously breathing patient. Later in the postoperative course, if the patient remains ventilated on PICU, sedation may be required to relieve the discomfort of lying still or tolerating an endotracheal tube. Large doses of opioids are unlikely to be needed at this stage.

It is clear from the literature that, when using a sedative/anaesthetic drug, there are a series of end points at different infusion rates of the individual drugs which define "depth of sedation". These end points are each associated with a dose-response curve and an ED 95%. For example, with propofol recall and awareness are eliminated at lower doses than those required to eliminate spon-

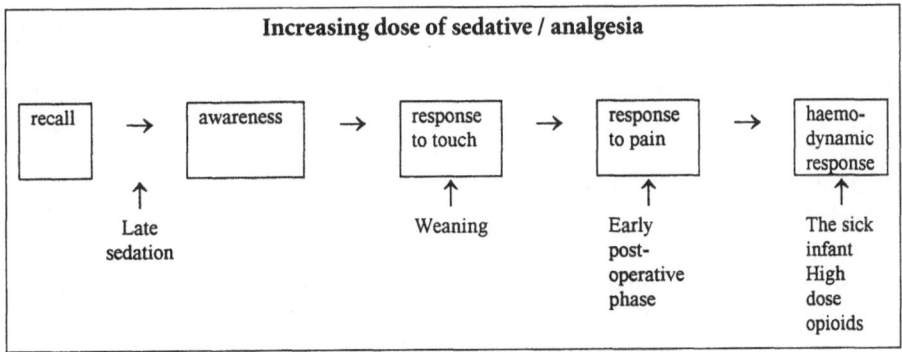

Fig. 2. Ideal levels of sedation at different perioperative stages

taneous movement or responses to stimulation. Higher doses will eliminate protective reflexes (eyelash response) and spontaneous motor responses to non-painful stimulation, but will not stop motor responses to painful stimuli. Higher doses still are required to anaesthetise the patient to painful stimuli and it is not until this dose is further increased that haemodynamic responses to nociception are abolished. Figure 2 demonstrates the effects of increasing doses of sedative/analgesic agents and the levels of sedation required at different stages in the course of a PICU stay.

When embarking on long-term sedation it is important not to oversedate the patient for the reasons explained above. If the patient is not in pain and is critically ill, low doses of sedative drugs will ensure lack of recall and awareness. At these low doses the patient may well try to move and may have some haemodynamic response to PICU procedures. This does not imply that sedation is inadequate, if there is no pain associated with the patients condition.

Paralysing drugs

The use of paralysing drugs opens up the issue of patients being paralysed and aware on intensive care. Paralysis is undesirable in the long-term PICU patient because it results in water retention/oedema, involution of the muscles of ventilation and difficulties in assessing the adequacy of sedation. However, in the sick patient or in the early phase of a PICU admission, it may be highly desirable. Prescribing sedative drugs at levels that are that are normally associated with lack of awareness may be a useful guide to managing the paralysed patient, but dosing requirements rise rapidly during intensive care stay due to both pharmacokinetic [7] and pharmacodynamic effects of prolonged exposure [8].

Drug combinations for PICU sedation

The scheme set out below attempts to use a rational choice of analgesic and sedation drugs in combination. In long-term sedation, the aim is to use different pharmacological groups of drugs in different weeks. Thus, an opioid (group 1) in combination with a phenothiazine (group 3) in "week 1" avoids the use of benzodiazepines, which can then be reserved for later use. Polypharmacy, the use of multiple drug combinations without any overall strategy, is bad practice because it uses up drug options. On the other hand, the use of large doses of a single agent for more than a few days promotes major drug tolerance, making subsequent weaning from the drug difficult.

– Week 1
- Analgesic drug: morphine infusion 0-40 µg/kg/per hour.
- Sedation drug: promethazine intravenous supplementation 0.5-1 mg/kg every 6 hours.

This combination should be used exclusively without additional agents. Effectiveness of the technique should be measured with formal and regular sedation assessment (see below).

– Week 2
- Analgesic drug: ketamine infusion 0-80 µg/kg/per minute.
- Sedation drug: midazolam 0-100 µg/kg/per hour.

By the second week morphine infusions may have been increased to 50 µg/kg/per hour or more as tolerance sets in. Morphine and promethazine should be replaced by ketamine and midazolam infusions, unless there is a specific contraindication (e.g., raised intracranial pressure). The midazolam avoids the risks of hallucinations associated with ketamine.

– Week 3
- Analgesic drug: clonidine infusion 0 1 - 1.0 µg/kg/per hour.
- Sedation drug: chloral hydrate 25 mg/kg orally or rectally.

As with the week 2 adjustment, ketamine should be replaced with clonidine and chloral hydrate on week 3, which represents a completely new group of pharmacological agents to which the patient has not developed tolerance.

– Week 4
- On week 4 the drugs are cycled back to the week 1 regimen of morphine and promethazine.

Propofol infusions in the PICU

If tolerance develops and it becomes necessary to withdraw a patient from the drugs, an infusion of propofol can be used to induce general anaesthesia. The infusion of 4-6 mg/kg/per hour will maintain anaesthesia and all other drugs can then be abruptly withdrawn. After an infusion of 72 h the propofol can usually be weaned off and a week 1, 2 or 3 regimen started. Propofol is now available as a more concentrated 2% solution which avoids the fat and water load associated with the standard preparation. It is important not to exceed the safe upper limits for propofol infusion, given the previous published experiences [10]. Paralysis may be useful during the propofol infusion once it has been established that the patient is comfortable.

Propofol is a useful drug in the PICU for procedures that require a short period of general anaesthesia (i.l., chest drain removal). It is not a good long-term drug for infusion in PICU because once the peripheral stores become saturated, recovery after the drug is discontinued may take a considerable time. Tolerance to propofol also occurs after several days.

Long-term weaning

Long acting, orally administered drugs are useful in long-term weaning after a protracted PICU stay. Drugs such as lorazepam, clonidine, chlorpromazine and oramorph all have use in this respect. A weaning regimen with one or more of these drugs should be set up with gradual dosage reduction over a 7- to 10-day period.

Monitoring analgesia and sedation

Optimising sedation to avoid both over- and underdosing can only be achieved effectively with regular assessment of adequacy of sedation. It is important for the nursing staff to be aware that non-movement and non-responsiveness is not the correct endpoint of PICU sedation. The overall plan is to use sedative drugs as sparingly as possible so that the patient remains comfortable and responsive to his/her surroundings. Figure 3 sets out the sedation and analgesia scoring system as used in the PICU at the Royal Hospital for Sick Children in Bristol. It is a version of the Objective Pain Scale [18, 19] modified to measure discomfort in both ventilated and non-ventilated patients on PICU. It uses both physiological and behavioural measurement in the score, with ideal values (neither over or undersedated) at 3 to 7 (Fig. 3).

Sedation scoring must be carried out hourly to monitor the adequacy of sedation and comfort. If the major component of the discomfort is judged to be pain, then the analgesic component of the drug combination should be increased (increase the morphine /ketamine/ clonidine infusion). If the major component is restlessness, then sedative drugs may be needed. Often simple nonpharmacological approaches alone are sufficient to calm a distressed infant (group 5).

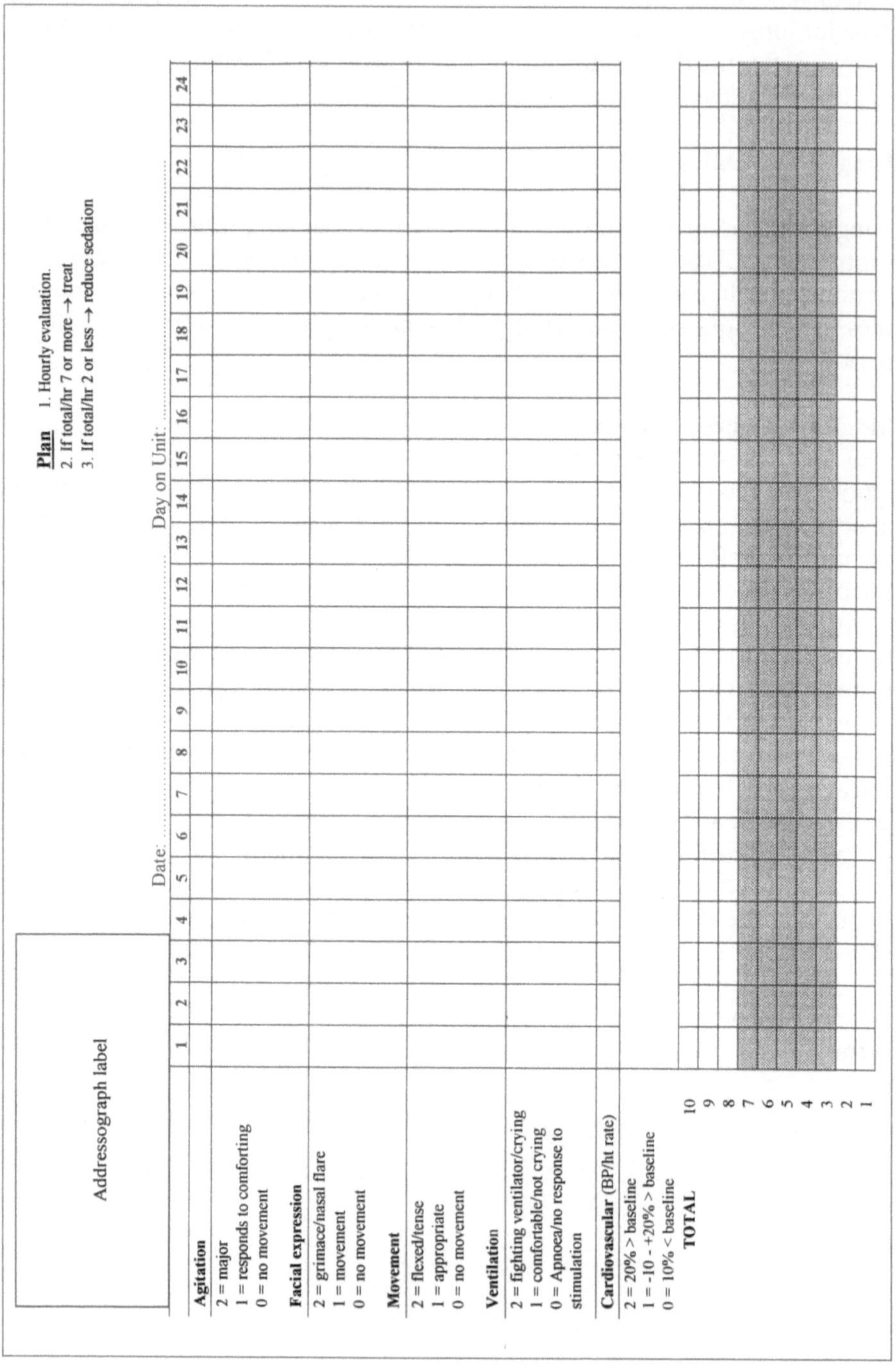

Addressograph label

Date: ....

Day on Unit: ....

	1	2	3	4	5	6	7	8	9	10	11	12	13	14	15	16	17	18	19	20	21	22	23	24

Agitation
2 = major
1 = responds to comforting
0 = no movement

Facial expression
2 = grimace/nasal flare
1 = movement
0 = no movement

Movement
2 = flexed/tense
1 = appropriate
0 = no movement

Ventilation
2 = fighting ventilator/crying
1 = comfortable/not crying
0 = Apnoea/no response to stimulation

Cardiovascular (BP/ht rate)
2 = 20% > baseline
1 = -10 - +20% > baseline
0 = 10% < baseline

TOTAL
10
9
8
7
6
5
4
3
2
1

Plan   1. Hourly evaluation.
2. If total/hr 7 or more → treat
3. If total/hr 2 or less → reduce sedation

Fig. 3. Sedation/analgesia chart

References

1. Wolf AR, Hughes D (1993) Pain relief for infants undergoing abdominal surgery: comparison of infusions of IV morphine and extradural bupivacaine. Br J Anaesth 70:10-16
2. McNeely JK, Farber NE, Rusy LM et al (1997) Epidural analgesia improves outcome following paediatric fundoplication. A retrospective analysis. Reg Anaesth 22:16-22
3. Olkkolo KT, Maunuksela EL, Korpela R et al (1988) Kinetics and dynamics of postoperative morphine in children. Clin Pharmacol Ther 44:123-136
4. Kart T, Christup LL, Rasnussen M (1997) Recommended use of morphine in neonates, infants and children based on a literature review. Part 1. Pharmacokinetics. Part 2. Clinical use. Paediatr Anaesth 7:5-13; 93-101
5. Wolf AR (1998) Neonatal analgesia. In: Rennie JM, Roberton NRC (eds) Textbook of neonatology, 3rd ed. Churchill Livingstone, London
6. Collins C, Koren G, Crean P et al (1985) Fentanyl pharmacokinetics and hemodynamic effects in preterm infants during ligation of patent ductus arteriosus. Anaesth Analg 64:1078-1080
7. Greeley WJ, Debruijn NP (1988) Changes in sufentanil pharmacokinetics within the neonatal period. Anaesth Analg 67:86-90
8. Arnold JH, Truog RD, Scavone JM et al (1991) Changes in the pharmacodynamic response to fentanyl in neonates during continuous infusion. J Pediatr 119:639-643
9. Mirski MA, Muffelman B, Ulatowski JA et al (1995) Sedation for the critically ill neurologic patient. Crit Care Med 23:2038-2053
10. Sinclaire ME (1992) Propofol infusion in children. Br Med J 305:17-20
11. Acolet D, Modi N, Giannakoulopoulos X, Bond C, Weg W, Clow A, Glover V (1993) Changes in plasma cortisol and catecholamine concentrations in response to massage in preterm infants. Arch Dis Child 68:29-31
12. Als H, Lawhon G, Brown E et al (1986) Individualized behavioural and environmental care for the very low birthweight preterm infant at high risk for bronchopulmonary dysplasia: neonatal intensive care unit and developmental outcome. Pediatrics 78:1123-1132
13. Haouari N, Wood C, Griffiths G, Levene M (1995) The analgesic effect of sucrose in full term infants: a randomised controlled trial. Br Med J 310:1498-1500
14. Editorial (1992) Pacifiers, passive behaviour and pain. Lancet 339:275-276
15. Lloyd Thomas AR, Howard RF (1994) A pain service for children. Paediatr Anaesth 4:3-15
16. Cook B, Grubb DJ, Aldridge LA et al (1995) Comparison of the effects of adrenaline, clonidine, and ketamine on the duration of caudal anaesthesia produced by bupivacaine in children. Br J Anaesth 75:698-701
17. Wolf AR (1991) The use of opioids in epidural analgesia. J Psychopharmacol 5:370-374
18. Norden J, Hannallah R, Getson P et al (1992) Concurrent validation of an objective pain scale for infants and children. Anaesthesiology 75:A934
19. Norden J, Hannallah R, Getson P et al (1991) Reliability of an objective pain scale in children. Anaesth Analg 72:S199

Chapter 20

Sedation and the paediatric patient

N.S. MORTON

The actual figures of mortality and morbidity in children under sedation are not known. In an analysis of sedation disasters in the United States 52 deaths and 27 cases of significant morbidity were reported which were directly attributed to sedation. These were mainly due to drug overdose, inadequate monitoring, inadequate training or premature discharge home. It is important to realise that hospitals and practitioners are being taken to task in court for inadequate sedation as well as for "sedation disasters".

Aims and problems

The aims of sedating children for diagnostic or therapeutic procedures are to relieve anxiety and stress, to provide pain relief, to induce appropriate sleep and to keep the child still enough to allow safe conduct of the procedure. The problems in achieving these aims are primarily the wide variability in the response of children to sedative agents in terms of both dose requirements and clinical effects. There is a continuum from the awake to the anaesthetised state, with loss of protective airway reflexes occurring unpredictably. Hypoventilation, apnoea and airway obstruction may occur with hypoxaemia and hypercarbia developing. This is particularly seen in younger infants or when combinations of sedatives and opioids are used. Cardiac output, heart rate and blood pressure may fall with the development of metabolic acidosis. Pulmonary, intracranial and intraocular pressures may rise primarily due to the effects of the sedative drug (i.e., ketamine) or secondarily to hypoxaemia and acidosis. Disinhibition, restlessness and movement can occur unpredictably and may be exacerbated by hypoxaemia. Progression of the depth of sedation after painful or stimulating procedures are finished is also commonly seen, particularly when long-acting agents are used. Achieving the aims of sedation while minimising the problems is difficult and in some children should not be attempted.

Sedation is defined as "a technique in which the use of a drug or drugs produces a state of depression of the central nervous system, enabling treatment to be carried out, but during which verbal contact with the patient is maintained throughout the period of sedation. The drugs and techniques used should carry a margin of safety wide enough to render unintended loss of consciousness unlikely". In the sedated state, protective reflexes are maintained, the airway is maintained independently and continuously and the child can respond to physical stimulation or verbal command [1].

In children it is difficult to achieve adequate anxiolysis, analgesia, sleep and lack of movement to allow the safe conduct of many diagnostic and therapeutic procedures if a state of sedation as defined in this way is used. Many children are, in fact, anaesthetised to achieve these aims. "Loss of consciousness is a state of anaesthesia with all its attendant risks". In the anaesthetised child, partial or complete loss of protective reflexes occurs, the airway cannot be maintained independently and continuously and the child is unable to to respond to physical stimulation or verbal command. Any attempt to differentiate light sedation, deep sedation and anaesthesia is fundamentally flawed because the states overlap unpredictably.

Principles of safe sedation of children

The standards of care of the sedated child should therefore be those of the child undergoing general anaesthesia. This requires careful selection and preparation of patients, exclusion of unsuitable patients, use of appropriate drugs, equipment, clinical and electronic monitoring by personnel appropriately trained in paediatric sedation and resuscitation, avoidance of the "operator-sedationist" and implementation of appropriate discharge criteria. This is the approach recommended in adult practice by the working party reports of several Royal Colleges (Physicians, Surgeons, Anaesthetists, Radiologists and Ophthalmologists) and in the published guidelines from the American Academy of Paediatrics [2]. A rational approach is to ask and answer the following key questions before undertaking the procedure:
 – Is the procedure going to be painful?
 – How long will the procedure last?
 – What is the medical status and age of the child?
 – Are there contraindications to sedation?
 – Has consent been obtained?
 – Has the child been fasted?
 – Who is going to look after the child during and after the period of sedation and what training does this person have?
 – When and by whom is the child going to be discharged?

It is preferable to use drugs with a rapid onset and short duration of action so that it is easier to titrate the dose to achieve the desired effect. The ability to pharmacologically antagonise any sedatives used is desirable. If the procedure is painful, use of local anaesthesia at the painful site applied topically in advance and /or infiltrated has an important "sedative-sparing" effect and often circumvents the need for opioids with all their potential adverse effects.

Patient selection

A full history and examination should be carried out and an active search made for contraindications to sedation and for significant underlying medical and surgical disorders [3, 4]. The past sedation history should be checked because previous failed sedation may warrant referral for a general anaesthetic. Small children merit particular caution and in some children the pharmacokinetics and dynamics of sedatives may be abnormal, for example in renal failure, hepatic failure, and in children with induced enzymes such as those on regular anticonvulsant drugs. Contraindications to sedation are:
– abnormal airway;
– raised intracranial pressure;
– depressed level of consciousness;
– history of sleep apnoea;
– respiratory failure;
– cardiac failure;
– gastro-oesophageal reflux;
– bowel obstruction;
– active infection;
– known drug allergy / adverse reaction;
– previously failed sedation.
   Particular caution is required with sedation in the following:
– neonates, especially if premature or ex-premature;
– infants and children age <5 years;
– renal impairment;
– hepatic impairment;
– epilepsy;
– on anticonvulsant therapy;
– asthma.

Patient preparation

Written informed consent should be obtained and this should include an explanation of the procedure and sedation technique to be used. Parents should be informed of the possibility that sedation may fail and that either the procedure may have to be abandoned or the child may require a formal general anaesthetic. The child should be fasted as for a general anaesthetic (6 h for solids or bottle milk, 4 h for breast milk, 3 h for clear fluids). Venous access should be secured under topical local anaesthetic cover, if at all possible prior to the administration of any sedation. Topical local anaesthesia should also be applied to the sites of any other needle punctures such as for lumbar puncture, bone marrow sampling or cannulation for interventional radiology or cardiology. The skin overlying these areas will be anaesthetised and the area can then be infiltrated with further local anaesthetic prior to the needling procedure. The sedative prescription should be double checked to ensure dosages are correct. Monitoring should be started from the time of administration of the sedative agent until discharge and must include the period when the patient is being transferred, for example, from ward to radiology department. Equipment for monitoring children and paediatric resuscitation drugs and equipment must be available throughout the period from the time the sedative is given until discharge. The staff undertaking this monitoring role must be properly trained and should be able to deliver basic life support measures and initiate advanced life support for children.

Checklist for safe paediatric sedation:
- check age, weight and identity;
- check consent;
- check fasting;
- check for contraindications;
- check past sedation history;
- check for significant underlying medical or surgical disorders;
- check for allergies;
- double check the sedation prescription and administration;
- check monitoring, resuscitation equipment and drugs;
- check the supervision of the child from pre-sedation to discharge.

Monitoring standards

The personnel undertaking monitoring of the sedated child must be appropriately trained in paediatric resuscitation, monitoring techniques and sedation techniques. These individuals may be nursing, paediatric medical, surgical, radiology or anaesthetic staff and should have as their sole duty the monitoring of the sedated child and should not take part in the procedure. They must be additional to and separate from the person carrying out the procedure whether this is diagnostic or therapeutic. In some countries the concept of monitored anaesthesia care has been developed for such situations and it may be that anaesthetists need to become more actively involved in the large numbers of such cases. The most important monitor is the trained person using observational and clinical skills and assisted by electronic monitoring as appropriate (i.e., pulse oximetry, ECG, non-invasive blood pressure device, temperature measurement and capnography).

The frequency and intensity of observations and assessments to be made should be matched to the child and the procedure and a balance must be struck between safety and practicality to allow the procedure to proceed without arousing the sleeping child and with the minimum of disruption. It is important for clinical and legal reasons that the observations are charted, something that is rarely done in many centres at present. The minimum monitoring standard should comprise regular assessments of the level of sedation, oxygen saturation by pulse oximetry, respiratory rate and pulse rate supplemented by temperature, ECG and blood pressure for infants, for prolonged procedures or when verbal contact with the child is lost. Monitoring should continue after the procedure and during transfer back to the recovery or ward area until discharge criteria are met. This is important because the depth of sedation may progress, particularly after the stimulus of a painful procedure has receded and especially if long-acting agents are used. A proactive check on the patency and stability of the airway should be made, protective reflexes should be intact, the child should be awake or back to his normal response level, hydration should be adequate and haemodynamics should be stable.

Recovery and discharge criteria are:
- airway patent and stable, unsupported;
- easily rousible;
- oxygen saturation >96% breathing air;
- haemodynamically stable;
- hydration adequate;
- returned to normal level of responsiveness and orientation for age and mental.status;
- can talk (age appropriately);
- can sit up unaided (age appropriately).

Recommended techniques

Single, short-acting sedative agents (i.e., midazolam) and appropriate use of local anaesthesia (topically applied and/or infiltrated) are preferred. Combinations of sedatives with opioids and use of long-acting agents are not recommended. Anaesthetic drugs such as propofol or ketamine should only be given by anaesthetists.

Nitrous oxide or Entonox

Nitrous oxide is a gas with analgesic and sedative properties which is taken up and eliminated very rapidly from the lungs. It is very insoluble in the blood so is delivered very quickly to the brain to produce an analgesic effect equivalent to intravenous morphine. Maximal pain relief is achieved after approximately 2 min of inhalation. Nitrous oxide can be given in oxygen in inspired concentrations up to 70% but this requires a special delivery system and such a concentration may lead to loss of verbal contact with the patient. It is more conveniently given in the form of "Entonox", which is a cylinder of premixed nitrous oxide in oxygen which automatically delivers 50% nitrous oxide and 50% oxygen. The cylinder contents are under pressure and a flow of gas to the patient is usually activated on demand by the patient taking a breath in via a special valve. Recently, the design of these valves has improved to a lightweight, child-friendly system with an opening pressure of 1-2 cmH$_2$O. The child can breath via a facemask, nasal mask or mouthpiece and the system is best regarded as a form of inhaled PCA with the child holding the mask or mouthpiece and con-

trolling the inhalation. This has an important safety function in maintaining sedation and thus verbal contact. It is not very suitable for children <3 years old and works best of all in co-operative children aged >5 years. Entonox can be used for a wide variety of procedures in paediatrics which require potent analgesia for a short time:
- suture insertion or removal;
- dressing removal or changes (including burns);
- drain or catheter removal;
- venepuncture or cannulation;
- lumbar puncture;
- physiotherapy;
- biopsies (skin, muscle, renal, bone marrow).

Nitrous oxide/Entonox is not suitable for all children and there are absolute contraindications to its administration:
- pneumothorax;
- bowel obstruction;
- abnormal airway;
- recent head injury (especially if intracranial air);
- chronic respiratory disease;
- uncorrected congenital heart disease;
- gastro-oesophageal reflux;
- age <3 years;
- cannot cooperate or understand technique;
- previous problems with Entonox;

Nitrous oxide is highly diffusable and will move more rapidly into an air pocket than the nitrogen in the air pocket moves out. The air pocket will therefore expand in volume or if in a confined space (i.e., within the chest or cranial cavities or within the lumen of the bowel) the pressure will increase. This tension effect is extremely dangerous, producing tension pneumothorax, ischaemia or shift of intracranial contents or bowel distension with risk of perforation.

Nitrous oxide produces a degree of sedation and potentiates the sedative effects of other central nervous system depressants so care is required when opioids, benzodiazepines or antihistamines have also been given. Nitrous oxide can also induce nausea and vomiting but if it is to be used as the sole sedative and analgesic, the incidence of emesis is very low and therefore fasting is not required. If, however, other sedatives or analgesics have been given, the child should be fasted as for a general anaesthetic (6 h for solids or milk, 3 h for clear fluids). Other adverse effects of nitrous oxide are the potential to oxidise vitamin B_{12} and affect erythropoiesis and disputed effects on personnel of prolonged or repeated exposure. It is important that nitrous oxide administration is performed in well ventilated areas and that, where possible, the expired gases are scavenged.

As with any sedative technique, consent, selection, preparation, monitoring and record-keeping should be as noted above and trained personnel should be in charge of administering and monitoring the child receiving nitrous oxide.

Midazolam

Midazolam is a water-soluble benzodiazepine which produces sedation, anxiolysis and amnesia but is not an analgesic. It can be administered by parenteral (i.v., i.m.), oral, sublingual, nasal or rectal routes. It is rapidly distributed and has an elimination half-life of 70-140 min but this is considerably prolonged in neonates.

Intravenous midazolam

The intravenous formulation of midazolam (2 or 5 mg/ml) is very acidic, with a pH of 3.3, and prior to administration to children it is advisable to dilute the drug with 5% dextrose or 0.9% saline to a minimum volume of 10 ml. There is no pain on injection and small increments of 0.05 mg/kg (50 mg/kg) given over 10-15 s will produce smooth induction of sedation whilst minimising respiratory depression or hypotension. The onset of action is slower than that seen with intravenous anaesthetic agents. This means that after each increment a delay of at least 60 s should be allowed for the effects of the drug to be seen. The incremental dose of 0.05 mg/kg can be repeated in this way, titrating the dose against the level of sleep up to a total dose of 0.3 mg/kg. A useful clinical endpoint for a safe level of sedation is ptosis (closure of the eyelids).

Occasionally, hypotension is seen when bolus doses are used in critically ill or very small infants and particular care is required in these cases. Respiratory depression may be seen, particularly when midazolam is given along with opioids or other sedative agents. Like all benzodiazepines, midazolam can produce a state of disinhibition or restlessness in up to 10% of children, especially in those under 5 years of age. This state does not respond to further increments of the drug and misinterpretation of this sign can lead to overdosage.

There is a wide interpatient variability in response to benzodiazepines, so titration with an upper dose limit is the safest approach. The intravenous midazolam technique must only be used in the context of careful patient selection, preparation and monitoring and children must be fasted as if they are having a general anaesthetic. This procedure must not be undertaken by untrained staff. The person giving intravenous midazolam must be fully trained in paediatric sedation and paediatric resuscitation and must have as their sole duty the sedation and monitoring of the child. They must not undertake the diagnostic or therapeutic procedure as well. Trained anaesthetic or medical staff or nurse specialists can all use this technique safely provided the selection and monitoring standards are implemented correctly.

Oral midazolam

Midazolam can be given orally and this route has been extensively researched as a method of premedication of children. The standard intravenous formulation is used but is very bitter tasting so a sweet vehicle is required as disguise. A variety of local-favourite formulations have been developed, including standard pharmaceutical syrup, cola, lemonade, sweet or iced fruit juices, paracetamol syrup or a Glasgow perennial "Irn-Bru"! Up to 1 ml/kg of any of these can be allowed as a diluent and a commercially produced formulation is under trial. The oral dose is ten times larger than the intravenous incremental dose because of extensive first-pass liver metabolism after gastrointestinal absorption. The most commonly used dose is 0.5 mg/kg, maximum 15 mg (although some workers recommend 0.75 mg/kg). The onset of effect is within 30 min and there is a further 30 min window of opportunity when sedation is at its maximum. Supplementary intravenous midazolam may be given, with the provisos noted above. For painful procedures, local anaesthesia supplementation should be used in preference to opioid supplementation to minimise the risk of respiratory depression. In some cases, nitrous oxide/Entonox analgesia may be more appropriate.

Recovery after these techniques is rapid and is usually complete within 2 h, allowing early return to oral intake of fluids and nutrition and prompt discharge home if appropriate.

Midazolam-based sedation techniques should be the first-choice technique in modern paediatric practice and a suggested scheme to cover most paediatric diagnostic and therapeutic procedures will be presented.

Antagonism of benzodiazepine sedation with flumazenil

In the event of overdosage with midazolam, basic and advanced life support measures are the priority (Airway, Breathing, Circulation, Oxygen) but the specific benzodiazepine antagonist flumazenil should also be considered. Flumazenil must be available immediately whenever midazolam is given to children. The incremental dose is 5 mg/kg, repeated every 60 s to a total of 40 mg/kg. In severe cases, an infusion of flumazenil may be needed as its effective half-life is shorter than that of most of the benzodiazepines (rate 10 mg/kg/h). Children receiving flumazenil may awaken very abruptly and may become acutely agitated, restless or even have seizures, and care must be taken to protect the child from injury if this occurs. The availability of flumazenil should not be an excuse for using excessive doses of benzodiazepines, and care is required when deciding when to discharge children if flumazenil has been used as resedation is a possibility.

Midazolam can also be given by the nasal, rectal or intramuscular routes but these are unpleasant and disliked by children, and cannot be recommended.

Temazepam

Temazepam can be used orally as anxiolytic and sedative premedication prior to procedures in a dose of 0.2-0.5 mg/kg to a maximum dose of 20 mg. It is best given 60-90 min in advance of the procedure and produces useful sedation for up to 2 h. The syrup (1 mg/ml) or tablet formulations can be used.

Diazepam

Diazepam can be useful as oral premedication in a dose of 0.2-0.3 mg/kg. As an emulsion formulation it can be titrated intravenously in increments of 0.1 mg/kg repeated at 60 s intervals up to a total maximum dose of 0.5 mg/kg or until ptosis is seen. Diazepam has a long-acting, active metabolite which may delay recovery. The effects of diazepam can be reversed by flumazenil as above.

Trimeprazine

Trimeprazine oral syrup is still commonly used as a paediatric sedative, antiemetic premedication. The recommended dose is 1-2 mg/kg, but many paediatric centres still use 3 mg/kg. Recovery may be prolonged after larger doses. Sedation is not reversible with flumazenil or naloxone.

Chloral hydrate

This syrup is used for sedative premedication prior to non-painful procedures. The recommended dose is 25-50 mg/kg but doses up to 100 mg/kg are sometimes used. The onset of sedation takes about 1 h and lasts about 1 h but residual effects may be evident for 24 h. Particular care is required when combined with other sedative agents. Gastric irritation, hypotension and excessive depth of sedation may occur and the sedation is not reversible with flumazenil or naloxone.

Barbiturates

Rectally or orally administered barbiturates (i.e., oral quinalbarbitone 5-10 mg/kg) have been used for paediatric sedation but produce variable depth and duration of sedation. They should not be used for painful procedures. There are no antagonists available.

Ketamine

Ketamine is an anaesthetic agent which can be given by the oral, intravenous or intramuscular route. It should only be administered by trained anaesthetists and children should be fasted as for a general anaesthetic. In low doses it is a potent analgesic and in higher doses it also produces a state of dissociative anaesthesia. Ketamine tends to cause sympathetic nervous system stimulation and so blood pressure tends to remain stable or increase, intracranial pressure increases and elevated pulmonary pressure may rise further. It should not be used in patients with systemic, intracranial or pulmonary hypertension. Ketamine induces dose-related respiratory depression and augments the respiratory depressant effects of other sedative agents. It also tends to stimulate salivation and airway secretions and this may induce coughing and laryngeal spasm.

These effects can be prevented by atropine premedication (orally 20-40 mg/kg or i.v. 10-20 mg/kg). Central nervous stimulation may lead to restlessness, nightmares and delirium but these effects can be reduced by premedication with a benzodiazepine as above. The new purified stereoisomer form of ketamine (S-ketamine) is as effective as ketamine without producing the CNS side effects.

Ketamine dosage schedule

- Oral: 10-20 mg/kg, 20-30 min in advance.
- Intramuscular: 2-10 mg/kg.
- Intravenous: 1-2 mg/kg, increments 0.5 mg/kg every 60 s or infusion 10-50 mg/kg/per minute.

Opioids

Opioids should only be used for painful procedures if local anaesthesia cannot be used or has failed. They should not be used as sedatives for non-painful procedures because of the risk of respiratory depression. Cocktails of sedatives with opioids given orally or intramuscularly should not be used as they are associated with a high risk of respiratory depression, loss of airway control, cardiovascular instability and prolonged recovery. Short-acting potent opioids such as fentanyl, alfentanil and remifentanil should only be used by anaesthetists or intensivists and should not be used outwith the operating room or intensive care unit. It is probably best to become familiar with titrating one opioid such as morphine given in small increments intravenously, for example 20 mg/kg, repeated every 5 min to the desired end-point. Morphine can be given orally but the sedative effect is unpredictable and it is difficult to titrate the dose to achieve the desired effect.

Antagonist for opioids: naloxone

The sedative, respiratory depressant and analgesic effects of opioids can be antagonised by naloxone 2-4 mg/kg i.v. repeated to 10 mg/kg. The duration of naloxone's effect is short and an infusion may have to be given to maintain reversal at a dose of 10 mg/kg/per hour. Naloxone can be given i.m. in an emergency in a dose of 10 mg/kg.

Conclusions

- Children undergoing sedation should be prepared and monitored as for a general anaesthetic.
- A separate trained person should monitor the child during and after sedation.
- The contraindications to sedation must be actively sought.

- An accurate record of the sedation procedure and monitored recordings should be made and filed in the case record.
- Single titratable antagonisable agents should be used and combinations with opioids avoided.
- Do not use opioids for non-painful procedures.
- Use local anaesthesia for pain control wherever possible.

References

1. Working Party on Training in Dental Anaesthesia (1981) The Wylie Report British Dental Journal 151:385-388
2. Committee on Drugs (1992) Guidelines for monitoring and management of pediatric patients during and after sedation for diagnostic and therapeutic procedures. Pediatrics 89:1110-1115
3. Morton NS (1998) Acute paediatric pain management: a practical guide. WB Saunders, London
4. Royal College of Paediatrics and Child Health (1997) Prevention and control of pain in children. BMJ Publishing Group, London

Chapter 21

Immediate postoperative considerations

P.A. Lönnqvist

Indications of the unglamorous nature of immediate paediatric postoperative care are the telling scarcity of published studies in this field and the very limited attention paid to these problems in paediatric anaesthesia textbooks. Despite the lack of flair this is indeed an important period in both the surgical and anaesthetic process. Here a review of the different problems that the paediatric anaesthesiologist might face are presented and, due to the relative lack of significant publications within this field, to a large extent mirror the views, opinions and patient populations encountered by the author. The review does not include specific problems that might occur following more advanced types of surgery for example, neonatal, cardiac, neuro- or maxillofacial surgery. For the best available overview of this topic the text by Berde and Todres [1] is recommended to the reader.

Standard treatment and monitoring

All patients should benefit from certain fundamental monitoring and basic therapies. Immediately on arrival to the recovery area the patient should receive supplemental oxygen and have a pulse oximeter probe put on [2, 3]. Whether additional monitoring, i.e., ECG and noninvasive blood pressure recording, is warranted depends on the extent of the surgical procedure or if any complications were experienced during anaesthesia. However, even following minor surgery or interventions, the patient's blood pressure should be checked at least once in the immediate postoperative period. The administration of supplemental oxygen is often not accomplished without some difficulties in children. Face masks and intranasal catheters are often poorly tolerated since the child will try to take them away as soon as they start to regain consciousness. Better options are usually nasal prongs or just to flood oxygen in front of the patient's face. Motion artifacts or frank dislodgment of the pulse oximeter probe, causing false alarms, are also frequent problems. If the patient has an epidural or some other sort of more extensive regional block which impairs the mobility of a limb, an excellent option is to put the probe on the blocked limb. This will not only ensure better stability of the probe but, since the block will also cause a sympathetic block, perfusion is good and the opportunity for a good pulse oximeter signal enhanced. However, since the patient will not be able to feel discomfort from the probe under these circumstances, care must be taken not to cause undue pressure when fixating the probe. Failure to do so has been found to cause incipient pressure sores or first degree burn injury (own unpublished observations). Of utmost importance is monitoring the patient's respiratory rate. This is a simple and effective way of avoiding hypoventilation and, thus, respiratory rate should be monitored in all patients that are not wide awake. If the patient has an intravenous catheter in place, an intravenous infusion should be started if not already running. This will ensure hydration of the patient who, despite new preoperative fasting guidelines, only too often will have had a prolonged period of fluid restriction prior to surgery. Inclusion of glucose in the postoperative solution might be of benefit for the general sense of well-being of the patient. The neuroendocrine reaction to surgery will cause a certain degree of water retention and, thus, the infusion rate does not have to be higher than the basic requirements of normal patients. Overenthusiastic infusion rates can increase the problem of postoperative urinary retention (see below). All patients delivered to the recovery room should have received some type of analgesia in advance and written orders for the recovery nurse should be readily available if the patient should experience breakthrough pain.

Postoperative hemorrhage

In contrast to adults, postoperative hemorrhage is uncommon following paediatric surgery since paediatric surgeons are usually very meticulous regarding hemostasis. Exceptions to this are patients who have been subjected to spinal (scoliosis), craniosynostosis or hip surgery or have undergone liver resections or tonsillectomies. These patients need to be followed very carefully regarding blood loss by checking surgical drains, haemodynamics and hematocrit levels. Despite the rarity of postoperative hemorrhage following paediatric surgery, it is prudent to check hematocrit levels at least once during the recovery room stay after anything but minor procedures. In view of potential infections (i.e., HIV, hepatitis C) and the negative effect on the immune system as well as the body's own erythropoesis, physicians are becoming more conservative regarding transfusions of packed red cells. It is therefore not possible to have a general target value below which the patient should be transfused. Before the administration of blood products it is therefore wise to consult with the surgeon in charge. Although low hematocrit levels might be tolerated without any major problems or drawbacks, it is vital that the patient is kept normovolemic. This can be accomplished by the administration of either crystalloids or colloids.

Respiratory problems

Respiratory problems are frequently encountered and range from simple snoring due to a slight runny nose to life-threatening airway obstructions. Some of the most frequent conditions causing respiratory problems are listed below together with a suggested cause of action to solve the problem.

- *Pulse oximeter desaturation alarm*: first, observe the patient and see whether he is obviously cyanotic and check that the supplemental oxygen is in place. Secondly, control that the pulse oximeter probe is still on the patient, that there is an adequate plethysmographic curve on the monitor, and that the perfusion indicator is adequate. If not, change the location of the probe. If the pulse oximeter still shows that the patient is desaturated, further action is required.

- *Postextubation stridor*: due to the specific anatomy of the paediatric airway, where the cricoid cartilage constitutes the narrowest part of the airway, postextubation stridor is a frequent problem [4]. The situation resembles pseudocroup, with inspiratory stridor and a barking cough, and is due to subglottic edema caused by either too large an endotracheal tube or a hypersensitive airway mucosa, most often due to recent pseudocroup or other airway infections. The best treatment is prophylaxis, using an endotracheal tube which will allow some leakage at inspiratory pressures of 20 cmH$_2$O or deferring anaesthesia and surgery for 6 weeks following an episode of pseudocroup. The use of a laryngeal mask airway might be a good alternative in this situation. However, if faced with this condition in the recovery room, inhalation of racemic epinephrine and intravenous administration of cortisone is usually effective. In severe cases, reintubation with a very small endotracheal tube might become necessary.

- *Bronchospasm*: this condition might present itself in already predisposed children or can occur as a part of the emergence from anaesthesia. Regurgitation with minor or major aspiration are other triggering factors. In contrast to the case in adults, pulmonary embolism is quite uncommon. However, pulmonary embolism can occur also in children and, if it does, the cause is usually air embolism. The symptoms of bronchospasm are the ordinary ones: expiratory stridor combined with wheezing on auscultation. Bronchospasm will most often respond well to inhalation of β2-agonists. If this does not ameliorate the condition, further treatment with intravenous theophylline and corticosteriods should be given. In more persistent cases inhalation of a helium – oxygen mixture can, in certain patients, prevent the necessity of deep sedation combined with reintubation and artificial ventilation.

- *Opioid-induced respiratory depression*: hypoventilation due to opioid overdose is quite frequently encountered in the immediate postoperative period. There are usually three different explanations for the occurrence of opioid-induced respiratory depression:
  - overdosage of opioids during the anaesthetic, necessitating the administration of naloxone at the end in order to regain spontaneous ventilation. If an subcutaneous dose of naloxone was not administered concomitantly with the intravenous dose, or if an insufficient subcutaneous dose was given, renarcotization can occur in the recovery room;
  - an overdose of opioids has been administered in the recovery room due to insufficient initial pain relief;

- intravenous opioids have been administered in a patient who has received epidural or intrathecal opioids.

The symptoms are classical: bradypnea and pinpoint pupils with or without concomitant desaturation. Treatment consists of manual ventilation followed by the administration of naloxone. Care should be taken not to be to overambitious with the dosage of naloxone since otherwise the patient can awake in excruciating pain.

- *Upper airway obstruction*: apart from postextubation stridor (see above) upper airway obstruction almost exclusively appears in patients who have undergone surgery in the airways (i.e., ENT surgery, cleft palate repair, bronchoscopy) or have some already known predisposing syndrome (i.e., Pierre Robin, Down's syndrome). The causative factors are mainly nasal congestion, swelling of the upper airways, residual anaesthetic effects leading to hypotonia of the pharyngeal muscles, or a foreign body (i.e., blood clot, mucus plug or a surgical swab/throat pack left behind). Immediate actions can range from a chin lift or inserting a nasopharyngeal airway to emergency laryngoscopy with reintubation, or, in the worst case scenario, tracheotomy, depending on the degree of the obstruction. In more severe cases the patient should be brought back to the operating room immediately and be re-anaesthetized, preserving spontaneous ventilation, and an ENT surgeon should be alerted in order to be ready to perform a tracheotomy should regular intubation fail to avert the problem.
- *Pertussis-induced, severe coughing*: during the acute phase of pertussis, coughing can be so severe that extubation will become virtually impossible. This predisposition to react with whooping-like cough to a common cold or to manipulations in the airway can persist for up to 6 months after the acute episode. If possible, elective surgery should, thus, be postponed until this risk is overcome. If previous pertussis infection is not identified during the preanaesthetic interview or if surgery has to be performed regardless of an acute pertussis infection, severe problems can occur during emergence from anaesthesia or sometimes as late as in the recovery room. This is a very problematic situation and deep sedation and reintubation are frequently required. On occasion, intravenous administration of lidocaine (1-2 mg/kg) may be helpful.
- *No obvious reason immediately apparent*: do not forget the possibility of pneumothorax, especially following central venous catheterization, intercostal blocks, upper abdominal surgery, bronchoscopy, or dilatation of an esophageal stricture. Major atelectasis can also be a cause of significant desaturation. A thorough physical examination and an emergent chest radiograph are fundamental to rapid diagnosis and treatment of these conditions.

Unsatisfactory pain relief

Unsatisfactory pain relief constitutes one of the most frequent complaints in the immediate postoperative period. In this regard age-appropriate pain scales are very useful tools for two reasons. First, postoperative pain can be repeatedly assessed and, secondly, the effects of supplemental analgesic administration can be evaluated. Satisfactory results can often be achieved by adequate administration of nonopioid analgesics, for example, paracetamol (initial dosage of 40 mg/kg has recently been proposed), regular nonsteroidal anti-inflammatory drugs (NSAIDs) (i.e., diclofenac 1 mg/kg following orthopedic procedures), or keterolac (0.1 mg/kg i.v.). Combinations of paracetamol and codeine (approx. 1 mg/kg) can also be helpful in this regard. Top-up dosing of continuous regional blocks might be effective but attention should be paid to maximum safe dosage (bupivacaine in neonates: 0.2 mg/kg per hour; in older children: 0.4 mg/kg per hour). Despite the actions outlined above opioids will often be needed either as single bolus injections, continuous infusions, or patient-controlled analgesia.

Postoperative confusion/agitation

As part of the emergence process quite a number of patients display a state of confusion or agitation. It is obviously of vital importance to rule out hypoxia as the cause of this condition but the use of pulse oximetry usually solves this issue. Urinary retention is another possible cause for this condition (see below). However, most often no specific cause can be found and, thus, frequently an unusual reaction to drugs administered in the preoperative period might be the causative factor. When midazolam was first introduced, recovery room nurses regularly complained about an increased frequency of this problem. The use of sevoflurane has also been associated with a brief period of adverse emergency reactions especially in preschool boys [5]. However, problems following sevoflurane anaesthesia might be attributed to inadequate pain relief due to the rapid emergence after sevoflurane anaesthesia and the problem is less pronounced if regional anaesthesia techniques have been used. The drug used for premedication can also affect the occurrence of unwanted emergence reactions after sevoflurane anaesthesia. In the author's experience such reactions are extremely rare if morphine, diazepam or clonidine has been used for premedication, whereas confusion/agitation is not infrequent if midazolam has been administered in the preoperative period. Thus, in the opinion of the author midazolam is overrated as a premedication in children and should best be avoided if sevoflurane is going to be used as the main anaesthetic.

Urinary retention

Urinary retention is usually not a main problem in the recovery room except following lengthy procedures during which quite a lot of intravenous fluid has been administered and a Foley catheter has not been placed. The patient only rarely complains about urgency to void or suprapubic pain but instead presents with agitation or confusion frequently mistaken for emergence delirium, pain, or possible hypoxia. Palpation and percussion will usually give the diagnosis but if the patient is very uncooperative, an ultrasonographic examination is very helpful. However, if the opportunity for an ultrasonographic examination is not readily available, a test catherization of the bladder should be performed if other reasons for the patient's problems have been ruled out.

Postoperative nausea and vomiting

Postoperative nausea and vomiting (PONV) present a very significant clinical problem. A multitude of risk factors have been identified which increase the likelihood of PONV, for example age >2 years, previous history of PONV or motion sickness, certain types of surgery (strabismus correction, ENT procedures, inguinal hernia repair), and perioperative use of opioids [6]. Regarding ambulatory surgery PONV is the most frequent factor causing unplanned overnight hospitalization of the patient. Three important issues regarding PONV will be discussed in some depth.

Currently used treatments for PONV

The new HT-3 blockers (i.e., ondansetron) have been found to be effective in the treatment of established PONV. However, most studies comparing the efficacy of ondansetron vs. low-dose droperidol have found droperidol as efficacious as ondansetron for the treatment of PONV. Since droperidol is much cheaper than ondasetron, droperidol currently appears to be the first choice. Small doses of propofol have also been suggested as an effective treatment of PONV. However, the results of initial paediatric studies regarding the use of propofol in this setting have been disappointing.

Need for preventive measures in patients with risk factors

Patients with risk factors should receive special attention in order to minimize the risk for PONV. Exclusion of any medication known to cause PONV, prophylactic administration of low-dose droperidol, clonidine or ondansetron, and the use of a propofol or sevoflurane anaesthetic should be considered. Prophylactic steroid administration in patients undergoing tonsillectomy has been shown to be effective in this regard. Central nerve blocks (i.e., spinal and epidural blockade) combined with light intravenous sedation have been reported to substantially reduce the incidence of PONV and should be considered in appropriate patients.

Use of opioids and nitrous oxide

Opioids are notoriously known to cause PONV. With the availability of new analgesic drugs (i.e., ketorolac), more appropriate use and dosage of existing analgesics (i.e., paracetamol and NSAIDs), and the increasing use of regional anaesthesia techniques, it should be possible to minimize the use of opioids. By excluding the use of opioids in our out-patient inguinal hernia repair cases we have been able to reduce the incidence of vomiting from 25% to approximately 5%, still with good quality pain relief postoperatively. Especially the uncritical use of small doses of fentanyl or alfentanil for the attenuation of brief intraoperative events (i.e., endotracheal intubation, peritoneal traction during inguinal hernia repair) instead of temporarily increasing the depth of sevoflurane or propofol anaesthesia should best be avoided. Nitrous oxide has been implicated as a factor causing PONV. However, a meta-analysis review on this topic has failed to substantiate this allegation. Thus, the role of nitrous oxide in regard to PONV is still not entirely clarified.

Hypothermia/shivering

Due to the unfavorable body surface/body mass relationship neonates, infants, and toddlers are prone to intraoperative heat loss. Despite the use of intraoperative temperature monitoring as well as warm intravenous fluids and forced hot air devices, postoperative hypothermia is still encountered too frequently at the end of surgery. In order to regain normal temperature the body needs to produce heat. The neonate is unable to produce heat by shivering and has to rely on increased metabolism in brown adipose tissue. However, older children will increase muscle activity by way of shivering. Both of these heat-producing mechanisms substantially increase oxygen consumption and oxygen demand. As outlined above, frank hypoxia or borderline hypoxia is not infrequently experienced in the immediate postoperative period for a number of reasons and, thus, increases in oxygen demand during the recovery room stay can be deleterious to the patient. Shivering is also frequently seen following volatile agent anaesthesia despite apparently normal body temperature. The initial treatment of hypothermic patients in the recovery room should consist of supplemental oxygen administration, warm blankets, or an overhead radiant heater. If shivering is pronounced and is deemed to require pharmacological intervention, either low-dose pethidine (approx. 0.2 mg/kg i.v.) or clonidine (1 µg/kg i.v.) are often useful.

Duration of recovery room stay

No consensus guidelines exist regarding duration of the recovery room stay. This is governed both by patient-related factors as well as the possibility for supervision and monitoring of the patients on the general ward. Patients with an unstable haemodynamic situation, patients with obvious or potential airway problems, or patients who have received epidural morphine should ideally stay overnight. In more normal postoperative patients, the recovery room stay can be individualized but should not ever be less than 30 min, except maybe after single-injection propofol anaesthesia/sedation for very minor procedures. In patients who have been endotracheally intubated a 2 h observation period is required in order to safeguard against the occurrence of postextubation stridor.

Discharge criteria

Prior to discharge the patient should be fully conscious with stable haemodynamics. No signs of respiratory problems should be allowed and, thus, if the patient displays any symptoms of stridor, respiratory distress or borderline oxygen saturation he should be kept for an extended period in the recovery room until these problems resolve or should be admitted to the intensive care unit for further observation and treatment. One very important issue that needs to be confirmed in these days of health care budget cuts and nursing staff limitations is that the receiving ward has appropriate staffing and monitoring capabilities to take care of the patient. The lack of such fundamental resources has provoked the necessity for the development of high-dependency units where patients can be cared for during an extended postoperative period.

References

1. Berde CB, Todres ID (1993) Recovery from anaesthesia and the postanaesthesia care unit. In: Coté CJ et al (eds) A practice of anaesthesia for infants and children. Saunders, Harcourt Brace Jovanovich, Philadelphia, pp 471-482
2. Motoyoma EK, Glazener CH (1986) Hypoxemia after general anaesthesia in children. Anesth Analg 65:267-272
3. Patel R, Norden J, Hannallah RS (1988) Oxygen administration prevents hypoxia during post-anaesthetic transport in children. Anaesthesiology 69:616-618
4. Koka BV, Jeon IS, Andre JM et al (1997) Postintubation croup in children. Anesth Analg 56:501-505
5. Aono J, Ueda W, Mamiya K et al (1997) Greater incidence of delirium during recovery from sevoflurane anaesthesia in preschool boys. Anaesthesiology 87:1298-1300
6. Baines D (1996) Postoperative nausea and vomiting in children. Paediatric Anaesthesia 6:7-14

PAEDIATRIC INTENSIVE CARE UNIT (PICU)

Chapter 22

Update on respiratory distress syndrome

D. VIDYASAGAR

Respiratory distress syndrome (RDS), also known as hyaline membrane disease (HMD), is the most common cause of mortality and morbidity in premature infants. Approximately 1% of all newborns world/wide develop RDS. In the USA about 5 000 neonatal deaths/year are due to RDS [1]. Over the last two decades mortality from RDS has dramatically decreased even for extremely premature newborns [2]. Several factors are attributable to improved outcome, and namely: 1) better understanding of lung maturation; 2) improved perinatal management; 3) postnatal use of surfactant as replacement therapy; 4) improved ventilatory management; 5) overall improvement in managing extremely low birth weight infants. This review will highlight the advances in these areas.

Respiratory distress syndrome: growth of body of knowledge

Recently, we reviewed all the articles related to neonatology published in "Paediatrics", the official journal of American Academy of Paediatrics during the last fifty (1948-1998) years [3]. Several interesting points were observed. The number of publications related to neonatology gradually increased from 1948 and peaked in 1970-80's; the golden era of neonatal medicine. The growth in the body of knowledge of neonatal pulmonary diseases showed the same trend. Table 1 shows time line of landmark papers that appeared in "Paediatrics" that contributed to the understanding of fetal/neonatal cardiopulmonary physiology, consequently leading to sound physiologically based treatments. The introduction of each new treatment modality was associated with a significant decrease in mortality. There were several other landmark publications that changed the natural history of RDS, which appeared in other journals and they are shown in this same table. Not all the publications listed in the table refer to pulmonary physiology alone. The new knowledge in other related areas contributed to improve overall management and therefore enhanced survival of infants with RDS.

Natural history of respiratory distress syndrome

The natural history of RDS/HMD is also very interesting to be followed (Fig. 1). In 1976 Farrel [4] estimated that over 10 000 infants died every year of

Table 1. A neonatology time line. Publications in "Paediatrics" which have changed clinical practice and our understanding of RDS in premature infants*

1948	1958	1968	1978	1988	1998
Causes of fetal and neonatal deaths (Miller 1950)	*Pulmonary function in the newborn (Nelson 1962)*	*Antepartum glucocorticoids for prevention of RDS (Liggins 1972)* *Tracheal surfactant/Fetal rabbit model- Enhorning* *NICU morbidity/ mortality <1000 g BW (Alden 1972)*	Cerebral flow velocity (Volpe 1982) IVH: pneumothorax (Hill 1982)	Pulse oximetry (Ramanathan 1987) (Jennis 1987)	
Angiographic studies of the human fetal circulation (Lind 1949)	*Alveolar lining layer (Avery 1962)*	*CNP-device, use in HMD (Vidyasagar 1971)* (Chernick 1972)	*Surfactant (Fujiwara 1980)*	Preventability of chronic lung disease (Avery 1987)	
Water and electrolytes/premature infants (Smith 1949)	Circulatory studies in RDS (Rudolph 1961) Physiology of respiration in RDS (James 1959)	Nasojejunal feeding tube (Rhea 1970)	*Surfactant for treatment of RDS (Enhorning 1980)*	Cryotherapy/ ROP (Palmer 1986)	
	Thermal environment/survival (Silverman 1958)	Aortic blood pressure in the newborn (Kitterman 1969) Umbilical artery catheterization (Cochran 1968)	*Head ultrasound (Bejar 1980)*	Dexamethasone/ BPD (Avery 1985)	
			Non-invasive cerebral blood flow measurement (Leahy 1979)	ROP international classification (Patz 1984)	
		Grunting in HMD (Harrison 1968)		Cost analysis of NICU care (Walker 1984)	

Cont. **Table 1.**

Neonatal anoxia/intellectual development (Apgar 1955)	BPD *(Northway 1967)*	Idomethacin/PDA (McCarthy 1978)	Bovine surfactant (Smyth 1983)
	Negative pressure ventilation *(Silverman 1967)*	ECMO (Kirkpatrick 1983)	High-frequency ventilation (Frantz 1983)
Birthweight/survival (Wegman 1954)	Pulmonary hyperfusion syndrome *(Chu 1965)*	Non-invasive ICP measurement (Vidyasagar 1977)	Growth/development of infants < 800 gms BW (Bennett 1983)
Thirty years experience/care of premature infants (Hess 1953)	Capillary blood samples *(Gandy 1964)*	Intracranial hemorrhage/CT sca (Krishnamoorthy 1977)	Human amniotic fluid surfactant (Hallman 1983)
	Adjustment of ventilation/acid-base balance, first day of life *(Prod'hom 1964)*	Hyperosmolality/NEC (Willis 1977)	
	IV glucose/NaHCO3 in RDS *(Usher 1963)*	PDA in LBW infants *(Siassi 1976)*	Outcomes/ELBW (Hack 1996)
	Intrauterine growth curves, *(Lubchenco 1963)*	Transillumination diagnosis of pneumothorax (Kuhns 1975)	
	Detection of PKU *(Guthrie 1963)*	Intravenous lipids in TPN (Heird 1975)	Nitric oxide/ PPHN (Kinsella 1993)
		Prevention of apnea/theophyllin (Shannon 1975)	
		Transcutaneous PO2 monitoring (Rooth, Fenner 1975)	Liquid ventilation (Greenspan 1990)
		L/S ratio (Gluck 1974)	

* Table shows landmark publications related to Hyaline Membrane Disease/Respiratory Distress Syndrome since 1948. Italics indicates publications in the journal Paediatrics an official journal of the American Academy of Paediatrics. Others were published elsewhere. For simplicity, only the years are given

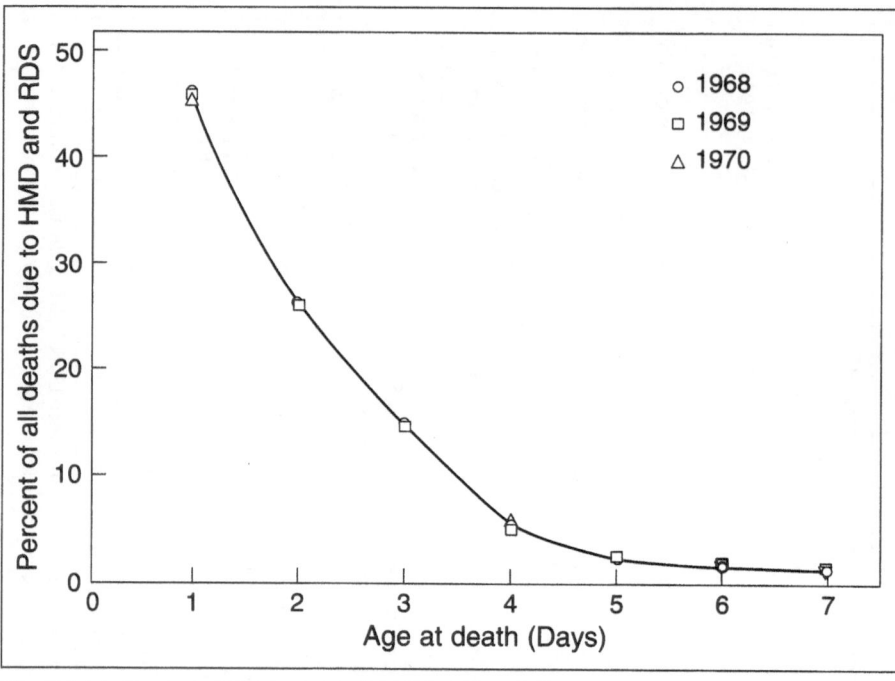

Fig. 1. Mortality from RDS 1968-70. (Modified from [4])

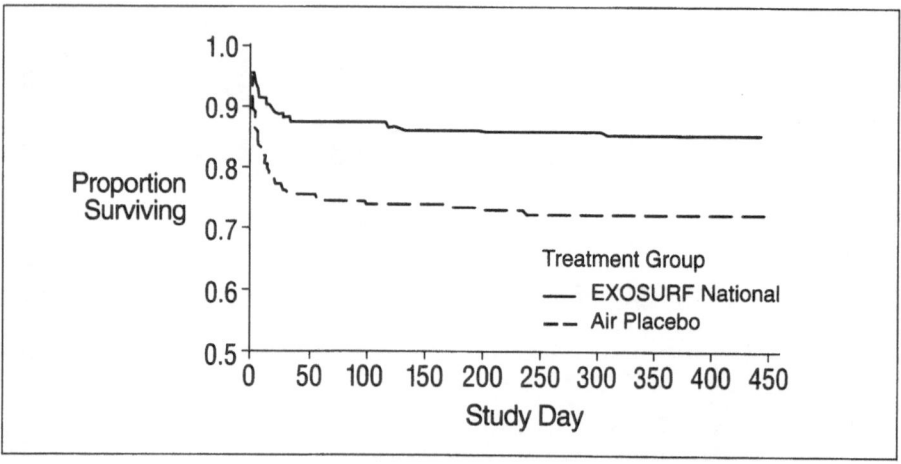

Fig. 2. Survival of infants treated with Exosurf or placebo through one year

HMD in USA. Further majority died within the first 3 days of life. It should also be noted that most survivors were <2 500 g in birth weight. The Kaplan
Meir survival curve from surfactant studies in 1990s shows a dramatic improvement in survival rates (Fig. 1) [5]. Almost 90% survive the disease if treat-

ed with surfactant, including infants of 700-1 100 g at birth. These data indicate a dramatic improvement when compared to those of the previous two decades. Further those who succumb die much later than 3 days of age. Only extremely immature infants die in <3 days of age. The change in the natural history of the disease is the reflection of the advances made in neonatal care over the last three decades.

Lung maturation

Since RDS is a manifestation of lung immaturity, it is critical to understand the process of lung development and lung maturation. The lung starts as a ventral outgrowth of primitive gut as early as 25 day old embryo. It begins to divide into two major bronchi as early as 12 weeks. By 22-24 weeks of gestation the tubular bronchi are divided down to small respiratory bronchioles with terminal alveoli. At this point the alveoli are simple hemispheres where gas exchange can take place. Further growth of lung into mesenchyme continues, with formation of multiple alveoli by 35 weeks of gestation and continues well after birth.

The basic alveolar morphology consists of alveolar lining of two types of cells: type I and type II cells. It is in type II cells that surfactant is produced stored and transported within the cells. The number of lamellar bodies in these cells increases with gestation. By term, lamellar bodies contain mature surfactant. Although, lamellar bodies are released into alveoli even in early gestation, the onset of breathing at birth causes a surge of release of lamellar bodies into the alveoli. The surfactant from the lamellar bodies is absorbed into the thin air liquid interface.

The presence of surfactant in the alveolar lining stabilizes the alveoli during expiration, since it lowers the surface tension at lower lung volume. This is fundamental to the evolution of infants ability to establish normal functional residual capacity (FRC) after the first breath, and normal ventilatory pattern after birth [6]. Since surfactant deficiency is a mark of immature lung, the prematurely born infant has difficulty in establishing a "physiologically normal first breath" thus a normal FRC; this leads to various degrees of atelectasis which clinically manifests as RDS/HMD.

Surfactant recovered from lungs contains 70% to 80% phospholipid, 10% protein and 10% neutral lipids [7]. Phosphatydyl choline is the predominant component of phospholipid (80%). Much of the protein in alveolar lavage is not specific to surfactant. However, four surfactant specific proteins have been identified [8].

Surfactant protein A: (SP-A). A water soluble protein coded on human chromosome 6 with 24 kDa. It is thought to be a regulator of the surfactant metabolism. A number of potential defense properties of SP-A are being recognized. It can suppress or activate macrophage function, facilitate phagocytosis, and bind to pathogens such as *Staphylococcus aureus*. SP-A protein deficient patients have not yet been identified.

Surfactant protein B: (SP-B). The gene is located on human chromosome 2. Translation product is 40 kDa. It is essential to surface tension lowering property. Infants with genetic deficiency have lethal RDS after term birth. Animals with antibodies to SP-B develop RDS. It seems to be most important surfactant protein.

Surfactant protein C: (SP-C). Its gene is on chromosome 8. It is a 22 kDa protein. Absence of SP-C in experimental model results in disrupted lung development. It helps adsorption of surfactant, no SP-C deficient lung disease has been identified.

Surfactant protein D: (SP-D). A 43 kDa protein similar to SP-A, it is thought to function as a host defense molecule, by binding pathogene and facilitating clearance.

Pathophysiology of respiratory distress syndrome

A normal term infant initiates lung inflation with generation of 40-60 cmH_2O pleural negative pressure and expands lungs to a volume of 40 ml/kg [6]. During expiration the lungs deflate only partially, establishing a FRC of 20-30 ml/kg, with the help of alveolar lining of surfactant. The final normal respiratory pattern consists of a tidal volume of 5-6 ml/kg with a transpulmonary pressure of 6 cmH_2O. A premature baby will also initiate breathing with a weak cry because of poorly compliant, surfactant-deficient lungs and a highly compliant chest wall. The initial lung expansion will lead to a considerably lower volume than that in a full-term lung. Furthermore, the high alveolar surface tension causes collapse of the alveoli on expiration. As such, the functional residual capacity falls to near-zero at the end of each breath. The clinical presentation of an infant with HMD demonstrates the attempted – but inadequate – compensation for these problems. Respiratory distress begins soon after birth and is manifested by sternal retractions (compliant chest, noncompliant lungs), expiratory grunting, and flaring of the nasal alae (an attempt to maintain the functional residual capacity). With nearly every breath there is progressive pulmonary atelectasis (the pathologic hallmark of HMD), with continued worsening of lung compliance.

A low, uneven ventilation-perfusion ratio compounded with physical fatigue leads to hypoventilation. Hypoxia and hypercapnia will lead to the development of acidosis.

Postnatal diagnosis

The clinical features of RDS are well recognized. They consist of tachypnea, retractions, cyanosis, grunting, and poor aeration of lungs [9]. Following are the major clinical features and their physiologic basis, which is important to understand (Table 2).

Table 2. Clinical respiratory distress scoring system. (From [9])

Clinical sign	Score		
	0	1	2
Respiratory rate (per minute)	60	60-80	>80 or apneic episode
Cyanosis	None	In air	In 40% O^2
Retractions	None	Mild	Moderate to severe
Grunting	None	Audible with stethoscope	Audible without stethoscope
Air entry* (crying)	Clear	Delayed or decreased	Barely audible

* Air entry represents the quality of inspiratory breath sounds as heard in the midaxillary line

Tachypnea and apnea

Tachypnea is the most frequent and easily recognized sign in infants; the normal rate in infants is 40 breaths per minute. Respiratory rates beyond 60/min are consistent with increasinghy compromised condition of the infant. Although infants with HMD initially have high respiratory rates, they eventually may show apnea denoting either accumulation of excess CO_2 or muscular exhaustion or terminal CNS hemorrhage.

Retractions

Chest wall retractions are associated with pulmonary or upper airway changes. Under normal conditions, the expansion of chest wall requires no energy beyond the normal tidal volume. However, an increased effort is made to expand the non-compliant lung via decreasing the pleural pressure. The thoracic cage is drawn in because of the very compliant nature of the neonatal rib cage. Thus, retractions indicate an increase in the efforts of the neonate to improve lung expansion. The degree of retraction correlates well with the degree of severity of the disease. However, retractions are also noted in conditions other than RDS. As previously mentioned, increased retractions lead to increased O_2 consumption, and hence, to muscular exhaustion. These contribute to the accumulation of lactic acid. In persistent hypoxemia, anaerobic metabolic pathways continue and add to metabolic acidosis.

Prenatal diagnosis

Prenatal diagnosis of infants at risk of developing RDS is based on the analysis of the amniotic fluid for the presence of pulmonary surfactant, namely, lecithin and sphingomyelin [10]. The relationship of the presence of these substances to the occurrence of RDS is best expressed by the L/S ratio at different gestational ages. Prior to 34 weeks gestation, the ratio is 1, which begins to increase thereafter. Various studies indicate that L/S ratios greater than 2.0 are associated with little risk of RDS, unless the mother has diabetes. When the ratio was 1.5 to 2.0, a 40% risk of RDS was seen. When the ratio was less than 1.5, 73% of infants developed RDS. On the other hand, when the L/S ratio was more than 2.5, the incidence of RDS was less than 1%. However, the relationship of L/S ratio to the development of RDS may be altered in the presence of maternal diabetes or erythroblastosis. Identification of phosphatidylglycerol (PG) in addition to L/S ratio has been recommended, since PG is only produced in fetal lungs. Amniotic fluid, L/S ratio assessment, and identification of PG are an essential part of the workup in the assessment of fetal maturity. This is indicated in pregnancies of uncertain dates, fetal growth assessment, and elective cesarean sections.

Grunting

Grunting is common in infants with RDS. It is produced by the passage of exhaled gases through narrowing vocal cords. The phenomenon has a significant physiologic implication. Through close approximation of vocal cords during expiration intra-alveolar pressure is generated, which in effect distends the collapsing alveoli. Since the hallmark of RDS is collapse of alveoli during expiration, this natural mechanism will improve distribution of ventilation. When grunting is eliminated by intubation, the arterial PO_2 drops immediately [11]. Similarly, when artificially adding end-expiratory pressure, the arterial PO_2 improves, hence, the importance of the presence of grunt in HMD.

Breath sounds

Auscultation in the neonate must be a part of routine examination. Breath sounds are described as decreased, poor or absent. However, because of the small thoracic cavity, such observations are, at best, only estimates. One has to be careful in assessing small differences that exist between the two sides of the chest and also the presence of breath sounds that might exist despite atelectasis or pneumothorax. When there is a discrepancy between clinical findings and physiologic states, one must attempt to further establish the underlying problem by X-ray.

Cyanosis

Oxygen desaturation in RDS is the end result of the basic lung pathophysiology. In neonates clinical cyanosis is commonly associated with arterial PO_2 levels less than 40 mmHg. Current technologies, which provide accurate and continuous methods of quantifying oxygenation of blood, include transcutaneous PO_2 measurements, intra-arterial PO_2 electrodes, and intra-arterial oximeters.

Radiologic diagnosis

Radiologic examination is the most important diagnostic procedure in infants with respiratory distress. The distinctive features of RDS have been well described in the literature. The common and earlier features consist of the so-called reticulogranular pattern. In a moderate-to-severe disease the chest X-ray shows air bronchogram extending beyond the cardiac shadow. In a severe form of the disease the X-ray of the chest is totally white, so that one cannot distinguish the cardiac silhouette from the overlying opaque lung. The prognosis of the disease correlates well with the severity of the changes seen in X-ray. One of the major differential diagnoses is group B streptococcal pneumonia. Other associated findings along with the typical findings already described are pneumothorax and pneumomediastinum, and pulmonary interstitial emphysema.

A normal chest film in the early course of the disease does not exclude RDS. Hence, in the presence of persisting respiratory distress, chest X-ray should be repeated. X-ray should be obtained at the bedside, using a portable machine because infants are too sick to be removed from the unit or from the bed. Procedures should be done with minimum disturbance to the infant. If the infant is in an oxygen hood or on the respirator, utmost care should be taken not to disrupt the therapy.

Laboratory findings

Acute hypoxia and hypovolemia are two clinical problems associated with RDS. Changes in these two physiologic variables can only be assessed by measuring arterial blood gases and blood pressure by intra-arterial line catheters [12]. Patency of umbilical artery in the immediate neonatal period provides an easy access to indwelling catheters. Catheters have been placed at other arterial sites as well (i.e., radial, temporal, and posterior tibia). Repeated blood sampling for blood gas tension and pH measurements can be made through these arterial lines or intermittent arterial punctures.

Capillary blood sampling from warmed heel in the neonate has been used for blood gas and pH monitoring in infants with RDS. However, there are limitations in interpretation. Capillary PO_2 correlates well within a range of 40 to 60 mmHg of PO_2 only.

More recently, noninvasive methods of monitoring blood gases have become routine [13]. The limitations of noninvasive blood gas monitoring are well understood. More important, the physiologic significance of transcutaneous PO_2 values in relation to PaO_2 values should be interpreted appropriately. Experience with transcutaneous monitoring in the neonate shows that both $PtcO_2$ and $PtcCO_2$ depend on blood PaO_2, $PaCO_2$, and blood flow. When flow is adequate, $PtcO_2$ follows PaO_2 when flow is compromised but PaO_2 is adequate, $PtcO_2$ tracks flow. When both saturation and flow are compromised, $PtcO_2$ and PaO_2 are low. $PtcO_2$ monitoring will obviate repeated arterial sampling. During the last 15 years, the use of O_2 saturation monitoring has become routine in all neonatal intensive care units [14].

Hypoxemia and acidosis with increasing respiratory distress are the primary findings in infants with RDS. Continuation of metabolic acidosis and superimposed respiratory acidosis due to hypoventilation are also evident. Initial PaO_2 may vary from 50 to 60 mmHg even while breathing high O_2 concentrations. In some infants even 100% O_2 does not increase PaO_2 beyond 100 mmHg, suggesting a major R → L shunt at both pulmonary and patent ductus arteriosus (PDA) level. Alveolar to arterial O_2 ($AaDO_2$) gradients will increase. Hypoventilation reflected by high $PaCO_2$ indicates muscular exhaustion. Metabolic acidosis is due to anaerobic metabolism and lactic acidosis. Hypoglycemia (blood glucose <40 mg/dl) may ensue unless intravenous glucose supplementation is started. Serum electrolytes show varying degrees of hyperkalemia (normal levels: K^+ 3.5 mEq/l), suggesting ongoing tissue catabolism. Other electrolytes remain within the normal levels unless the clinical course is complicated by dehydration (caused by excessive insensible water loss or overhydration caused by excess fluids or decreased renal functions.

Since premature infants also have low hemoglobin levels, blood workup should include a complete blood cell count (CBC), including reticulocyte count. When hematocrit is <40% or hemoglobin <13 g/dl, the infant needs a blood transfusion. Since premature infants do not have the ability to handle bilirubin, hyperbilirubinemia is not uncommon. Serum bilirubin levels should be measured on a daily basis, and treated with phototherapy. Very rarely infants would require exchange transfusion.

Intracranial hemorrhage is known to occur frequently. Although the incidence and degree of intraventricular hemorrhage (IVH) is steadily decreasing. A baseline assessment of the head using a bedside ultrasound should be made early in the course of the disease. The ultrasound should be repeated to document the presence, absence, or degree of progress of the hemorrhage because, if present, this information will be useful for assessing the prognosis.

Principles of management

The birth of infants at risk of developing RDS can be anticipated by evaluation of amniotic fluid L/S ratio [10]. A paediatrician or a neonatologist should be in attendance at premature births and high-risk deliveries to provide proper care.

Prenatal management

Since the basis of RDS is the birth of premature infant, the goal should be either to prevent premature birth, (i.e. to delay labor) or to accelerate lung maturation to minimize the risk of developing RDS. It could be unequivocally said that the major advance made in perinatal medicine is the management of fetal surveillance, fetal steroid treatment and management of preterm labor, using tocolytic agents.

The pathogenesis of preterm labor is not well understood. It is multifactorial in origin. Among the many causes chorioamnionitis has gained considerable importance as a cause of preterm labor. The bacteria in lower genital tract gain access in amnion and amniotic fluid leading to inflammatory reaction and release of prostaglandin PGE2 which initiates labor. Management of preterm labor consists in preventing the initiation of labor, and inhibiting the preterm labor [15]. Overall improvement in antenatal care of at risk mother, bed rest and supportive therapy and treatment of underlying causes may ameliorate initiation of preterm labor. Once the preterm labor sets in, tocolysis and management by expert perinatal care are required. A variety of tocolytic agents, including β-adrenergic agonist ritodrine, prostaglandin synthetase inhibitor, oxytocin agonists and $MgSO_4$. Despite these agents and bed rest premature labor may progress. Thus the management of preterm labor includes treatment with glucocorticoid to enhance lung maturation [16].

Maternal corticosteroid therapy

The majority of published reports have demonstrated the effectiveness of antenatal steroid therapy in reducing the incidence of RDS in prematurely born infants. A meta-analysis of randomized controlled placebo/steroid treatment showed a decrease of 50% in RDS with no adverse later outcome even at 12 years of age [17]. Based on these findings, the National Institute of Health (NIH) consensus panel strongly recommend that:
- all fetuses 24-34 week gestation at risk of premature delivery be considered for antenatal corticoid treatment;
- the optimal benefit of treatment is 24 hours after initiation of therapy and lasts for 7 days;
- the treatment consists of two 12-mg doses of betamethasone 1m given at 24-h interval or 6 mg given at 12-h interval [18].

The overall benefits of antenatal corticosteroid are far more outreaching. It also reduces mortality and morbidity, such as necrotizing enterocolitis, periventricular hemorrhage and patent ductus arteriosus. In addition, it shortens hospital stay leading to a decrease in cost. It is estimated to save $200 000 to 500 000 per 100 infants treated, with an annual saving of 61 million dollars according to cost analysis in USA [19]. Risks of antenatal corticosteroid treatment include potential increase in infections and loss of diabetic control moreover, multiple therapies prior to delivery may have adverse effect on fetal brain growth. An attempt to use corticosteroid in combination with thyroid releasing hormone to enhance lung maturation has not proved to be beneficial. Overall antenatal corticosteroid treatment has been steady from a low 18% in 1990 to 66% in 1996 (Table 3) in infants who were born with birth weight of <1 500 g. Overall use may be higher if all preterm deliveries are considered.

Table 3. Fetal exposure to antenatal steroids in less than 1500 g infants during 1990-1996 (From Vermont Oxford Data, Burlington, USA)

%	1990	1991	1992	1993	1994	1995	1996
None	81	76	73	67	53	41	34
Partial	6	7	8	9	15	19	21
Complete	12	17	19	24	32	40	45

Use of surfactant therapy

Since 1959, when Avery and Meade first reported that surfactant deficiency is the underlying cause of RDS [20] extensive investigations have been made to study the surfactant synthesis, its isolation and possible replacement treatments. Fujiwara [21] successfully demonstrated the effectiveness of exogenous surfactant in treating infants with severe RDS. Since then, multiple controlled trials have confirmed its effectiveness in reducing the severity of RDS, mortality and complications from RDS [22, 23]. The details on surfactant therapy are given elsewhere in this symposium.

There is a proven benefit of combined use of prenatal steroid and postnatal surfactant therapy [24]. The effects are additive. Antenatal steroids induce structural maturation of lung along with enhancement of surfactant synthesis. A controlled trial of prior steroid or placebo in infants later treated with surfactant showed that antenatal steroids reduced pulmonary morbidity and periventricular leukomalacia. Postnatal surfactant therapy clearly made a difference in the natural history of RDS [5].

Respiratory distress syndrome: bronchopulmonary dysplasia-chronic lung disease

Bronchopulmonary dysplasia (BPD), or chronic lung disease (CLD), is the most vexing residual problem of RDS. Twenty per cent to 40% of infants with RDS go on to develop BPD/CLD [25]. The improved survival in extremely premature infants increases the number of infants developing BPD/CLD. The effects of BPD are both of medical (i.e., recurrent infections, cardiopulmonary compromise) and economic concern because of the cost of caring prolonged O_2 or ventilator-dependent infants.

The focus of research on BPD has been a part of overall investigation on RDS. Since Northway's [26] first description of BPD, the clinicians' view point consisted of 4 major underlying factors: immaturity, O_2 toxicity, barotrauma and time [27]. Extensive studies imply that O_2 induced inflammatory reaction is the triggering factor in the pathogenesis of BPD. This model offers opportunity to explore the biochemical basis of pulmonary injury following O_2 exposure. Series of events lead to the ultimate lung injury [28].

In the preterm infant lungs show greater alveolar capillary membrane permeability leading to protein leakage. The proteins in the pulmonary oedema fluids inactivate surfactants, exaggerating the primary surfactant deficiency.

Neonatal lungs exposed to O_2 injury also show influx of neutrophils, which contain variety of toxic elements affecting phagocytosis. Along with these activities many oxyradicals, proteases and platelet activity factors are released which damage the lung tissue. In addition, premature infants are subject to a variety of ischemia-reperfusion events. These events are associated with bursts of superoxide anion production by xanthine oxidase. Premature infants are also deficient in antioxidants (i.e., low levels of superoxide dismutase (SOD) enzyme levels). All these deficiencies lead to cascade of events causing lung damage.

Therapeutic approaches

Several attempts have been made to reduce oxygen toxicity by administering antioxidants Vitamin E [29], Vitamin A [30, 31], and SOD [32, 33]. Steroids have also been used to suppress inflammation [34-36]. Steroid postnatal treatment of 2-4 week-old infants with BPD have shown ability to wean off O_2 and to allow early extubation. Now steroids are routinely used to wean BPD infants. Steroid treatment has been shown to decrease markers of lung inflammation, neutrophil count, elastase/L, protease inhibitor ratio, free elastase activity, albumin and fibrinectin concentration [37]. Levels of urinary hydroxyproline also decreased with steroid treatment thus implicating decreased collagen synthesis [38].

In a recent randomized study some investigators used steroids within 12 h of birth on infants with severe RDS [39]. They found that steroid treated infants with chronic lung disease had lower concentration of LTB_4, 6-ketoPGF, α-1 protein and cell count in the tracheal aspirate than control patients, all suggesting anti-inflammatory action of steroids. The steroid treated infants had transient higher BP and blood glucose levels and cardiac septal hypertrophy. There was no increase in mortality, IVH, ROP or NEC neither in steroid nor in control groups. However, caution is indicated in advancing the early treatment with steroids.

Vitamin E [29]

Premature infants are deficient in α-tocopherol levels. This deficiency causes lipid peroxidation of the cell membrane. Unfortunately, treatment with Vitamin E has not proven to be beneficial in reducing BPD.

Vitamin A [30, 31]

Retinol (Vitamin A) promotes differentiation of various epithelial cell populations. Preterm infants have low levels of Vitamin A. There is a correlation between Vitamin A deficiency and the development of BPD. One controlled interventional study with supplementation of Vitamin A showed a decreased incidence of BPD; however, subsequent studies failed to confirm previous findings. There is a need for further well controlled studies.

Superoxide dismutase treatment

Number of studies show deficiency of SOD in premature lungs [32, 33]. It may be postulated that exogenous SOD helps reduce BPD. Since SOD has a very short half-life (4 min), SOD capsulated within liposomes or conjugated to polyethylene glycol has been tried. Subsequently SOD was delivered intratracheally. The later study results are yet to be published. Though being a logical antioxidant enzyme (with potential benefits) SOD has not yet found to be ready for clinical use to prevent oxygen induced by injury.

In summary, the bronchoalveolar inflammatory response leads to release of many enzymes that are injurious to lung. Understanding these mechanisms allows clinicians to develop newer approaches to prevent, ameliorate and treat BPD. Prenatal steroids, postnatal surfactant and steroid treatment at the moment seem to be most effective in preventing BPD.

Advances in ventilatory management

Initiation of mechanical assisted ventilation in infants with RDS in the late 1950's and early 1960's was a major step forward [20]. However, the limiting factor was the lack of appropriate technology for neonatal use. In mid 60's the survival of ventilated infants was only 30%-35%. Introduction of constant positive airway pressure (CPAP) independent of assisted mechanical ventilation or in conjunction with it (PEEP) in 1970 made a dramatic improvement in survival [40].

Early use of CPAP in RDS has reduced need for subsequent mechanical ventilation. A single dose of surfactant in infants with moderate RDS followed by CPAP has shown to improve gas exchange. There are many techniques of delivering CPAP.

Conventional mechanical ventilation

During the last four decades conventional mechanical ventilation (CMV) in the neonate has improved to a great deal. Besides building ventilators to meet the physiologic limits of the extremely small infants, various new modes of ventilation are also being introduced. Recently patient-triggered ventilation has been utilized to trigger the ventilator by the infant's inspiratory effort. This technique allows improved Vt, and blood gases [41, 42].

Synchronized IMV allows the infant to trigger the ventilator only on a fraction of respiratory effort. In clinical trials these techniques reduced duration of assisted ventilation and facilitated weaning [43]. Proportional assisted ventilation is a technique which amplifies the flows generated by the patient in proportion to his respiratory effort with the purpose of normalizing ventilation.

Advantages include: patient comfort, less peak airway pressure, less need for sedation. Obviously, presence of patient effort is critical to initiating the inspiration. This new technique is still under study. Several clinical trials have compared different ventilators. The results show no definitive superiority of one ventilator over the other, or one ventilatory mode over the other. Clinicians must get acquainted with the ventilator they intend to use, and also understand all the technicalities involved.

Negative pressure ventilation

Negative pressure ventilation was used for neonates with respiratory failure during 1960's-1980's [44-46]. It has been used as both intermittent and constant negative pressure ventilator. An advantage of this ventilation is that it does not require intubation. A disadvantage is its limitation of use for extremely small infants. Because of this, negative pressure ventilation has not been used routinely. In recent years a few investigators are beginning to recognize certain advantages of negative pressure ventilation, but overall it has limited use.

High-frequency ventilation

It is the mode of ventilation that employs respiratory frequencies of 150-600 breaths per min. These ventilators, jet as well as oscillatory, have been used in number of clinical trials [47-49].

Controlled trials of jet ventilation in RDS infants demonstrated adequately improved gas exchange, lower PIP and mean airway pressure lower than conventional ventilation. Early use have not resulted in reduction of mortality or morbidity. In infants with interstitial emphysema it helps to resolve the air leak. Other advantages include: less cardiovascular compromise, help in bronchopulmonary fistula, and in persistant pulmonary hypertension of newborn (PPHN). Problems are associated with appropriate humidification.

High-frequency oscillatory ventilation is different since the expiration is actively generated. It generates extremely small volumes at high rates of 600-900 breaths per min.

Controlled studies showed that incidence of BPD or mortality was not improved, but was associated with grade III & IV IVH. Recent studies using higher mean airway pressure are showing improved results. Overall meta-analysis of various studies of high-frequency ventilation (HFV) have not shown any superannuity over CMV in reducing mortality or morbidity.

Other methods of ventilation: liquid ventilation

This technique uses inert per fluorocarbon liquid which has high solubility for oxygen. Lung is filled with liquid and ventilated using conventional mechanical ventilation. Another technique is to only to instill the lung equivalent to FRC [50]. Extensive animal studies have shown the effectiveness of liquid ventilation in oxygenation. Clinical experience in a few small infants has shown dramatic advantages [51]. However, clinical trials to study advantages of liquid ventilation over CMV still have to be made. Liquid ventilation can also be used to deliver drugs into alveoli; it may be used in conjunction with HFV and surfactant therapy. We need to wait for more information regarding the benefits of liquid ventilation.

Although extrocorporal membrane oxygenation (ECMO) [52] and nitric oxide [53] have been used extensively in the management of difficult to ventilate term infants. Infants with RDS rarely need these alternate approaches.

Complications of respiratory distress syndrome

The natural history of RDS has changed considerably over the last thirty years. Before 1960's most infants either survived within the first three days or succumbed to death, the severe ones dying before any complications occurred. With the advent of oxygen therapy, assisted ventilation, correction of biochemical abnormalities, and introduction of vascular invasive techniques, the natural history has been punctuated with numerous complications while still in the hospital. These can be classified as acute complications and late complications. The major acute complications consist of pulmonary barotrauma, intraventricular hemorrhage, and patent ductus arteriosus (PDA). The late complications consist of bronchopulmonary dysplasia and retinopathy of prematurity (ROP). Complications that are noticed after discharge and during follow-up consist of neuro-developmental delays and difficulties in schooling. Vast experience over the years shows that most acute complications have been minimized through more skilled medical and nursing personnel and improved technology. The complications of pulmonary barotrauma have been significantly reduced since the introduction of surfactant replacement therapy. The incidence of pneumothorax and pulmonary interstitial emphysema (PIE), which was in the range of 25%-30% in the 60's, has been reduced to less than 5%. The incidence of BPD has been somewhat slow to be reduced. The incidence of PDA has not been affected by surfactant therapy, neither was IVH. There is some increase in the incidence of pulmonary hemorrhage following surfactant therapy. Besides decreasing the incidence of RDS, antenatal steroid therapy has also reduced the severity of the disease and its associated complications.

In general, the neuro-developmental and scholastic achievements of these infants are more related to birth weight and gestational age than to RDS itself. One can foresee that the birth weight of survivors will continue decreasing reaching lower than 500 g. Such immature infants will continue to pose challens to neonatologists in the next decade. This presentation covers various aspects of the complications from RDS. Although good prenatal care, antenatal steroid therapy followed by surfactant therapy, supportive intensive care, and ventilatory care would decrease mortality and morbidity from RDS, its economic and social burden will remain a main concern.

Life after surfactant

Surfactant treatment has changed the life in numerous ways. There is a definitive decrease in mortality in each of 100 g birth weight groups starting from 600 g upwards, following the routine use of surfactant (Tables 4 and 5). Schwartz et al. [54] have shown decreased utilization of resources. Cost analysis also shows decreased overall cost per survivor. This was particularly evident in infants with birth weight >1250 g. This group of infants recover faster, are extubated earlier, thus requiring shorter hospital stay. Utilization of hospital resources (i.e., laboratory tests, X-rays, etc.) are also decreased, leading to savings of dollars.

Paradoxically but expectedly, the saving of lifes (improved survival) in extremely low birth weight infants, adds cost because of extended hospital stay. Prolonged hospital stay in this group of infants is primarily due to immaturity (i.e., limitations in meeting nutritional needs, and associated complications of parenteral nutrition). Low gestation also makes the infant susceptible to multiple infections.

BPD/CLD, the sequelae of RDS, although minimized continue to be major factors for prolonged hospital stays. Various home health care programs have been developed to facilitate discharge of infants who are ventilator and/or O_2 dependant. These newly emerging diseases require that community physicians and health care workers become acquainted with the special needs of these infants.

All controlled and randomized studies have clearly shown that complications of RDS, particularly air leaks, have significantly decreased from 20% prior to surfactant to 10% or less post surfactant era. However, the incidence of BPD and CLD has not decreased significantly. The incidence of IVH has also decreased during the last decade. The incidence of grade III/IV IVH being as low as 5% in infants <1500 g birth weight.

Long term outcome has shown no difference in infants treated with or with-

Table 4. Incidence of RDS and surfactant treatment and mortality by weight. (From Vermont Oxford Data, Burlington, USA)

	600	700	501/ 800	601/ 900	701/ 1000	801/ 1100	901/ 1200	1001/ 1300	1101/ 1400	1201/ 1500
RDS %	90	90	86	84	78	69	62	52	48	42
Surfactant %	82	84	80	75	70	68	52	41	36	30
Overall survival %	38	64	80	85	91	94	95	96	97	97

Table 5. Incidence of RDS and surfactant treatment and mortality by gestational age. (From Vermont Oxford Data, Burlington, USA)

GA weeks	<23	23	24	25	26	27	28	29	30	31	32
Survival %	4	18	56	74	84	90	92	94	96	96	96

GA, gestational age

out surfactant. Outcome variables were more related to lower birth weight, lower gestational age and existence of neurologic problems (i.e., intraventricular hemorrhage). Children who were followed for 10-12 years after steroid exposure showed advantage of prenatal steroids in lowering neurologic abnormalities and no difference in psychomotor scores [57].

Conclusions

Since the early description of HMD in German literature in 1903 [55] numerous landmark laboratory investigations and clinical observations were followed by new and improved therapeutic interventions which altered the course of RDS/HMD. This century has seen the "rise and fall" of respiratory distress syndrome. There was maximum scientific activity in this field during the decades of 1970's and 1980's. This evolution was important not only from the perspective of RDS/HMD but also for the development of the new field of neonatal medicine.

Comroe [56] termed the early years of neonatal pulmonary investigation as "premature science and immature lungs". Today we continue to deal with "mature science and very immature lungs!". The closure of the chapter on RDS will depend on prevention (improving social problems) on one hand and on genetic engineering (molecular bases of diagnosis and treatment) on the other hand.

References

1. Wegman ME (1996) Infant mortality: some international comparisons. Pediatrics 96:1020-1027
2. Liechty EA, Donovan E, Purohit D et al (1991) Reduction of neonatal mortality after multiple doses of bovine surfactant in low birth weight neonates with respiratory distress syndrome. Pediatrics 88:19-28
3. Vidyasagar D, Bickers RO, Butterfield J (1998) Publication trends in the field of neonatology. A review of first half century. Pediatr Res 43:329A
4. Farrell PM, Wood RE (1976) Epidemiology of hyaline membrane disease in the United States: analysis of national mortality statistics. Pediatrics 58:167-183
5. Corbet A, Bucciarelli R, Goldman S et al (1991) Decreased mortality among small premature infants treated at birth with a single dose of synthetic surfactant, a multicenter controlled trial. J Pediatr 118:277-284
6. Karlberg P, Cherry RB, Escardo FE, Koch G (1962) Respiratory studies in newborn infants, II. Pulmonary ventilation and mechanics of breathing in first minutes of life, including onset of respiration. Acta Paediat Scand 51:121-26
7. Klaus MH, Clements JA, Havel RJ (1967) Composition of surface active material isolated from beef lung. Proc Natl Acad Sci 47:1858
8. Hagwood S, Shiffer K (1991) Structures and properties of the surfactant-associated proteins. Ann Rev Physiol 53:375-394
9. Downes JJ, Vidyasagar D, Morrow GM et al (1970) Respiratory distress syndrome of newborn infants. New clinical scoring system with acid-base and blood gas correlations. Clin Pediatr 9:325-331

10. Gluck L, Kulovich MV, Borer RC et al (1971) Diagnosis of respiratory distress syndrome by amniocentesis. Am J Obstet Gynecol 109:440-445

11. Harrison VC, Heese H de V, Klein M (1968) The significance of grunting in hyaline membrane disease. Pediatrics 41:549-559

12. Cochrane WD (1976) Umbilical artery catheterization. Report of the 69th Ross Conference on Pediatric Research. Iatrogenic problems in neonatal intensive care. Columbus Ross Laboratories

13. Huh R, Huch A, Albani M et al (1976) Transcutaneous PO_2 monitoring in routine management of infants and children with cardiopulmonary problems. Pediatrics 57:681-690

14. Jennis MS, Peabody JR (1987) Pulse oximetry: an alternative method for the assessment of oxygenation in newborn infants. Pediatrics 79:524-528

15. ACOG Technical Bulletin (1995) Preterm labour. Int Gynecol Obstet 50:303

16. Liggins GC, Howie RN (1972) A controlled trial of antepartum glucocorticoid treatment for prevention of the RDS in premature infants. Pediatrics 50:515

17. Crowley P (1995) Antenatal corticosteroid therapy: a meta analysis of randomized trials, 1972 to 1994. Am J Obstet Gynecol 173:322-334

18. NIH Consensus Conference (1995) Effect of corticosteroids for fetal maturation on perinatal outcomes. JAMA 273:413-418

19. Simpson KN, Lynch SR (1995) Cost savings from the use of antenatal steroids to prevent respiratory distress syndrome and related conditions in premature infants. Am J Obstet Gynecol 173:316-321

20. Avery ME, Meade J (1959) Surface properties in relation to atelectasis and hyaline membrane disease. Am J Dis Child 97:517-523

21. Fujiwara T, Chida S, Watabe YJ et al (1980) Artificial surfactant therapy in hyaline membrane disease. Lancet 1:55-59

22. Jobe AH (1993) Pulmonary surfactant therapy. N Engl J Med 328:861-868

23. Halliday HL (1997) Clinical trials of surfactant replacement in Europe. Biol Neonate 71(Suppl 1):8-12

24. Jobe AH, Mitchell BR, Grunkel JH (1993) Beneficial effects of the continued use of prenatal corticosteroid and postnatal surfactant on preterm infants. Am J Obst Gynecol 168:508-513

25. Northway WH, Rosan RC, Porter DY (1967) Pulmonary disease following respiratory therapy of hyaline membrane disease: bronchopulmonary dysplasia. N Engl J Med 176:357-368

26. Northway WH (1992) Bronchopulmonary dysplasia: twenty-five years later. Pediatrics 89:969-973

27. Philip AGS (1975) Oxygen plus pressure plus time: the etiology of bronchopulmonary dysplasia. Pediatrics 55:44-50

28. Zimmerman JJ (1995) Broncho alveolar inflammatory pathophysiology of bronchopulmonary dysplasia. Clin Perinatol 22:429-456

29. Saldana RL, Cepeda EE, Poland RL (1982) The effect of vitamin E prophylaxis on the incidence and severity of bronchopulmonary dysplasia. J Pediatr 101:89-93

30. Shenai JP, Chytil F, Stahlman MT (1985) Vitamin A status of neonates with bronchopulmonary dysplasia. Pediatr Res 19:185-189

31. Shenai JP, Kennedy KA, Chytil F et al (1987) Clinical trial of vitamin A supplementation in infants susceptible to bronchopulmonary dysplasia. J Pediatr 111:269-277

32. Rosenfeld W, Concepcion L (1986) Endogenous antioxidant defenses in neonates. Free Radic Biol Med 2:295-298

33. Rosenfeld W, Evans H, Concepcion L (1984) Prevention of bronchopulmonary dyspla-

sia by administration of bovine superoxide dismutase in preterm infants with respiratory distress syndrome. J Pediatr 105:781-785

34. Avery GB, Fletcher AB, Kaplan M et al (1985) Controlled trial of dexamethasone in respiratory dependent infants with bronchopulmonary dysplasia. Pediatrics 75:106-111
35. Cummings JJ, D'Eugenio DB, Gross SJ (1989) A controlled trial of dexamethasone in preterm infants at high risk for bronchopulmonary dysplasia. N Engl J Med 320:1505-1510
36. Yeh TF, Torre JA, Rastogi A et al (1990) Early postnatal dexamethasone therapy in premature infants with severe respiratory distress syndrome: a double-blind, controlled study. J Pediatr 117:273-282
37. Gerdes JS, Harris MC, Polin RA (1988) Effect of dexamethasone and indomethacin on elastosis, L proteinase inhibitor and fibrinectin in bronchoalveolar lavage fluid from neonates. J Pediatr 113:727-731
38. Co E, Chari G, McCulloch K et al (1993) Dexamethasone treatment suppresses collagen synthesis in infants with bronchopulmonary dysplasia. Pediatr Pulm 16:36-40
39. Yeh TF (1996) Prevention of chronic lung disease in premature infants with early dexamethasone therapy procedure of 9th Congress of the Federation of the Asia & Oceania Perinatal Societies. Monduzzi, Bologna
40. Avery ME, Mead J (1959) Surface properties in relation to atelectasis and hyaline disease. Am J Dis Child 97:517-523
41. Gregory GA, Kitterman JA, Phibbs RH et al (1971) Treatment of idiopathic respiratory distress syndrome with continuous positive airway pressure. N Engl J Med 284:1333-1340
42. Mehta A, Wright BM, Callen K et al (1986) Patient triggered ventilation in the newborn. Lancet 2 (8497):17-19
43. South M, Morley CJ (1986) Synchronous mechanical ventilation of the neonate. Arch Dis Child 61:1190-1195
44. Bernstein G, Mannino FL, Heldt GP et al (1996) Randomized multicenter trial comparing synchronized and conventional intermittent mandatory ventilation in neonates. J Pediatr 128:453-463
45. Vidyasagar D, Chernick V (1972) Continuous positive airway pressure in hyaline membrane disease. Pediatrics 49:144
46. Chernick V, Vidyasagar D (1972) Continuous negative chest wall pressure in hyaline membrane disease: one-year experience. Pediatrics 49:753-760
47. Cvetnic WG, Cunningham MD, Sills JH et al (1990) Reintroduction of continuous negative pressure ventilation in neonates. Two-year experience. Pediatr Pulm 8:245-253
48. HIFI Study Group (1989) High frequency oscillatory ventilation compared with conventional mechanical ventilation in the treatment of respiratory failure in preterm infants. N Engl J Med 320:88-93
49. Ogawa Y, Miyasaka K, Kawano T, Imura S, Inukai K et al (1993) A multicenter randomized trial of high frequency oscillatory ventilation as compared with conventional mechanical ventilation in preterm infants with respiratory failure. Early Human Development 32:1-10
50. HIFO Study Group (1993) Randomized study of high frequency oscillatory ventilation in infants with severe respiratory distress syndrome. J Pediatr 122:609-619
51. Greenspan JS, Wolfson MR, Rubenstein D et al (1990) Liquid ventilation of human preterm neonates. J Pediatr 117:106-111
52. Leach C, Greenspan JS, Rubenstein SD et al (1996) Partial liquid ventilation with perflubron in premature infants with severe respiratory distress syndrome. N Engl J Med 335:761-767
53. Bartlett RH (1990) Extracorporeal life support for cardiopulmonary failure. Curr Probl Surg 27:621-705

54. Kinsella JP, Ivy DD, Abman SH (1994) Inhaled nitric oxide improves gas exchange and lowers pulmonary vascular resistance in severe experimental hyaline membrane disease. Pediatr Res 36:402-408
55. Schwartz RM, Luby AM, Scanlon JW, Kellogg RJ (1994) Effect of surfactant on morbidity, mortality, and resource use in newborn infants weighing 500 to 1500 g. N Engl J Med 330:1476-1480
56. Stahlman MT (1984) The history of hyaline membrane disease: hyaline membrane disease pathogenesis and pathophysiology. Grun & Stratton, New York, pp 1-16
57. Comroe JH (1977) Retrospectroscope. Insights into medical discovery. Von Gehr Press, Menlo Park, California

Chapter 23

High frequency ventilation

J.H. Arnold

Acute respiratory failure remains a major cause of morbidity and mortality in both paediatric and adult populations. The reported annual incidence in the United States may be as high as 150 000 cases, with published mortality rates generally ranging between 50% and 70% [1]. Although there is some indication that there have been improvements in outcome recently [2], the underlying pathophysiology responsible for the clinical syndrome is not precisely targeted by continuing modifications of conventional therapy. Although progress has recently been made, particularly regarding the role of the cytokines and adhesion molecules as essential components of the inflammatory cascade in acute lung injury [3], the use of nonconventional modes of supporting gas exchange is becoming increasingly popular in many centers [4]. One of the most promising alternative modes, high frequency ventilation, has been examined in a number of animal models of lung injury as well as in several human populations.

History

The effects of rapid ventilatory rates on gas exchange were first described in 1915 by Henderson and Chillingworth and Jack Emerson was the first to patent a high frequency device for clinical use in 1952 [5]. The theoretic advantages of high frequency ventilation include: a) smaller phasic volume and pressure change; b) gas exchange at significantly lower airway pressures; c) less depression of endogenous surfactant production. The mechanisms of gas exchange involved during high frequency ventilation have been reviewed in detail elsewhere [5]. To summarize, the mechanisms of gas exchange that are most important during high frequency ventilation are bulk axial flow, interregional gas mixing, and molecular diffusion. Previous work on an animal model has shown convincingly that the phenomenon of interregional gas mixing ("pendelluft") is greatly enhanced during high frequency oscillatory ventilation in particular [6].

Animal data

There is an emerging recognition that mechanical ventilation-induced lung injury is related to cyclic volume change. In a classic study, Webb and Tierney showed that ventilating normal rats with peak inspiratory pressures of 45 cmH$_2$O produced significant perivascular edema and an increase in lung weight [7]. In addition, these investigators showed that an end expiratory pressure of 10 cmH$_2$O was protective, suggesting that the absolute level of inspiratory pressure is not as important as the volume change exerienced by the lung during the duty cycle. It has also been shown in a normal animal that binding of the chest and abdomen, with restriction of chest wall movement, prevented lung injury during ventilation with peak inspiratory pressures of 45 cmH$_2$O [8]. This study provided important evidence that microvascular permeability is related not to pressure but to volume change. Dreyfuss et al. have provided similar data in rats, demonstrating that volume is a much more significant contributor to lung injury and than is absolute pressure level, and that PEEP may well be protective in an animal model of mechanical ventilator-induced lung injury [9].

Mathieu-Costello and West have shown that large cyclic volume changes during conventional ventilation are associated with a significant increase in the disruption of the alveolar capillary, and have elegantly documented breaks in the capillary, endothelium that are produced by large tidal volumes [10]. Their research convincingly demonstrates that pulmonary edema is an important component of mechanical ventilator-induced lung injury. Fluid and protein in the alveolar space are well-known inhibitors of surfactant function and thereby act synergistically to decrease lung compliance and further the cycle of repetitive cyclic overdistention and further lung injury.

In a series of experiments in a saline-lavaged rabbit model, Froese et al. [11-15], have demonstrated that lung volume maintenance with minimization of alveolar pressure and volume change using a piston oscillator device is associated with the least degree of mechanical ventilator-induced lung injury. McCulloch et al. [12] demonstrated that high frequency oscillatory ventilation (HFOV) using an optimal lung volume strategy designed to reverse atelectasis resulted in significant improvements in oxygenation and minimized histopathologic evidence of lung injury when compared with a conventionally ventilated group or when compared to animals treated with HFOV and a low lung volume strategy. More recently, Sugiura et al. [15] have shown in the saline-lavaged rabbit that HFOV results in significantly less activation of pulmonary neutrophils, as evidenced by both chemiluminescence and chemotaxis. These findings have been confirmed by a separate group of investigators using luminol-dependent chemiluminescence [16]. Furthermore, it has also been convincingly demonstrated that high frequency oscillatory ventilation prevents the release of thromboxane B$_2$ and PAF, which are important chemical mediators of inflammatory lung injury [17].

There is compelling animal evidence that HFOV may be most effective when used early in the course of respiratory failure in both premature baboons [18, 19] and adult surfactant-depleted rabbits [12]. Furthermore, despite the conceptual appeal of providing gas exchange at reduced airway pressures, there is abundant evidence that an optimal lung volume during HFOV is best achieved utilizing an aggressive volume recruitment strategy with relatively high mean airway pressures [11, 20]. It should also be noted that despite the use of high proximal airway pressures there is an important difference between measurements made at the proximal airway, the trachea and the alveolus. There is a clinically important gradient in both peak and mean airway pressures from ventilator to alveolus [21] which results in limited volume change in the alveolus, which may well be the most important variable in producing mechanical ventilator-induced lung injury [22].

Clinical data

The initial clinical experience with HFOV in premature infants with hyaline membrane disease raised significant concerns about adverse effects on cerebral haemodynamics and the ductus arteriosus as well as an increased incidence of air leak [23]. However, the methods used in that study have been criticized [24], and the conclusions reached by this multicenter collaborative effort regarding the utility of HFOV in this population should be viewed with some skepticism. Clark et al., in a single-center study using a uniform ventilator strategy, have demonstrated that premature infants treated with HFOV have a significantly reduced incidence of chronic lung disease [25]. A recent study in premature infants with severe hyaline membrane disease has shown a significant improvement in oxygenation and a reduced incidence of air leak syndromes in the infants managed with HFOV [26]. In a large multicenter, prospective examination of early intervention with HFOV using a lung recruitment strategy following surfactant administration, Gerstmann et al. demonstrated improved short- and long-term outcomes as well as a significant reduction in total hospital costs attributable to early institution of HFOV [27]. Interestingly, a large, multicenter randomized study of high frequency jet ventilation (HFJV) in preterm infants showed the best pulmonary and neurologic outcomes in the HFJV patients managed with an optimal lung volume approach rather than a low lung volume approach [28].

These data suggest that for preterm infants the volume recruitment approach is beneficial, independent of the high frequency device utilized. A well-conducted meta-analysis of nine studies comparing HFV and conventional ventilation failed to demonstrate a significant increase in the incidence of intraventricular hemorrhage [29]. In most neonatal centers, current ventilatory options include some form of HFV as well as the recognition that aggressive volume recruitment using either incremental increases in mean airway pressure or intermittent, sustained inflation maneuvers are essential to success.

There is limited published information available regarding the use of HFOV in paediatric patients. We have previously described our rescue experience in a small group of paediatric patients with weights ranging from 3 to 42 kg [30]. We utilized an aggressive approach to rapidly attain and maintain optimal lung volume. This typically requires an increase in mean airway pressure of 5-8 cmH$_2$O when converting from conventional to HFOV. Interestingly, despite significant increases in mean airway pressure, haemodynamic compromise as indicated by cardiac index or oxygen delivery does not appear to be an important problem when using this "ideal lung volume" strategy. We have recently completed a prospective, multicenter, randomized clinical study comparing HFOV and conventional mechanical ventilation in paediatric patients with either diffuse alveolar disease or air leak syndrome [31]. These data demonstrate that HFOV offers rapid and sustained improvements in oxygenation without adverse effects on ventilation. The increase in mean airway pressure utilized during use of HFOV does not result in an increase in the incidence of barotrauma and the oxygenation index declines significantly during the first 72 h of HFOV. Despite the use of higher mean airway pressures, the optimal lung volume strategy used in this study was associated with a lower incidence of barotrauma, as indicated by the requirement for supplemental oxygen at 30 days and improved outcome compared with conventional mechanical ventilation. When ventilator subgroups were compared, the patients managed with high frequency oscillation-only had significantly better ranked outcomes than patients managed with conventional ventilation-only and the patients who crossed over from conventional to high frequency ventilation had significantly better ranked outcomes than patients crossed over from high frequency to conventional ventilation.

Given the success of high frequency oscillation in improving outcome, time-sensitive predictors of survival in patients managed with high frequency oscillation would be quite helpful in developing a step-wise ventilatory approach to the patient with acute lung injury. Specifically, are there precise predictors of HFOV failure that would identify the population of patients who may benefit from alternative modes of respiratory support such as extracorporeal membrane oxygenation [32] or liquid ventilation [33]? In our prospective, randomized clinical trial [31], the oxygenation index in survivors was significantly lower than in nonsurvivors during the first 72 h of therapy; furthermore, there was a significant association between time and a decreasing oxygenation index in survivors as well as time and a rising oxygenation index in the nonsurvivors. An oxygenation index of ≥ 42 at 24 h predicted mortality with an odds ratio of 20.8, a sensitivity of 62%, and a specificity of 93%. There is also evidence that early institution of HFOV in the paediatric population is associated with a lower incidence of barotrauma in the patients who survive. In our prospective, randomized study, patients who were treated with HFOV within 72 h of intubation had a significantly lower incidence of chronic lung disease; specifically, the odds ratio for chronic lung disease in surivors was 25.2 in patients who received more than 72 h of conventional ventilation prior to institution of HFOV.

The adult experience with high frequency techniques is difficult to interpret. The only prospective, randomized study thus far published examined the use of a high frequency jet ventilator in 309 adults with respiratory failure [34]. This study included both immunocompetent as well as immunocompromised patients and did not have a standardized measure of severity of illness for inclusion into the study. The patients managed with HFJV achieved similar oxygenation and ventilation at lower airway pressures. However, duration of ICU stay and mortality were not significantly different between the two groups and the authors concluded that HFJV was equivalent, but not superior to, conventional volume-cycled ventilation. A subsequent, uncontrolled report of HFJV at higher frequencies showed improved gas exchange at lower airway pressures following initiation of HFV [35]. However, effects on outcome cannot be evaluated in the absence of concurrent controls and the authors also reported a 15% incidence of mucous dessication, raising significant concerns about the adequacy of humidification in the device studied. A recent, uncontrolled study of high frequency oscillatory ventilation in 17 adults with severe acute respiratory distress syndrome (ARDS) (mean PaO_2/FiO_2 ratio at entry 66) showed a significant increase in the PaO_2/FiO_2 ratio over the first 48 h after initiation of HFOV [36]. The nonsurvivors in this cohort were treated with conventional ventilation for a longer period and had a higher pre-HFOV oxygenation index than the survivors. Several centers are currently collaborating in a prospective, randomized study of HFOV vs CMV in adults with ARDS.

Conclusions

In summary, recognition that lung injury (and lung mechanical properties) in patients with ARDS is inhomogenously distributed and that repetitive cyclic overdistention of the compliant (predominantly nondependent) areas of lung produce lung injury can lead to significant improvements in supportive care in this patient population. In order to make sense of the complex interactions between repetitive cyclic stretch of the acutely injured lung, transpulmonary pressure amplitude, and the tremendous shear stresses generated during alveolar reexpansion, it is useful to keep in mind three important variables:
– the relationship between end expiratory pressure and the critical opening pressure of lung units (the so-called "lower inflection point");
– the magnitude of cyclic stretch forces applied during tidal conventional ventilation;
– the relationship between end inspiratory lung volume and the upper "deflection point" of the pressure-volume curve.

Recently, a prospective, randomized study of adults with ARDS demonstrated that minimizing cyclic parenchymal stretch with titration of PEEP according to the lower inflection point produces better oxygenation, lung compliance, and a higher weaning rate [37]. These investigators have also recently reported that this approach produces significant improvements in survival [38].

In practical terms, it will in most settings be simpler to avoid the lower and upper inflection points as well as minimize cyclic stretch injury by using HFV. Our data suggest that early institution of HFOV in paediatric patients with acute lung injury is associated with a lower incidence of chronic lung disease. Furthermore, ranked outcome analysis of these data demonstrates improved outcomes in patients who are managed with HFOV either primarily or following a failure of conventional mechanical ventilation. The ideal ventilatory approach in patients with hypoxemic respiratory failure may be early institution of an "open lung" strategy using high frequency oscillation with rapid identification of patients who are not likely to survive in order to allow institution of other modes of gas exchange prior to the onset of irreversible lung injury.

References

1. Bernard GR, Artigas A, Brigham KL et al (1994) The American-European consensus conference on ARDS. Am J Respir Crit Care Med 149:818-824
2. Milberg JA, Davis DR, Steinberg KP et al (1995) Improved survival of patients with acute respiratory distress syndrome (ARDS): 1983-1993. JAMA 273:306-309
3. Strieter RM, Kunkel SL (1994) Acute lung injury: the role of cytokines in the elicitation of neutrophils. J Invest Med 42:640-651
4. Ring JC, Stidham GL (1994) Novel therapies for acute respiratory failure. Pediatr Clin North Am 41:1325-1363
5. Wetzel RC, Gioia FR (1987) High frequency ventilation. Pediatr Clin North Am 34:15-38
6. Lehr JL, Butler JP, Westerman PA et al (1985) Photographic measurement of pleural surface motion during lung oscillation. J Appl Physiol 59:623-633
7. Webb HH, Tierney DF (1974) Experimental pulmonary edema due to intermittent positive pressure ventilation with high inflation pressures: protection by positive end-expiratory pressure. Am Rev Respir Dis 110:556-565
8. Hernandez LA, Peevy KJ, Moise AA et al (1989) Chest wall restriction limits high airway pressure-induced lung injury in rabbits. J Appl Physiol 66:2364-2368
9. Dreyfuss D, Soler P, Basset G et al (1988) High inflation pressure pulmonary edema: respective effects of high airway pressure, high tidal volume, and positive end-expiratory pressure. Am Rev Respir Dis 137:1159-1164
10. Mathieu-Costello OA, West JB (1994) Are pulmonary capillaries susceptible to mechanical stress? Chest 105: S102-S107
11. Hamilton PP, Onayemi A, Smyth JA et al (1983) Comparison of conventional and high-frequency ventilation: oxygenation and lung pathology. J Appl Physiol 55:131-138
12. McCulloch PR, Forkert PG, Froese AB (1988) Lung volume maintenance prevents lung injury during high frequency oscillatory ventilation in surfactant-deficient rabbits. Am Rev Respir Dis 137:1185-1192
13. Byford LJ, Finkler JH, Froese AB (1988) Lung volume recruitment during high-frequency oscillation in atelectasis-prone rabbits. J Appl Physiol 64:1607-1614
14. Bond DM, Froese AB (1993) Volume recruitment maneuvers are less deleterious than persistent low lung volumes in the atelectasis-prone rabbit lung during high-frequency oscillation. Crit Care Med 21:402-412
15. Sugiura M, McCulloch PR, Wren S et al (1994) Ventilator pattern influences neutrophil influx and activation in atelectasis-prone rabbit lung. J Appl Physiol 77:1355-1365
16. Matsuoka T, Kawano T, Miyasaka K (1994) Role of high-frequency ventilation in surfactant-depleted lung injury as measured by granulocytes. J Appl Physiol 76:539-544
17. Imai Y, Kawano T, Miyasaka K et al (1994) Inflammatory chemical mediators during conventional ventilation and during high frequency oscillatory ventilation. Am J Respir Crit Care Med 150:1550-1554
18. DeLemos RA, Coalson JJ, Meredith KS et al (1989) A comparison of ventilation strategies for the use of high-frequency oscillatory ventilation in the treatment of hyaline membrane disease. Acta Anaesthesiol Scand Suppl 90:102-107

19. Meredith KS, DeLemos RA, Coalson JJ et al (1989) Role of lung injury in the pathogenesis of hyaline membrane disease in premature baboons. J Appl Physiol 66:2150-2158
20. Froese AB (1989) Role of lung volume in lung injury: HFO in the atelectasis-prone lung. Acta Anaesthesiol Scand Suppl 90:126-130
21. Gerstmann DR, Fouke JM, Winter DC et al (1990) Proximal, tracheal, and alveolar pressures during high-frequency oscillatory ventilation in a normal rabbit model. Pediatr Res 28:367-373
22. Sykes MK (1991) Does mechanical ventilation damage the lung? Acta Anaesthesiol Scand Suppl 95:35-38
23. HIFI Study Group (1989) High-frequency oscillatory ventilation compared with conventional mechanical ventilation in the treatment of respiratory failure in preterm infants. N Engl J Med 320:88-93
24. Bryan AC, Froese AB (1991) Reflections on the HIFI trial. Paediatrics 87:565-567
25. Clark RH, Gerstmann DR, Null DM Jr et al (1992) Prospective randomized comparison of high frequency oscillatory and conventional ventilation in respiratory distress syndrome. Paediatrics 89:5-12
26. HiFO Study Group (1993) Randomized study of high-frequency oscillatory ventilation in infants with severe respiratory distress syndrome. J Pediatr 122:609-619
27. Gerstmann DR, Minton SD, Stoddard RA et al (1996) The Provo Multicenter early high-frequency oscillatory ventilation trial: improved pulmonary and clinical outcome in respiratory distress syndrome. Paediatrics 98:1044-1057
28. Keszler M, Modanlou HD, Brudno DS et al (1997) Multicenter controlled clinical trial of high-frequency jet ventilation in preterm infants with uncomplicated respiratory distress syndrome. Paediatrics 100:593-599
29. Clark RH, Dykes FD, Bachman TE et al (1996) Intraventricular hemorrhage and high-frequency ventilation: a meta-analysis of prospective clinical trials. Paediatrics 98:1058-1061
30. Arnold JH, Truog RD, Thompson JE et al (1993) High frequency oscillatory ventilation in paediatric respiratory failure. Crit Care Med 21:272-278
31. Arnold JH, Hanson JH, Toro-Figuero LO et al (1994) Prospective randomized comparison of high frequency oscillatory ventilation and conventional mechanical ventilation in paediatric respiratory failure. Crit Care Med 22:1530-1539
32. Moler FW, Palmisano J, Custer JR (1993) Extracorporeal life support for paediatric respiratory failure: predictors of survival from 220 patients. Crit Care Med 21:1604-1611
33. Fuhrman BP (1993) Perfluorocarbon liquids and respiratory support. Crit Care Med 21:951
34. Carlon GC, Howland WS, Ray C et al (1983) High-frequency jet ventilation: a prospective, randomized evaluation. Chest 84:551-559
35. Gluck E, Heard S, Patel C et al (1993) Use of ultrahigh frequency ventilation in patients with ARDS: a preliminary report. Chest 103:1413-1420
36. Fort P, Farmer C, Westerman J et al (1997) High-frequency oscillatory ventilation for adult respiratory distress syndrome: a pilot study. Crit Care Med 25:937-947
37. Amato MBP, Barbas CSV, Medeiros DM et al (1995) Beneficial effects of the "open lung approach" with low distending pressures in acute respiratory distress syndrome: a prospective randomized study on mechanical ventilation. Am J Respir Crit Care Med 152:1835-1846
38. Amato MBP, Barbas CSV, Medeiros DM et al (1998) Effect of a protective-ventilator strategy on mortality in the acute respiratory distress syndrome. N Engl J Med 338:347-354

Chapter 24

Surfactant in respiratory distress syndrome

D. Vidyasagar

Great deal of progress has been made since the first successful report of the use of surfactant in respiratory distress syndrome (RDS) by Fujiwara in 1980 [1]. Since then scores of randomized clinical trials involving thousands of infants in different countries have been conducted. Indeed the science of clinical research of multicentered trials evolved during the last 20 years, thanks to interest in RDS.

In parallel with these clinical studies we also saw development of a number of new surfactant products. With experience gained we have learnt a great deal about surfactant and its effect on RDS as well as its effect on other organ systems and its overall impact on natural history and outcome. One could say that after the introduction of ventilation, surfactant replacement therapy has made a major impact on RDS and therapy on the overall neonatal mortality and morbidity. It has also made an impact on infant mortality. The purpose of this lecture is to review the information in regard to surfactant therapy in RDS.

Since the first preparation of surfactant by Fujiwara (surfactant TA) [1] several other new preparations have been introduced. Although similar, there are distinct biochemical differences among them. Surfacten, Survanta, Curosurf, are all derived from minced bovine or porcine lungs. Infasurf, Alveofact, are made from lung washing, Pneumactant and Exosurf are solely synthetic compounds without any surfactant proteins (Table 1).

The biochemical composition of pulmonary surfactant is given in (Table 2). All natural surfactants contain surfactant proteins B and C. None of the commercial surfactants contain surfactant protein A. Only amniotic fluid derived surfactant contains surfactant protein A, which cannot be industrially made (Table 3).

The biochemical and biophysical properties of pulmonary surfactant have been extensively studied [2-4]. Surfactant derived from alveolar wash have less contaminants than those prepared from lung minces. Biophysically, the presence of surfactant proteins particularly show important differences in vitro [5].

With better understanding of surfactant preparation and surfactant properties, newer genetically designed surfactant preparations are being synthesized. KL_4 a synthetic peptide which mimics the sequence of SP-B protein in aqueous solution leads to surface active property similar to natural surfactant [6]. In vitro KL_4 resists inhibition by plasma proteins and oxidants released during the lung inflammation. Clinical trials using the new surfactant are in progress.

Table 1. Available commercial surfactant

Surfactant		Preparation	Manufacturer
Generic name	*Trade name*		
• Beractant	Survanta	Bovine lung mince extract with added DPPC, tripalmitin, and palmitic acid	Abbott Laboratories (USA)
• Surfactant-TA	Surfacten	Bovine lung mince extract with added DPPC, tripalmitoglycerol, and palmitic acid	Tokyo Tanabi (Japan)
• Porcine surfactant	Curosurf	Porcine lung mince; chloroform-methanol extract; liquid-gel chromatography	Chiesi Pharmaceuticals (Italy)
• Calf lung surfactant extract (CLSE)	Infasurf	Bovine lung wash; chloroform-methanol extract	Forrest Laboratories (USA)
SF-RI 1	Alveofact	Bovine lung wash; chloroform-methanol extract	Boehringer (Germany)
• Artificial lung expanding compound (ALEC)	Pneumactant	DPPC and phosphatidyl glycerol in 7:3 ratio	Britannia Pharmaceuticals (UK)
• Colfosceril palmitate, hexadecanol, tyloxapol (CPHT)	Exosurf	DPPC with 9% hexadecanol and 6% tyloxapol	Burroughs Wellcome Co. (USA)
• Peptide (KL$_4$)	Surfaxin	KL$_4$ Peptide	Acute Therapeutics USA

DPPC, dipalmityl phosphatidylcholine

Surfactant theraphy

Premature infants with hyaline membrane disease

In hyaline membrane disease (HMD), surfactant is present in insufficient quantity to perform the functions. Surfactant deficiency results in the widespread atelectasis, poor compliance, oedema, and haemorrhage that characterize the lungs of infants with HMD. The feasibility of administering surfactant to compensate for the deficiency in HMD has been of great interest to physiologists and clinicians. Initial clinical trials of exogenous artificial surfactant in human infants with HMD used aerosolized dipalmityl phosphatidylcholine (DPPC) and were

Table 2. Biochemical composition of pulmonary surfactant

• Lipid	85%-90%
• Phospholipids	75%-85%
• PC	60%-70%
• DSPC	40%-45%
• PG	
• PI ⎫	10%-15%
• PE ⎭	
• Lyso-PC ⎫	5%-10%
• SM ⎭	
• Neutral lipids	5%-10% (predominantly cholesterol)
• Protein	5%-10%
• Carbohydrate	5%

PC, phosphatidylcholine; DSPC, disaturated phosphatidylcholine; PG, phosphatidylglycerol; PI, phosphatidylinositol; PE phosphatidylethanolamine; Lyso-PC, lysophosphatidylcholine; SM, sphingomyelin; DPPC, dipalmitoyl phosphatidylcholine

Table 3. Surfactant proteins

Type	Monomer size (Da)	Predominant oligomer
SP-A	28 000-36 000	Trimer
SP-B	8 000	Dimer
SP-C	3 800	Dimer
SP-D	43 000	Trimer

not successful, probably because of the poor adsorption velocity of pure DPPC. Two other exogenous artificial surfactants, a dry mixture of DPPC and phosphatidyl-glycerol (PG) in a 7:3 ratio and a mixture of DPPC and high-density human serum lipoprotein in a 10:1 ratio, produced inconsistent results, again probably as a result of adsorption rates inferior to natural surfactant [7, 8]. In premature animal models of HMD, excellent therapeutic effects were demonstrated with direct tracheal instillation of natural surfactant isolated by centrifugation of bronchoalveolar lavage (BAL) fluid from mature lungs. Successful clinical trials in human infants with HMD have used exogenous natural surfactant from the following sources: human amniotic fluid [9]; bovine lung homogenate supplemented with PG or with DPPC, palmitic acid, and tripalmitoylglycerol (surfactant TA) [1]; neonatal bovine BAL fluid (calf lung surfactant extract (CLSE), and Infasurf) and porcine lung homogenate [10]. Survanta is a bovine lung-derived, reconstituted surfactant. Efforts to develop an effective synthetic surfactant continued because of concern about possible immune sensitization of infants to foreign animal proteins present in heterologous natural surfactant. Clinical trials using a synthetic surfactant consisting of DPPC supplemented with hexadecanol and tyloxapol (Exosurf) have shown good results [11].

Immediate beneficial effects of surfactant therapy include improved oxygenation, lowered mean airway pressure, and improved aeration on chest radiographs [12]. Response to treatment occurs in about 80% of infants. Causes for treatment failure include extreme prematurity, pre-existing severe hypoxia, hypotension and acidosis. Meta-analyses of the outcome differences between surfactant-treated and control infants, from the reports of randomized controlled trials, revealed that surfactant was associated with a 30% to 40% reduction in neonatal mortality, a marked decrease in the occurrence of pneumothorax, and a decrease in the combined outcomes of bronchopulmonary dysplasia (BPD) or death at 28 days. However, there were no overall decreases in the incidence of bronchopulmonary dysplasia, patent ductus arteriosus, or intracranial haemorrhage [13]. The incidence of pulmonary haemorrhage, a rare problem in premature infants, is increased by about 50% in infants who receive surfactant and autopsy evaluations have shown extensive intra-alveolar haemorrhage to be approximately four times more common in surfactant-treated infants than in untreated control infants [14, 15].

Although there had been concern that improved survival in premature infants with HMD might be associated with increased long-term morbidity, several follow-up studies have shown that surfactant treatment is associated with similar or improved late pulmonary and neurodevelopmental function in comparison with untreated controls. Serum samples from infants treated with bovine lung derived surfactant have contained no detectable antibodies to SP-B or SP-C at 6 and 12 months of adjusted age (Table 4) [16, 17].

Table 4. Clinical outcomes of surfactant trials for hyaline membrane disease* (prophylaxis and rescue; synthetic and natural)

Mortality	+++
BPD or death at 28 days	++
BPD	+–**
Pneumothorax	–
PDA	no effect
IVH	no effect
SP-B, SP-C antibodies	not found
Long-term morbidity	no effect

BPD, bronchopulmonary dysplasia; PDA, patent ductus arteriosus; IVH, intraventricular hemorrhage; SP, surfactant-associated protein
* Cumulative data from 35 clinical trials [18, 19] expressed in a simplified way
** Although the combination of BPD or death at 28 days was definitely influenced by surfactant replacement, a reduction in BPD alone was not found consistently in all trials analyzed

Surfactant therapy in USA [18]

USA was first to conduct number of surfactant clinical trials using multiple centers. Over 10 000 infants were enrolled in studies of Survanta and Exosurf from 1985 to 1990. These studies led to the Food and Drug Administration (FDA) approval of two surfactant products for clinical use in 1989/90. Since then surfactant has been used routinely. In USA it is estimated that over 50% of very low birth weight cases (<1500 g) are treated with surfactant. Extensive use of surfactant has been identified with a decrease in neonatal and infant mortality.

The earliest clinical trials of exogenous surfactant involved administering it to infants in whom the diagnosis of severe HMD had already been established. Studies using this therapeutic approach have been termed treatment or rescue trials. However, animal studies showed that instillation of surfactant before the onset of ventilation resulted in better outcomes.

Thus, in clinical trials, surfactant was administered in birthing areas to infants at high risk of developing HMD. Studies using this treatment strategy are called prophylaxis or prevention trials. In prophylaxis studies, the incidence of HMD among treated infants becomes an outcome variable. Because not all at-risk infants actually develop HMD, the prophylaxis approach leads to unnecessary treatment of some infants, the proportion increasing with gestational age. However, using the treatment strategy, (Rescue) HMD may be quite advanced and infants may receive significant exposure to high oxygen concentrations and ventilator trauma before surfactant is given.

The earlier studies of surfactant therapy involved single-dose treatment, but because only transient improvement often occurred, later studies usually allowed multiple doses. Trials that have compared single versus multiple dose treatments indicate lower mortality and morbidity in infants who receive multiple doses [12, 18, 19]. However, whether retreatment should be scheduled or based on severity of symptoms remains unresolved.

Surfactant therapy for HMD has usually been administered to infants already receiving mechanical ventilation. A randomized non-blinded trial compared early initiation of nasal continuous positive airway pressure (NCPAP) alone and early NCPAP plus brief endotracheal intubation for tracheal instillation of a single dose of Curosurf in premature infants with moderate or severe HMD. Surfactant treatment was associated with a significantly higher mean ratio of arterial to alveolar oxygen tension 6 h after randomization and lower mean incidence of subsequent mechanical ventilation [20].

In the United States, two surfactant preparations were approved for open trials. Exosurf was licensed for treatment of HMD in 1990, and Survanta (a modified bovine surfactant) in 1991. During 1990, the United States infant mortality rate decreased by 6%. This was twice the annual average rate of decrease that occurred between 1980 and 1989. The large decrease in 1990 resulted from a 36% decrease in the mortality from HMD, which in turn was attributed to the widespread clinical use of surfactant therapy [21].

A multicenter randomized trial in mechanically ventilated premature infants with HMD compared Survanta and Exosurf in 652 and 644 infants, respectively. Survanta was associated with more rapid improvement in respiratory condition. The incidence of pneumothorax was significantly higher in the group that received Exosurf. However, the combined outcomes of BPD or death at 28 days of age were similar in the two treatment groups [22].

Clinical trials in Europe [23]

Number of clinical trials also took place in Europe in the 1980s. Initial studies used dry artificial surfactants, then were followed by natural surfactants Alveofact and Curosurf. Survanta, and Exosurf were also tested in clinical trials in Europe. A number of 9 942 infants were included in a surfactant trial coordinated in Oxford. Number of other trials have been conducted in Europe. One of the controversial use of surfactant was administration to human fetus via amniocentesis. This approach is very invasive and needs scrutiny before major clinical trials are undertaken. Recently Halliday summarized results of 12 randomized comparative trials [23]. The results show that natural surfactant had a better result over synthetic surfactant.

Surfactant was also used in conjunction with continuous positive airway pressure (CPAP), and nebulization. Method of administration has also been tested. Effects of nebulization lasted for a short period. Larger amount of surfactant was required. Comparison of two natural surfactants was also studied.

It was indicated that the overall survival in early years of introduction of therapy (1987) was 59% but four years later it increased to 86%. The most noticeable improvement was in 500-999 g infants, suggesting that improvement was due to experience gained in the use of surfactant. It may also be possible that other factors (i.e., improved antenatal care, improved management of preterm labor and steroid) were responsible for the enhanced outcome.

In Latin America [24] it was shown that surfactant use although decreased mortality and morbidity was higher suggesting surfactant use requires expertise as well as additional resources to manage extremely small preterm infants who otherwise would have died.

Surfactant therapy in developing countries [25-27]

The ready availability of surfactant have increased expectations of using surfactant globally. However, some practical considerations are to be made.

Cost

The cost of surfactant ($800-$1000 per vial) is high even for developed countries. This may indeed be twice the pro capite income in some countries (i.e., indian per capita income $350/year). Thus making it least cost effective. The aspect has been well studied in some countries where a development of policy for selective and restrictive use has been proposed. Similarly, other developing countries should develop such strategies. Alternately pharmaceutical industries should make efforts to produce low-cost surfactant.

Surfactant use and availability of appropriate technology

Use of surfactant presupposes the ready availability of trained personnel to manage neonatal ventilation and facilities to provide "total" intensive care. This in itself is a major undertaking. To establish a *de novo* NICU bed may cost $50 000 in equipment alone. Space utilization, availability of personnel (nursing, technicians), etc. will add up to the cost. In developed countries per day cost of such operation exceeds $1500/NICU bed, obviously high-tech care is highly expensive. One should be fully aware of such cost analysis prior to introducing NICU in a hospital. Best alternative is to develop preventive strategies, (improved prenatal care, antenatal steroids) and a regionalized system to pool resources, and to implement policies for treatment.

Introduction of surfactant in NICUs in developing countries

Number of Neonatal Intensive Care Units have been established in developing countries, Asia, Africa and Latin America by dedicated groups of neonatologists. These units have been providing excellent ventilatory support and intensive care. However a recent study from South America by Diaz J.L., Diaz R. (CLAP) (Personal Communication) has shown that surfactant use (in spite of high cost compared to countries' per capita income) has decreased overall mortality. However, there was an increase in complications, for example infections, lack of nutritional support, intraventricular haemorrhages (IVH). These complications were attributed to lack of skilled personnel or capabilities to minimize infections or improve nutritional support of extremely small weight infants who survived for longer time after surfactant therapy. These observations indicate that surfactant therapy alone without proper supporting measures will increase burden of disease and prove to be less cost effective.

Can surfactant be used without subsequent ventilator support?

In view of the above observations one might consider treating infants with surfactant either by aerosol (which will still require intubation) or use "single intubation" for surfactant instillation followed by nasal CPAP. Studies of aerosol treatment of surfactant are in progress but not yet available for clinical use. Single intubations for surfactant treatment followed by CPAP have been reported by a few investigators. There is a limited use specifically in larger infants. The need for superb nursing care of these infants must be clearly recognized.

Pulmonary and non pulmonary effects of surfactant

Circulatory effects [28]

Number of investigators have looked into the cardiovascular effects of surfactant therapy. It can be expected that since surfactant instillation will improve lung compliance, it leads to a decrease in pulmonary vascular resistance and to an increase in pulmonary blood flow. The clinically observed patent ductus arteriosus

(PDA) following surfactant treatment is thought to be due to the drop in pulmonary vascular resistance (PVR). We showed in premature baboons an increase in pulmonary blood flow following surfactant therapy [29]. Others have shown a drop in mean arterial blood flow following treatment. Pulmonary artery pressure (PAP) decreased by 20% and blood flow increased after Exosurf treatment in infants. Although there is a demonstrable decrease in PVR and an increase in PAP and pulmonary blood flow and consequent development of PDA, there is decreasing incidence of PDA with better management suggesting surfactant per se is not the cause for the PDA.

Cerebral circulation [28]

Both decrease and increase in cerebral blood flow velocity (CBFV) have been reported in the literature. Overall there is no significant changes occur with surfactant therapy.

Porcine surfactant decreased mean arterial blood pressure (MABP) by inducing vasodilation. The effect is dose dependant. This vasodilation is inhibited by NO synthetase by (L NAME). With Curosurf MABP and CO left ventricular output increased about 29%, other studies did not show consistent results.

Effects on patent ductus arteriosus

Increased incidence of PDA following surfactant therapy has been widely reported [29, 30]. A meta-analysis of 6 117 infants from 28 studies showed no overall increase in PDA after treatment.

Pulmonary functions

Pulmonary functions have been studied in infants treated with surfactant [31-33]. In Exosurf treated infants compliance improved 24 h after treatment, functional residual capacity (FRC) got better 12 h after treatment. Improvement in oxygenation is not followed by improvement in compliance. The immediate improvement may be due to increase in ventilation perfusion ratio.

In a controlled study of prophylactic therapy in the delivery room, pulmonary function test (PFT) was studied 1 h before, 24, 48 and 72 after treatment, leading to no significant differences in dynamic compliance (Cd), total pulmonary resistance, and tidal volume between surfactant and control, before and one hour after. However, dynamic compliance CL was 50% higher in surfactant group at 24 h. The difference increased to 94% at 7 days of age. Oxygenation was significantly greater in surfactant group during the first 72 h. Mean airway pressure was less than in control at all times. Compliance improved during first 48 h of life. Beneficial effect was not seen immediately. We also showed that significant improvement in blood gases preceded improvement in lung compliance during mechanical breathing. The study of Bowen et al. showed two patterns of response to surfactant treatment. One pattern gave a significant response in PaO_2 within 2 h of treatment. The second group had a fall in PaO$_2$, which improved after 2 h of treatment. Neither of them showed significant A-a differences in O$_2$/CO$_2$/or N$_2$. The data show that improvement that follows treatment occurs by recruitment and stabilization of alveoli without adding physiologic dead space.

Effects on renal function [34]

Onset of spontaneous diuresis was evaluated in 19 infants (12 surfactant treated, 7 control) with HMD, in a double blind controlled study. There was no difference in the time of onset of diuresis output >80% of intake. GFR was similar in surfactant and controls during the first 3 days of life. Fe, Na were higher in placebo at 24 h and 36 h. Placebo group had higher negative. Na balance than the treated grp. Ventilator status improved soon after surf Rx. The data suggested ventilatory status improvement was not due to diuresis. Other factors may be responsible.

Role of surfactant in host defenses [35]

Surfactant proteins A and D are being increasingly identified as important factors in host defense of lung. Surfactant protein A, binds, and opsonizes the bacteria, including group B streptococcal bacteria, *Pseudomonas* and *Pneumococci*. It agglutinates herpes, and influenza virus, and binds with lipo poly saccharide (LPS) endotoxin. SP-A deficient mice are susceptible to GBS infection. SPA concentrations are low in lavage fluid from premature infants. It is decreased by infection from respiratory synlitial virus (RSV), bacteria, LPS and tumor necrosis factor (TNFX). SP-A also activates macrophages, and polymorphonucleocytes (PMNs) enhancing bacterial killing. Surfactant protein D- synthesized by bronchiolar, tracheal-bronchial and alveolar epithelial cells. It binds bacteria, *E. coli*, *Salmonella*, *Klebsiella*, enhances uptake and killing of bacteria. It also agglutinates virus, and binds with LPS. Concentrations in bronchi alveolar lavage are low in prematurity. Thus natural surfactants play neither to unknown roles which are very critical to survival of immature infants.

Timing and method of administration

Considerable discussion surrounds regarding the timing of surfactant therapy. Since bronchiolar damage can be seen in animals exposed to oxygen and mechanical ventilation even for a short period of time, surfactant treatment soon after birth (prophylactic) has been proposed. It is also shown that the absence of surfactant and resultant atelectasis leads to protein leak which inhibits and inactivates surfactant. These consideration strongly support prophylactic treatment. However, long term benefits did not differ. It is estimated that routine administration of surfactant to at risk infants prior to first breath would lead to unnecessary treatment of 30% of infants; with increasing use of antenatal steroids even extremely low birth weight infants escape the need for surfactant and avoid developing of RDS. Routine surfactant administration in the delivery room may delay resuscitation and lower Apgar scores may be noted. It can be recommended that prophylactic administration of surfactant should be given in at risk infants <30 week of gestation, soon after resuscitation and establishment of endotracheal intubation. A large multi center randomized trial comparing treatment at 2 h versus treatment for severe RDS at 3 h showed small but significant (6%) risk for death or O_2 dependency [36].

Dosage

Most products recommend 100 mg/kg of phospholipid. The available information regarding multiple doses is based on earlier trials [37]. However, since the availability of drug timing and dosing has varied, doses beyond 3 do not seem to have much benefit. Exogenous surfactant is rapidly reutilized, it may also be inactivated by inhibitors necessitating redosing. Additional doses may not reach the previously atelectatic alveoli. We prefer to give maximum of 3 doses if infants continue to remain ventilator dependant requiring MAP>7 cmH$_2$O and FiO$_2$>40%.

Technique of treatment

The recommended techniques have differed from surfactant to surfactant. The manufactures of Survanta recommend a complicated procedure based on original advice of Fujiwara to assure distribution of surfactant to all portions of lung; others recommend minimal positioning to right and left sides [1, 37]. Most now recommend bolus injection with endotracheal tip left in midtrachea. Since administration requires disconnection of ventilator, special adopters with side part have been used for some surfactants. Studies comparing bolus versus drip treatment may preferentially go to dependent areas hence a bolus injection will have better distribution. Aerosol administration is under investigation. It requires sophisticated delivery system, it will require larger doses and distribution may be unhomogenous.

When given by instillation it is delivered in aliquotes with intermittent bagging in between. Noted complications include, bradycardia, cyanosis, and hypotension, all transient responses. Inappropriate management of ventilation following surfactant treatment may lead to the development of air leaks. There is a need to improve skills of personnel in the proper use of surfactant.

A study from Latin America also showed that although surfactant usage improved oxygenation and survival, there was an increase in associated complications (i.e., air leaks, infections and inadequate nutrition of surviving VLBW infants). These observations indicate the need for development of full support system in the NICU prior to initiating surfactant replacement therapy.

Pretransport surfactant use

Administration of surfactant prior to neonatal transport showed that it was safe but did not confer any advantage over post-transport treatment [38, 39]. It is also feared that pretransport administration by the transport team may cause delay. However, this practice may be recommended if infant's condition allows intubation and ventilation. Surfactant must be administered by skilled personnel to give the benefit prior to the arrival of the team. This suggestion presupposes that physician administering has the knowledge and skills of modulating ventilator settings according to response.

Use of surfactant in conditions other than respiratory distress syndrome

Surfactant therapy by virtue of its ability to maintain alveolar stability should be useful in all the conditions that produce alveolar alectasis. Consequently surfactant has been used in infants with pneumonia and meconium aspiration syndrome, pulmonary haemorrhage, diaphragmatic hernia.

Among these conditions the use of surfactant in meconium aspiration syndrome has been gaining clinical importance [40-42]. Some clinical studies have shown improved oxygenation following surfactant instillation therapy but have not been consistent in results. Recently a new method of surfactant treatment (i.e., bronchial lavage with surfactant) has been reported to be clinically beneficial [43, 44].

The difference in response between tracheal administration alone and lavage needs to be studied. Tracheal administration alone may not be as effective since the surfactant may be inactivated by meconium. Thus removal of meconium may be equally important. In lung washing surfactant may act as detergent. In animal and clinical studies using Survanta as well as KL$_4$ investigators have shown improvement in oxygenation; as regards compliance, these observations need to be studied more extensively.

Surfactant has also been used in neonatal group B βstreptococcus (GBBS) infection and adult RDS [45, 46]. The pathophysiology appears to involve increased microvascular permeability and pulmonary oedema. Surfactant is actively inhibited by oedema fluid. Although earlier observations with natural surfactant preparations were successful in the ARDS, multicenter controlled studies with synthetic surfactant in ARDS failed to show improved survival [47, 48]. In addition, multiple large doses required to treat adult lungs may prove to be costly.

Practical questions regarding surfactant therapy

What are the indications for surfactant therapy?

Surfactant replacement is being used primarily for neonatal surfactant deficiency states (i.e. HMD in the premature infant). The benefit of such therapy in other clinical states such as "shock lung" and ARDS is yet to be studied. It is suggested that surfactant therapy be withheld in the presence of pneumothorax because it may be drained through the chest tube. Shock and severe acidosis also should be corrected prior to initiating surfactant therapy for optimal results. Surfactant has been used in meconium aspiration syndrome both as a replacement, and more recently as a lavage.

Which is the best surfactant?

A review of the literature indicates that purified and reconstituted natural surfactant have had superior results in improving lung function and blood gases (oxygenation). Synthetic surfactant are also effective. Naturally derived and reconstituted surfactant are superior in improving blood gases rapidly.

How is surfactant supplied? How is it administered?

There are various surfactant preparations available in the global market. Clinicians should become familiar with these products. All surfactants are administered intratracheally. Bolus rather than drip technique of administration is recommended for better distribution. Clinicians should follow instructions of each product. Avoiding prolonged unnecessary interruption during administration will be important.

When to treat?

Physiologically, it is rational to treat the at risk infant at birth, prior to the first breath. Nevertheless, a large proportion of those at risk (up to 30% in one study) may not develop HMD and hence may be treated unnecessarily. It is suggested that for practical reasons, treatment immediately after intubation and full resuscitation is recommended in infants of less than 30 weeks of gestation.

What is the dose of surfactant therapy?

The dose of surfactant in various studies has ranged from 50 mg to 200 mg/kg. Most manufacturers recommend 100 mg of phospholipid/kg suspended in 3-5 ml of saline. One should follow the recommendations of each product.

How many doses are required?

The suggested regimen of doses and number of recommended treatments are all based on trials conducted prior to release of drugs. They varied from a single dose to 4 doses. We believe most of the times maximum of 2-3 doses will be adequate to overcome surfactant deficiency, to get even spread and to overcome inactivation by inhibitors. Doses are repeated for 6-8 h if there is no improvement in a/A ratio, or deteriorating status.

Can surfactant be given prior to transport?

At risk infants born at level II hospitals should be treated as early as possible. This presupposes that physician at the hospital has "intubation and ventilation" skills. It will be important to train such personnel if the expected travel time for transfer is long (i.e. hours). In metropolitan cities of USA where trained neonatologists manage level II hospitals, infants with RDS are routinely intubated, resuscitated and treated with surfactant prior to transport as per indication. Infants are well stabilized prior to the arrival of transfer team. We found it to be extremely helpful to treat as early as possible. If treatment is initiated by transport team after arrival at the hospital, they should allow additional time for instillation, stabilization and making changes in ventilatory settings.

Can surfactant be given when no ventilatory support is available?

As discussed in this chapter, surfactant has been used with "one intubation" followed by treatment with nasal CPAP, with good results. Such approach is warranted only in these areas where ventilatory support is out of reach. Cost effectiveness of routine use in a given country must be studied prior to routine use. Paediatricians, neonatologists must develop practical guidelines for their institutions and governments for proper use of surfactant. On the other hand, manufacturers must make drug available at reasonable cost.

Conclusions

In summary, since the report of successful clinical use of surfactant by Fujiwara, scores of randomized clinical trials in USA, Europe, and other countries were conducted. Thousands of infants were studied. These studies were not limited to changes in clinical status of RDS alone. Secondary effects on various organ systems have also been studied extensively. To date surfactant therapy has changed the course of RDS in more than one way: improved disease status, lowered complications, improved overall survival.

Exogenous surfactant therapy is a landmark in the history of clinical medicine. It is a major milestone of 20th century.

References

1. Fujiwara T, Chida S, Watabe YJ et al (1980) Artificial surfactant therapy in hyaline membrane disease. Lancet 1:55-59
2. King RJ (1982) Pulmonary surfactant. J Appl Physiol 53:1-8
3. Harwood JL (1987) Lung surfactant. Prog Lipid Res 26:211-256
4. Haagsman HP et al (1991) Synthesis and assembly of lung surfactant. Ann Rev Physio 53:441-464

5. Hawgwood S, Shiffer K (1991) Structures and properties of the surfactant associated proteins. Ann Rev Physiol 53:375-394

6. Cochrane CG, Revak SD, Merritt TA et al (1996) The efficacy and safety of KL_4 surfactant in preterm infants with RDS. Am J Resp Crit Care Med 153:404-410

7. Morley CJ, Bangham AD, Miller N et al (1981) Dry artificial surfactant and its effect on very premature babies. Lancet 1:64-68

8. Halliday H, McClune G, Reid MC et al (1984) Controlled trial of artificial surfactant to prevent respiratory distress syndrome. Lancet 1:476-478

9. Hallman M, Merritt TA, Jarvenpoa AL et al (1985) Exogenous human surfactant for treatment of severe respiratory distress syndrome. A randomized prospective clinical trial. J Pediatr 106:963-969.

10. Robertson B (1988) Surfactant replacement therapy for severe RDS. An international randomized clinical trial. Collaborative European Multicenter Study Group. Pediatrics 82:683-691

11. Long W, Corbet A, Colton R et al (1991) A controlled trial of synthetic surfactant in infants weighing 1250 g or more with respiratory distress syndrome. N Engl J Med 325:1696-1703

12. Raju TNK, Vidyasagar D, Bhat R et al (1987) Double blind controlled trial of single dose treatment with bovine surfactant in severe hyaline membrane disease. Lancet 1:651-656

13. Jobe AH (1993) Pulmonary surfactant therapy. N Engl J Med 328:861-868

14. Raju TNK, Langenberg P (1993) Pulmonary hemorrhage and exogenous surfactant therapy. A meta analysis. J Pediatr 123:603-610

15. Pappin A, Shenker N, Hack M et al (1994) Extensive intra alveolar pulmonary hemorrhage in infants dying after surfactant therapy. J Pediatr 124:621-626

16. Ferrara TB, Hoekstra RE, Couser RJ et al (1994) Survival and follow-up of infants born at 23 to 26 weeks of gestational age: effects of surfactant therapy. J Pediatr 124:119-124

17. Survanta Multidose Study Group (1994) Two-year follow-up of infants treated for neonatal respiratory distress syndrome with bovine surfactant. J Pediatr 124:962-67

18. Soll RF (1997) Surfactant therapy in the USA: trials and current routines. Biol Neonate 71(Suppl 1):1-7

19. Corbet A, Gerdes J, Long W et al (1995) Double-blind, randomized trial of one versus three prophylactic doses of synthetic surfactant in 826 neonates weighing 700-1100 grams: effects on mortality rate. J Pediatr 126:969-978

20. Verder H, Robertson B, Greison G et al (1994) Surfactant therapy and nasal continuous positive airway pressure for newborns with respiratory distress syndrome. N Engl J Med 331:1051-1055

21. Centers for Disease Control (1993) Infant mortality-United States in 1990. MMWR 42:161-165

22. Vermont-Oxford Neonatal Network (1996) A multicenter, randomized trial comparing synthetic surfactant with modified bovine surfactant extract in the treatment of neonatal respiratory distress syndrome. Pediatrics 97:1-6

23. Halliday HL (1997) Clinical trials of surfactant replacement in Europe. Biol Neonate 71(Suppl 1):8-12

24. Rossello JD, Hayward PE, Martell M, Del Barco M, Margotto P, Grandzoto J, Bastida J, Pena J, Villaneuva D (1997) Hyaline membrane disease (HMD) therapy in Latin America: impact of exogenous surfactant administration on newborn survival, morbidity and use of resources. J Perinat Med 25(3):280-287

25. Davies VA, Ballot DE, Rothberg AD (1995) The cost and effectiveness of surfactant replacement therapy at Johannesburg Hospital, November 1991-December 1992. S Afr Med J 85(7):649

26. Ballot DE, Rothberg AD, Davies VA (1995) The selection of infants for surfactant replacement therapy under conditions of limited financial resources. S Afr Med J 85(7):640-643
27. Davies VA, Rothberg AD, Ballot DE (1995) The introduction of surfactant replacement therapy into South Africa. S Afr Med J 85(7):637-640
28. Moen A (1997) Circulatory effects of surfactant therapy. Biol Neonate 71(Suppl 1):18-22
29. Vidyasagar D, Maeta H, Raju TNK, John E, Bhat R, Go M et al (1985) Bovine surfactant (surfactant TA) therapy in immature baboons with hyaline membrane disease. Pediatrics 75:1132-1142
30. Fujiwara T, Konishi M, Chida S et al (1990) Surfactant replacement therapy with a single postventilatory dose of a reconstituted bovine surfactant in preterm neonates with respiratory distress syndrome. Final analysis of a multicenter, double-blind, randomized trial and comparison with similar trials. Pediatrics 86:753-764
31. Todd DA, Choukroun ML, Fayon M, Kays C, Guenard H, Galperine I, Demarquez JL (1995) Respiratory mechanics before and after late artificial surfactant rescue. J Paediatr Child Health 31(6):532-536
32. Sandberg KL, Lindstrom DP, Sjoqvist BA, Parker RA, Cotton RB (1997) Surfactant replacement therapy improves ventilation inhomogeneity in infants with respiratory distress syndrome. Pediatr Pulmonol 24:337-343
33. Bhat R, Dziedzic K, Vidyasagar D (1990) Effect of single dose surfactant TA on pulmonary function. Crit Care Med 18:590-595
34. Bhat R, John E, Diaz-Blanco J, Ortega R, Fornell L, Vidyasagar D (1989) Surfactant therapy and spontaneous diuresis. J Pediatr 114:443-447
35. Weaver TE (1991) Surfactant proteins and SP-D. Am J Respir Cell Mol Biol 5:4-5
36. The OSIRIS Collaborative Group (1992) Early versus delayed neonatal administration of synthetic surfactant – the judgement of OSIRIS. Lancet 340:1363-1369
37. Corbet A, Gerdes J, Long W et al (1995) Double-blind, randomized trial of one versus three prophylactic doses of synthetic surfactant in 826 neonates weighing 700 to 1100 grams: effects on mortality rate. J Pediatr 126:969-978
38. Costakos D, Allen D, Krauss A, Ruiz N, Fluhr K, Stouvenel A et al (1996) Surfactant therapy prior to the interhospital transport of preterm infants. Am J Perinat 13(5):309-316
39. Bhuta T, Walker K, Jones N, Halliday R, Berry A (1995) Surfactant administration by newborn emergency transport service. Proceedings of the thirteenth annual Congress of the Australian Perinatal Society, Auckland
40. Khammash H, Perlman M, Wojtulewicz J et al (1993) Surfactant therapy in full-term neonates with severe respiratory failure. Pediatrics 92:135-139
41. Halliday HL, Speer CP, Robertson B (1996) Treatment of severe meconium aspiration syndrome with porcine surfactant. Eur J Pediatr 155:1047-1051
42. Findlay RD, Taeusch HW, Walther FJ (1996) Surfactant replacement therapy for meconium aspiration syndrome. Pediatrics 97:48-52
43. Paranka MS, Walsh WF, Stancombe BB (1992) Surfactant lavage in a piglet model of meconium aspiration syndrome. Pediatr Res 31:625-628
44. Revak SD, Cochrane CG, Merritt TA (1997) The therapeutic effect of bronchoalveolar lavage with KL4-surfactant in animal models of meconium aspiration syndrome. Pediatr Res 41:A265
45. Herting E, Jarstrand C, Rasool O et al (1994) Experimental neonatal group B streptococcal pneumonia: effect of a modified porcine surfactant on bacterial proliferation in ventilated near-term rabbits. Pediatr Res 36:784-791
46. Sherman MP, Campbell LA, Merritt TA et al (1994) Effect of different surfactant on pulmonary group B streptococcal infections in premature rabbits. J Pediatr 125:939-947

47. Walmrath D, Gunther A, Ghofrani HA et al (1996) Bronchoscopic surfactant administration in patients with severe adult respiratory distress syndrome and sepsis. Am J
Respir Crit Care Med 154:57-62
48. Anzueto A, Baughman RP, Guntupalli KK (1996) Aerosolized surfactant in adults with
sepsis-induced acute respiratory distress syndrome. N Engl J Med 334:1417-1421

Chapter 25

Liquid ventilation: recent concepts

J.H. Arnold

History of liquid ventilation

Perfluorocarbon (PFC) liquids were first demonstrated to be suitable as an alternative respiratory medium by Clark and Gollan in 1966 and are characterized by the unique combination of high solubility for O_2 and CO_2, low surface tension, high spreading coefficient, and high density. However, attempts to utilize liquid media to enhance gas exchange significantly predate the development of perfluorochemical compounds. In the 1920s, saline lavage was utilized to treat victims of gas attacks during World War I and directly stimulated an interest in the use of liquid ventilation to support gas exchange during saline lavage. Evaluation of the feasibility of liquid ventilation was propelled further by U.S. government-sponsored research efforts involving ultradeep diving and the potentially fatal physiologic changes associated with rapid descent and subsequent ascent. Physiologic studies of the saline-filled lung demonstrated alveolar recruitment, increase in lung compliance and a homogenization of the distribution of regional pulmonary blood flow. In 1966, Kylstra [1] performed the first liquid breathing experiment using saline in a hyperbaric chamber and was able to support gas exchange in animals for 60 min. Subsequently, a biochemical search began to identify liquids with low surface tension, high solubilities for O_2 and CO_2, as well as immiscibility and nontoxicity. In 1966, Clark and Gollan performed the first liquid breathing experiment under normobaric conditions using a perfluorocarbon [2]. Shaffer developed the first demand-controlled total liquid ventilator in 1974 and in the 1970s and 1980s, total liquid ventilation was examined in a number of animal models of lung injury. In 1989, Greenspan et al. reported the first human use of total liquid ventilation in three neonates using a gravity-dependent delivery system [3]. In 1991, Fuhrman et al. were the first to report the use of partial liquid breathing, whereby gas tidal volumes are delivered to the perfluorocarbon-treated lung using a conventional mechanical ventilator [4]. In 1995, Hirschl et al. reported the first partial liquid breathing trial in humans who were being supported with extracorporeal membrane oxygenation (ECMO) at the time of study [5].

Total liquid ventilation

Full-tidal or total liquid ventilation (TLV), which utilizes PFC tidal volumes delivered to the PFC-filled lung, has been shown to enhance gas exchange and improve pulmonary mechanics in animal models of preterm surfactant deficient lungs [6] and mature, acutely injured lungs [5, 7]. Improved gas exchange during TLV in pre-term human neonates has also been reported [3].

TLV is possible with PFC liquids because PFCs have high solubility for both oxygen and, importantly, carbon dioxide. In addition, bulk flow of PFC liquid to support ventilation can be achieved at acceptable intrapulmonary pressures due to the density and viscosity relationships of these compounds. In addition, PFCs are nontoxic to the lung and it has been shown that animals can resume gas breathing without difficulty. A complex device to deliver PFCs in precisely determined volumes is necessary and the initial gravity-dependent PFC delivery methods have evolved significantly. At present, an ECMO-like circuit in which the PFC fluid is oxygenated, purged of CO_2, and warmed is utilized. Problems in the development of TLV have arisen from the technical issues related to the design of devices which produce tidal movement of liquid. Although this technology is not invasive, it is expensive and unapproved by the FDA. Furthermore, the priming volumes for the liquid ventilator are large and potentially expensive.

The physiology underlying improved gas exchange and lung mechanics during TLV and its salutary effects on pulmonary mechanics in the surfactant-deficient and the injured lung have been extensively studied. Because of the combination of properties mentioned above, replacement of the air/alveolar interface with a PFC/alveolar interface leads to a reduction in interfacial tension and an increase in compliance and supports the re-establishment or "normalization" of functional residual capacity in states of reduced lung compliance [8-10]. In models of acute lung injury and surfactant deficiency due to prematurity, investigators have documented a reduction in shunt fraction [9] and, additionally, attributed improved gas exchange to improved ventilation/perfusion matching [9-11]. Quantification of ventilation/perfusion relationships has not been applied during TLV; however, analysis of pulmonary blood flow distribution during TLV in an isolated lung preparation [12] and in preterm meconium-stained lambs [9] demonstrated attenuation of the regional blood flow gradient, favoring the dependent regions of the gas-filled lung with a shift in flow from dependent to nondependent regions. This pattern has been attributed to the formation of an alveolar pressure gradient that, because of the dense nature of PFC liquids (specific gravity =1.76), exceeds the hydrostatic pressure gradient in the pulmonary vascular tree [12]. There is also interesting evidence that perfluorochemical compounds may attenuate the inflammatory response to acute lung injury. Liquid ventilation with the perfluorochemical, perflubron (perfluoro-octyl bromide, perflubron, Liquivent, Alliance Pharmaceutical Corp., San Diego, CA), has been associated with a marked reduction in inflammatory change in the lung in animal models in acute lung injury [7, 13, 14]. Although the precise mechanism by which perflubron alters immune responses is not clear, the compound clearly interferes with functions of macrophages [15, 16], lymphocyte function [17], and neutrophil response [18, 19].

Partial liquid ventilation

During the technical development of TLV, it was discovered that animals with PFC-filled lungs could be supported with a conventional ventilator: the ventilator produced tidal gas ventilation of the fluorocarbon-filled lung and both oxygenation and ventilation were noted to be enhanced. This technique [4] has become known as partial liquid ventilation (PLV) and has been shown to improve gas exchange and lung mechanics in a variety of animal models.

Likewise, the physiology of gas exchange during PLV has been extensively investigated. Although PLV in the normal lung is known to impair the efficiency of gas exchange [4, 20] and has been shown to increase intrapulmonary shunt and ventilation/perfusion heterogeneity [21], PLV has been shown to improve the efficiency of gas exchange and lung mechanics of injured lungs in models of premature [11, 22] and injured lungs [23, 24] and in preliminary human trials [25-27]. When PLV is initiated with a PFC volume equivalent to estimated functional residual capacity, lung recruitment is believed to be promoted by the reduction of interfacial tension and by bulk distension of alveoli with a noncompressible medium. This produces an increase in the alveolar/capillary surface area participating in gas exchange and thus reduces shunt fraction in injured lungs [20, 28].

It has also been suggested that the alveolar hydrostatic pressure generated by intrapulmonary PFC during PLV shifts regional blood flow within the lung in a manner similar to that during TLV. This would potentially lead to the normalization of disorganized regional ventilation/perfusion relationships within the injured lung, improving the efficiency of gas exchange [11]. We have recently demonstrated that during PLV, regional blood flow redistribution patterns in the vertical plane vary dramatically on the basis of transverse section location along an apical-diaphragmatic axis [29]. We found flow shunted away from diaphragmatic lung irrespective of location in the vertical plane and away from dependent lung in the hilar region. As part of this pattern, flow is augmented in nondependent hilar lung and in apical lung in general. In as much as we did not find an increase in overall pulmonary vascular resistance, it seems likely that the change in regional pulmonary vascular resistance responsible for the shift in flow away from dependent and diaphragmatic lung must be accompanied by a reciprocal fall in pulmonary vascular resistance in nondependent and apical lung. These blood flow redistribution data suggest that with matched changes in regional ventilation, PLV may enhance gas exchange in the injured lung by improving disorganized regional ventilation/perfusion matching.

PLV: preclinical and clinical studies in lung injury

Leach et al. described their experience with PFC-associated gas exchange in a premature animal model of respiratory distress syndrome [11]. Dynamic lung compliance increased three fold within 15 min of beginning PLV, and the PO_2 increased from a mean of 59 mmHg during conventional ventilation to 250 mmHg during PLV. Improvements in oxygenation and lung compliance persisted throughout the 60 minutes of study. Also of note was the fact that the PCO_2 decreased significantly and the pH increased significantly during PLV as compared with values obtained during conventional ventilation. Recent studies using perfluorooctyl bromide (perflubron) have shown PLV to result in improved oxygenation and lung mechanics in premature lambs with respiratory distress syndrome [30], neonatal piglets with gastric acid aspiration [13], saline-lavaged rabbits [14], oleic acid-injured dogs [23] and saline-lavaged, oleic acid-injured sheep [29]. The first human report of the use of PFCs in supporting gas exchange appeared in 1990 and involved the administration of warmed, preoxygenated Rimar 101 to three preterm infants using a system designed to provide total liquid ventilation [3]. More recently, Gauger et al. [25] reported a series of six paediatric patients with severe respiratory failure treated with perflubron for periods ranging from 3 to 7 days. The patients in this series were profoundly hypoxemic and all met the institution's criteria for institution of extracorporeal life support (ECLS). The mean alveolar/arterial oxygen gradient at the time the patients were studied was 635 torr. The patients ranged in age from 8 weeks to 5½ years and five of the six were less than 1 year. Perflubron was administered between 37 and 236 h following initiation of ECLS and all were on extracorporeal life support (ECLS) at the time they were treated with perflubron. The mean PaO_2 during separation from ECLS increased from 39 mmHg to 92 mmHg and this increase was statistically as well as clinically significant. In addition, the mean static lung compliance increased from 0.12 ml/cmH$_2$O/kg to 0.28 ml/cmH$_2$O/kg, which was also significant. All six patients were ultimately weaned successfully from ECLS and survived to hospital discharge. Two patients did manifest small pneumothoraces during administration of perflubron and both resolved spontaneously.

More recently, Leach et al. have reported their experience using PLV in a series of premature infants with severe respiratory distress sydrome [27]. In a phase I, open-label study 13 severely ill premature infants (mean BW 1 057 g) who had failed surfactant therapy were treated with perflubron with an inital mean dose of 15 ml/kg for a mean duration of 42 h. Ten infants responded and manifested a significant reduction in oxygenation index (65%) as well as a dramatic improvement in lung compliance (61%). The adverse events reported included endotracheal tube obstruction and hypoxia. Eight of the infants survived and these encouraging data have stimulated significant interest in controlled trials of PLV in this premature population with a high predicted mortality.

There is also exciting new evidence that liquid ventilation when compared with conventional mechanical ventilation decreases the histological evidence of lung injury in an oleic-acid treated animal model [32]. Appropriate application to older patient populations with acute hypoxia and respiratory failure or syndromes not associated with surfactant deficiency need to be carefully examined. In the absence of unforeseen problems with toxicity, it is likely that PFC will assume a dominant role in the management of respiratory failure over the next several years.

Interface between PLV and high frequency ventilatory techniques

The combination of high frequency oscillatory ventilation and partial liquid breathing offers the possibility of partitioning the physiologic changes associated with positive pressure ventilation. Perflubron is clearly distributed preferentially to dependent lung due to its density relative to water [25, 26, 33-35]. Dependent lung regions have the greatest degree of atelectasis in both animal models of lung injury [36] as well as adults with acute respiratory distress syndrome (ARDS) [37]. Perflubron, therefore, produces rapid expansion of atelectasis-prone lung while high frequency oscillation offers an effective modality of lung volume maintenance [38]. Perflubron has surface tension-reducing properties that may be most effectively distributed with high frequency oscillatory ventilation [39]. The viscosity of perflubron also alters the distribution of gas ventilation to the perflubron-treated lung [40] with the non dependent lung receiving the largest portion of the gas tidal volume.

Several investigators have examined the combination of high frequency ventilation and perfluorochemical administration in animal models of lung injury. Baden et al. examined sequential dosing of perflubron during high frequency oscillatory ventilation of neonatal piglets with saline lavage-induced lung injury [41]. Animals were all treated with the same mean airway pressure during high frequency oscillatory ventilation with no attempts to optimize lung volume during the period of study. Initial dosing of the injured animals with 3 ml/kg of perflubron produced a significant increase in oxygen tension compared with animals managed with high frequency ventilation alone. Subsequent dosing, to a total administered dose of 30 ml/kg of perflubron, did not produce statistically significant improvements in oxygenation. However, the absence of attempts to optimize lung volume, particularly as lung mechanics were altered with each successive dose of perflubron, as well as the sequential study design make these data difficult to interpret.

Smith et al. described the combination of perflubron administration and a variety of high frequency devices in neonatal piglets treated with saline lavage [42]. After induction of lung injury, perflubron was instilled to achieve a visible meniscus within the endotracheal tube at zero airway pressure, resulting in a mean dose of 36 ml/kg. Ventilator settings were manipulated to optimize oxygenation using a conventional ventilator, high frequency jet ventilation, high frequency oscillatory ventilation as well as high frequency flow interruption with a multiple crossover design to allow comparison of different ventilator types after initial administration of perflubron. The complex design of this study makes the precise effects of combined high frequency oscillation and perflubron administration on gas exchange difficult to interpret. It was clear, however, that dosing to a visible meniscus did not produce significant improvements in oxygenation.

In an important follow-up study, the same group of investigators examined the effect of combined high frequency ventilation and perflubron administration on lung pathology in lavaged neonatal piglets [43]. In this 20 h study, which included attempts to optimize lung volume with perflubron dosing to achieve a visible meniscus, the combination of high frequency oscillation with perflubron administration produced the lowest combined lung injury scores. Furthermore, there was evidence of enhanced lung protection in both dependent and non-dependent lung regions. One interpretation of these two studies [42, 43] is that the optimal dose for enhancement of oxygenation is not the same as for provision of lung protection. Unfortunately, these data are incomplete as there are currently no data available describing histopathologic evidence of lung protection during the combination of high frequency oscillation and partial liquid breathing at varying doses of perflubron.

In a recent study in larger animals, we described the effects of perflubron administration during high frequency oscillatory ventilation on gas exchange, haemodynamic function, and lung histopathology [44]. Healthy swine underwent repetitive saline lavage and were then randomized to high frequency oscillation or combined high frequency oscillation and partial liquid ventilation with perflubron (HFO-PLV). Lung volume was not optimized in either treatment group and the HFO-PLV animals received a dose of 30 ml/kg of perflubron. There were no differences in the two groups of animals regarding gas exchange or haemodynamic function. However, the animals treated with the combination of high frequency oscillation and perflubron manifested significantly less severe atelectasis that was apparent after 2 h [44].

We have recently completed a dose-ranging study using high frequency oscilloatory ventilation applied to groups of animals treated with 5, 15, and 20 ml/kg of perflubron after saline lavage and optimization of lung volume on HFO. These data, which describe the dose/response relationships for gas exchange and haemodynamic function, suggest that the optimal dose for oxygenation efficiency, as quantified by the lowest oxygenation index, is in the range of 5-15 ml/kg. Furthermore, the perflubron-treated animals achieved adequate oxygenation within the specified target ranges for FiO_2 and PaO_2 with the lowest possible mean airway pressure during high frequency oscillation.

In summary, the results of a number of preclinical studies suggest that the combination of high frequency oscillatory ventilation and perflubron administration may offer an important advance in the treatment of acute lung injury and ARDS. We suggest that the dependent distribution of perflubron maximally reduces surface tension and recruits lung volume in the most severely affected lung regions. Simultaneously, high frequency oscillation of the perflubron-treated lung allows optimal lung volume maintenance with reduction of cyclic alveolar volume changes in the more compliant lung regions that are predominantly nondependent and primarily gas-filled during HFO-PLV. Our data suggest that the optimal dose of perflubron to achieve the lowest oxygenation index during HFO-PLV is between 5 and 15 ml. High frequency oscillation of the perfluorochemical-treated lung may well represent the sentinel advance in nonconventional support of the acutely injured lung that will significantly impact morbidity and mortality in the clinical setting.

References

1. Kylstra JA, Paganelly CV, Lantieri CJ (1964) Pulmonary gas exchange in dogs ventilated with hyperbarically oxygenated liquid. J Appl Phys 21:177-184
2. Clark LC, Gollan F (1966) Survival of mammals breathing organic liquids equilibrated with oxygen at atmospheric pressure. Science 152:1755-1756
3. Greenspan JS, Wolfson MR, Rubenstein SD et al (1990) Liquid ventilation of human preterm neonates. J Pediatr 117:106-111
4. Fuhrman BP, Paczan PR, DeFrancisis M (1991) Perfluorocarbon-associated gas exchange. Crit Care Med 19:712-722
5. Hirschl RB, Pranikoff T, Gauger P et al (1995) Liquid ventilation in adults, children, and full-term neonates. Lancet 346:1201-1202
6. Shaffer TH, Rubenstein SD, Moskowitz D et al (1976) Gaseous exchange and acid-base balance in premature lambs during liquid ventilation since birth. Pediatr Res 10:227-231
7. Hirschl RB, Parent A, Tooley R et al (1995) Liquid ventilation improves pulmonary function, gas exchange, and lung injury in a model of respiratory failure. Ann Surg 221:79-88
8. Kylstra JA, Schoenfisch WH (1972) Alveolar surface tension in fluorocarbon-filled lungs. J Appl Physiol 33:32-35
9. Shaffer TH, Lowe CA, Bhutani VK et al (1984) Liquid ventilation: effects on pulmonary function in distressed meconium-stained lambs. Pediatr Res 18:47-52
10. Wolfson MR, Greenspan JS, Deoras KS et al (1992) Comparison of gas and liquid ventilation: clinical, physiological, and histological correlates. J Appl Physiol 72:1024-1031
11. Leach CL, Fuhrman BP, Morin F III et al (1993) Perfluorocarbon-associated gas exchange (partial liquid ventilation) in respiratory distress syndrome: a prospective, randomized, controlled study. Crit Care Med 21:1270-1278
12. Lowe CA, Shaffer TH (1986) Pulmonary vascular resistance in the fluorocarbon-filled lung. J Appl Physiol 60:154-159
13. Nesti FD, Fuhrman BP, Steinhorn DM et al (1994) Perfluorocarbon-associated gas exchange in gastric aspiration. Crit Care Med 22:1445-1452
14. Tütüncü AS, Faithfull NS, Lachmann B (1993) Comparison of ventilatory support with intratracheal perfluorocarbon administration and conventional mechanical ventilation in animals with acute respiratory failure. Am Rev Respir Dis 148:785-792
15. Smith TM, Steinhorn DM, Thusu K et al (1995) A liquid perfluorochemical decreases the in vitro production of reactive oxygen species by alveolar macrophages. Crit Care Med 23:1533-1539
16. Thomassen MJ, Buhrow LT, Wiedemann HP (1997) Perflubron decreases inflammatory cytokine production by human alveolar macrophages. Crit Care Med 25:2045-2047
17. Nesti FD, Fuhrman BP, Ballow M et al (1995) Modulation of PHA responsiveness with perflubron in acid aspiration pneumonitis. Crit Care Med 23:A213
18. Varani J, Hirschl RB, Dame M et al (1996) Perfluorocarbon protects lung epithelial cells from neutrophil-mediated injury in an in vitro model of liquid ventilation therapy. Shock 6:339-344
19. Lowe KC, Edwards CM, Röhlke W et al (1997) Perfluorochemical effects on neutrophil chemiluminescence. Adv Exp Med Biol 428:495-499
20. Tütüncü AS, Faithfull NS, Lachmann B (1993) Intratracheal perfluorocarbon administration combined with mechanical ventilation in experimental respiratory distress syndrome: dose-dependent improvement of gas exchange. Crit Care Med 21:962-969

21. Mates EA, Hildebrandt J, Jackson JC et al (1997) Shunt and ventilation-perfusion distribution during partial liquid ventilation in healthy piglets. J Appl Physiol 82:933-942
22. Tarczy-Hornoch P, Hildebrandt J, Mates EA et al (1996) Effects of exogenous surfactant on lung pressure-volume characteristics during liquid ventilation. J Appl Physiol 80:1764-1771
23. Curtis SE, Peek JT, Kelly DR (1993) Partial liquid breathing with perflubron improves arterial oxygenation in acute canine lung injury. J Appl Physiol 75:2696-2702
24. Tütüncü AS, Lachmann B, Faithfull NS et al (1992) Dose-dependent improvement of gas exchange by intratracheal perflubron (perfluorooctylbromide) instillation in adult animals with acute respiratory failure. Adv Exp Med Biol 317:397-400
25. Gauger PG, Pranikoff T, Schreiner RJ et al (1996) Initial experience with partial liquid ventilation in pediatric patients with the acute respiratory distress syndrome. Crit Care Med 24:16-22
26. Hirschl RB, Pranikoff T, Wise C et al (1996) Initial experience with partial liquid ventilation in adult patients with the acute respiratory distress syndrome. JAMA 275:383-389
27. Leach CL, Greenspan JS, Rubenstein SD et al (1996) Partial liquid ventilation with perflubron in premature infants with severe respiratory distress syndrome. N Engl J Med 335:761-767
28. Hernan LJ, Fuhrman BP, Kaiser RE et al (1996) Perfluorocarbon-associated gas exchange in normal and acid-injured large sheep. Crit Care Med 24:475-481
29. Doctor A, Ibla JC, Grenier B et al (1998) Pulmonary blood flow distribution during partial liquid ventilation. J Appl Physiol 84:1540-1550
30. Leach CL, Fuhrman BP, Morin FC III et al (1993) Perfluorocarbon-associated gas exchange (partial liquid ventilation) in respiratory distress syndrome: a prospective, randomized, controlled study. Crit Care Med 21:1270-1278
31. Hirschl RB, Tooley R, Parent AC et al (1995) Improvement of gas exchange, pulmonary function, and lung injury with partial liquid ventilation. Chest 108:500-508
32. Hirschl RB, Overbeck MC, Parent A et al (1994) Liquid ventilation provides uniform distribution of perfluorocarbon in the setting of respiratory failure. Surgery 116:159-168
33. Kazerooni EA, Pranikoff T, Cascade PN et al (1996) Partial liquid ventilation with perflubron during extracorporeal life support in adults: radiographic appearance. Radiology 198:137-142
34. Garver KA, Kazerooni EA, Hirschl RB et al (1996) Neonates with congenital diaphragmatic hernia: radiographic findings during partial liquid ventilation. Radiology 200:219-223
35. Meaney JFM, Kazerooni EA, Garver KA et al (1997) Acute respiratory distress syndrome: CT findings during partial liquid ventilation. Radiology 202:570-573
36. Broccard AF, Shapiro RS, Schmitz LL et al (1997) Influence of prone position on the extent and distribution of lung injury in a high tidal volume oleic acid model of acute respiratory distress syndrome. Crit Care Med 25:16-27
37. Gattinoni L, Pesenti A, Bombino M et al (1988) Relationships between lung computed tomographic density, gas exchange, and PEEP in acute respiratory failure. Anaesthesiology 69:824-832
38. McCulloch PR, Forkert PG, Froese AB (1988) Lung volume maintenance prevents lung injury during high frequency oscillatory ventilation in surfactant-deficient rabbits. Am Rev Respir Dis 137:1185-1192
39. Froese AB, McCulloch PR, Sugiura M et al (1993) Optimizing alveolar expansion prolongs the effectiveness of exogenous surfactant therapy in the adult rabbit. Am Rev Respir Dis 148:569-577

40. Cox PN, Morris K, Frndova H et al (1996) Relative distribution of gas and perfluoro-carbon (PFC) during partial liquid ventilation. Pediatr Res 39:45A
41. Baden HP, Mellema JD, Bratton SL et al (1997) High-frequency oscillatory ventilation with partial liquid ventilation in a model of acute respiratory failure. Crit Care Med 25:299-302
42. Smith KM, Bing DR, Meyers PA et al (1997) Partial liquid ventilation: a comparison using conventional and high-frequency techniques in an animal model of acute respiratory failure. Crit Care Med 25:1179-1186
43. Smith KM, Mrozek JD, Simonton SC et al (1997) Prolonged partial liquid ventilation using conventional and high-frequency ventilatory techniques: gas exchange and lung pathology in an animal model of respiratory distress syndrome. Crit Care Med 25:1888-1897
44. Doctor A, Mazzoni MC, Del Balzo U et al (1998) High frequency oscillatory ventilation of the perfluorocarbon-filled lung: preliminary results in an animal model of acute lung injury. Crit Care Med (in press)

Chapter 26

Hemopurification in paediatric intensive care

G. Zobel, S. Rödl, E. Ring, B. Urlesberger

Acute renal failure is defined as the cessation of renal function with or without changes in urinary output. The incidence of acute renal failure in paediatric intensive care units is highly variable, ranging from 2%-8% [1]. Acute renal failure in infants and children is often associated with severe medical or surgical illness. If conventional therapy fails to control fluid and metabolic balance, extracorporeal renal replacement therapy has to be instituted [2]. Intermittent hemodialysis and peritoneal dialysis are not always feasible in critically ill patients for both technical and clinical reasons [1]. Continuous hemofiltration, either driven in the arteriovenous or venovenous mode, is an alternative continuous renal replacement therapy (CRRT) to control fluid and metabolic balance [3, 4]. In 1977, Kramer et al. first described continuous arteriovenous hemofiltration (CAVH) for extracorporeal renal support in oliguric adults with diuretic-resistant fluid overload [5]. Recently, this technique has been used in critically ill paediatric patients [6-12]. During CAVH the blood is driven through the hemofilter by the arteriovenous pressure gradient. Fluid and solutes are removed by convective transport. The great advantage of CAVH is its simplicity, safety, and excellent clinical tolerance. However, arterial cannulation carries the risk of arterial thrombosis or thromboembolism. In addition, low efficiency and frequent hemofilter clotting are the disadvantages of CRRT. A variety of techniques, such as suction support, predilution, or intermittent or continuous hemodialysis, have been described to increase the efficacy of CAVH [13-16]. Suction-supported CAVH increases the ultrafiltration rates but decreases filter running time by increasing blood viscosity inside the filter. Predilution increases filter running without significantly increasing ultrafiltration rates. Continuous hemodiafiltration (CHDF) increases urea clearance rates without influencing the hemofilter running time and is an alternative to CAVH in critically ill patients with hypercatabolism. Recently, blood pumps have been increasingly used for hemofiltration both in adult and paediatric patients [4, 17, 18]. Continuous venovenous hemofiltration (CVVH) allows constant blood flow rates, produces higher ultrafiltration rates and prolongs filter running time.

Methods

Schematic graphs of spontaneous and pump-driven hemofiltration and hemodiafiltration are given in Fig. 1.

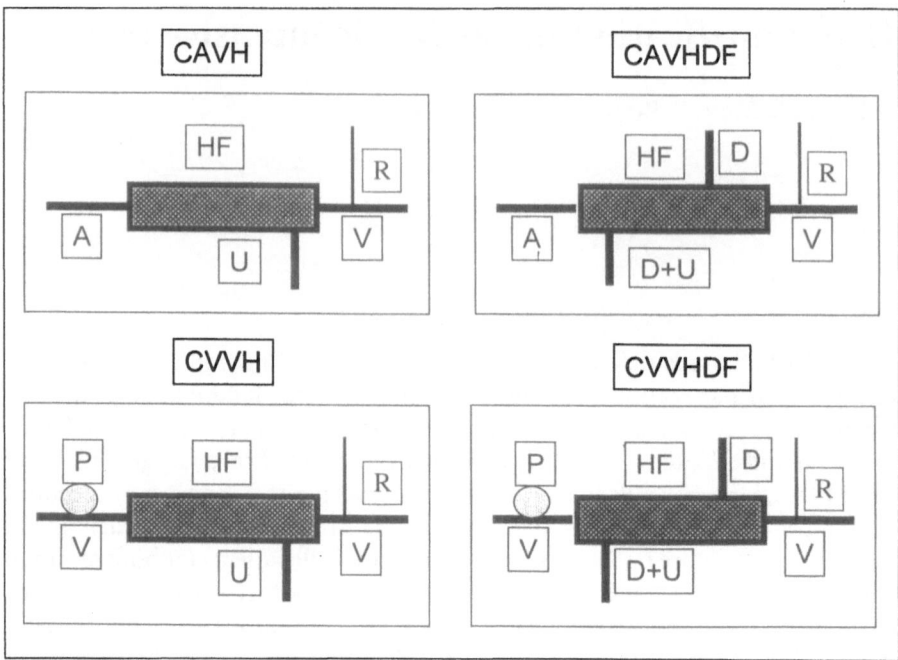

Fig.1. Schematic graphs of different techniques of continuous renal replacement therapies. *A*, artery; *V*, vein; *HF*, hemofilter; *U*, ultrafiltrate; *R*, replacement fluid; *D*, dialysate; *P*, pump; *CAVH*, continuous arteriovenous hemofiltration; *CAVHDF*, continuous arteriovenous hemodiafiltration; *CVVH*, continuous venovenous hemofiltration; *CVVHDF*, continuous venovenous hemodiafiltration

Extracorporeal circuit

Different hemofilter systems (Amicon Minifilter, Amicon Minifilter Plus, Amicon Diafilter D-20, Amicon Corp., Lexington, MA; Miniflow 10, Multiflow 60, Hospal Lyon, France; Gambro FH 22, Gambro Corporation, Hechingen, Germany) were used for CRRT in neonates, infants, and children. The hemofilter characteristics are given in Table 1. The membrane surface area ranges from 0.015 m^2 to 0.6 m^2 and the priming volume from 3.7 to 48 ml. The low end-to-end pressure drop of the Amicon filters is ideal for CAVH in small infants.

The blood lines should be as short as possible to minimize the resistance to blood flow. The arterial line needs one port for continuous heparin infusion and one for pressure tracings and blood sampling, and on the venous line there should be one port for the infusion of the replacement fluid and one for pressure tracings. The ultrafiltrate collection bag should be placed 70-100 cm below the hemofilter to exert a negative pressure on the hemofilter membrane.

The hemofilter system was rinsed with 1 l 0.9% saline solution containing 5 000 IU of heparin. In small infants the system was primed with heparinized blood (3 IU/ml) immediately before starting the procedure. Hemofilters were exchanged

Table 1. Characteristics of hemofilters for neonates, infants and children

Material	Polysulfone	Polyacrilonitrile	Polysulfone	Polyamide	Polysulfone	Polyacrilonitrile
	Minifilter old/new	*Miniflow 10*	*Minifilter Plus*	*FH-22*	*Diafilter D-20*	*Multiflow 60*
Length of fibers (cm)	8/12.7	21	12.7	11.5	12.5	15
Diameter of fibers (µm)	1 100/1 100	240	570	220	250	240
Surface area (m^2)	0.015/0.021	0.042	0.08	0.2	0.4	0.6
Filling volume (ml)	6/7.6	3.7	15	13	38	4.8
Number of fibers	60/60	264	450	2 400	5 000	6 000

when ultrafiltration rates had decreased to 60%-70% of the initial mean value.

Vascular access

Adequate vascular access is extremely important for CAVH in neonates and infants. The catheters have to be short with a relatively large inner diameter to minimize the resistance to blood flow. Vascular access for both the arteriovenous and venovenous techniques are given in Table 2. The umbilical vessels can be used for blood access in neonates during the first week of life. However, the resistance of standard umbilical catheters is rather high [19]. Short 20-22 G cannulas inserted into the radial or brachial arteries usually provide adequate blood flow in newborns. The femoral artery is not the first choice of vascular access in neonates, but is routinely used in older infants and children. Radial and brachial arteries are punctured directly. All other catheters are placed percutaneously using the Seldinger technique. The internal jugular vein should be used for blood return because its cannulation is safe and easy in small infants. The venous catheter should be short with a large inner diameter to optimize blood flow through the circuit. We now use 4-F catheters (Medcomp, Medical Components Inc., Harleysville, USA) for blood return in neonates and small infants. All venous catheters are placed with standard Seldinger technique.

For pump-driven hemofiltration we prefer the use of two 5-F single-lumen catheters in neonates. The tip of the catheter has to be placed into the middle of the right atrium to provide adequate drainage of venous blood. In infants older than 6 months, we routinely use double-lumen catheters from 7.5-9 F.

Table 2. Vascular access for continuous arteriovenous and venovenous hemofiltration in infants and children

	Artery	Catheter	Vein	Catheter-SL	Catheter-DL
Neonates	Umbilical	3.5-5 F	Umbilical	5 F	6-7F
	Radial	20-22 G	Internal jugular	4 F	6-7 F
	Brachial	20 G	Femoral	4 F	6-7 F
Infants	Radial	20 G	Internal jugular	5-6 F	7-8 F
	Brachial	18-20 G	Femoral	5-6 F	7-8 F
	Femoral	18 G			
Children	Femoral	4-5 F	Femoral	8 F	9-11 F
			Subclavian	8 F	9-11 F
			Internal jugular	8 F	9-11 F

SL, single-lumen; DL, double-lumen; F, french; G, gauge

Anticoagulation

Anticoagulation was usually achieved with unfractionated heparin. Patients with a normal coagulation status initially received a heparin bolus of 50-100 IU/kg followed by a continuous infusion of 10-20 IU/kg per hour into the arterial line of the extracorporeal device. Heparinization was controlled by partial thrombo-plastin time (PTT) measurements in the systemic circulation three to four times a day. PTT was maintained at 20-30 s over baseline. In patients at high risk of bleeding prostacyclin (Flolan, Welcome, London, UK) was given at a rate of 5-20 ng/kg per minute as the sole antithrombotic agent or in combination with low-dose heparin (2.5 IU/kg per hour).

Fluid balancing and replacement fluid

The ultrafitrate was partially or totally replaced according to the clinical situa-tion. The ultrafiltrate substitution was either based on lactate or bicarbonate and was warmed by a fluid warmer system (Hotline, Level 1 Technologies Inc., Rockland, MA, USA) before infusion. The lactate-based solution consists of 142 mmol/l sodium, 110 mmol/l chloride, 1.75 mmol/l calcium, 0.75 mmol/l mag-nesium, and 35 mmol/l lactate. Potassium was added up to 4 mmol/l according to the serum potassium levels. In all neonates and in children with multiple or-gan system failure, the ultrafiltrate substitution fluid was based on bicarbonate (Hemosol BO, Hospal Lyon, France). This solution consists of 140 mmol/l sodi-um, 109 mmol/l chloride, 1.75 mmol/l calcium, 0.5 mmol/l magnesium, 3 mmol/l lactate, and 32 mmol/l bicarbonate. Fluid in- and output were either controlled by the nurses on an hourly basis or continuously by a microproces-sor-controlled fluid balance system (Amicon Equaline system, Amicon Corp., Lexington, MA, USA) using the weight change program. The ultrafiltrate, the re-placed ultrafiltrate substitution fluid, and the fluid balance were continuously displayed on the control panel.

Continuous arteriovenous hemofiltration

During CAVH blood is driven through the highly permeable hemofilter by the patient's arteriovenous pressure gradient, producing an ultrafiltrate that is par-tially or totally replaced with an appropriate replacement solution.

Slow continuous ultrafiltration

Slow continuous ultrafiltration (SCU) is a form of CAVH/CVVH not associated with fluid replacement.

Continuous venovenous hemofiltration

Blood is driven through a highly permeable hemofilter by a roller pump. In CVVH the ultrafiltrate produced is partially or totally replaced according to the clinical requirements. For pump-driven hemofiltration we use a roller pump (Gambro AK 10 blood monitor, Gambro Corporation, Hechingen, Germany) and small blood lines. The roller pump has two exchangeable pump headings which enabled blood flow rates from 12 to 300 ml/min. Pressure tracings were performed immediately before the roller pump and after the hemofilter. Recently, we started with one of the newly designed machines (Prisma machine, Hospal Lyon, France) equipped with integrated safety alarms, pressure monitoring and pumps for fluid balancing control and the capability to perform hemofiltration, hemodialysis, or hemodiafiltration. However, these machines are not yet adapted for use in neonates and small infants.

Continuous hemodiafiltration

During CHDF the CAVH or CVVH circuit is modified by the addition of slow countercurrent dialysate flow into the ultrafiltrate-dialysate compartment of the hemofilter. CHDF can be driven in the spontaneous or pump-driven mode. The bicarbonate-based dialysate consists of 140 mmol/l sodium, 109 mmol/l chloride, 1.75 mmol/l calcium, 0.5 mmol/l magnesium, 3.0 mmol/l lactate, and 32 mmol/l bicarbonate. Potassium was added as required up to 4 mmol/l. The dialysate was administered by the Equaline system, using the infusion mode. The dialysate and ultrafiltrate flows were continuously displayed on the control panel of the Equaline system. During continuous hemodiafiltration, the ultrafiltrate was replaced by a volumetric pump. Now the Prisma machine is used in infants and children with a body weight of more than 10 kg to run the different techniques of renal replacement therapies.

Serum and ultrafiltrate/dialysate concentrations of urea and creatinine were determined routinely three times a day. Urea clearance was calculated as: dialysate effluent urea/serum urea × volume/time. Pre- and postfilter hematocrit and plasma protein were determined twice daily to calculate blood flow rate and filtration fraction during CAVH according to formulas described by Lauer et al. [3].

Data are given as mean±SEM. Student's t-test for unpaired samples and analysis of variance were used for comparison of the mean values.

Results

From June 1985 to June 1998, 98 critically ill infants and children with a mean age of 3.5±0.5 years and a mean body weight of 14.9±1.8 kg underwent continuous arteriovenous or venovenous renal support at the paediatric ICU of the Children's Hospital, University of Graz, Austria. The demographic data of the patients are given in Table 3. Twenty-five percent of the patients developed acute renal failure (ARF) after open heart surgery, 32% had severe sepsis, and only 12% a primary renal disease. Eighty-nine percent were on mechanical ventilation and 86% needed vasopressor support. The majority of the patients was on parenteral nutrition with a protein and caloric intake of 1.25 to 2.0 g/kg per day and 50-80 kcal/kg per day, respectively. Indications for continuous extracorporeal renal support were: acute renal failure, multiple organ system failure, diuretic resistant hypervolemia, metabolic crisis in inborn errors of metabolism, and low cardiac output.

Table 3. Clinical features of critically ill infants and children with continuous renal replacement therapy (n=98; mean±SEM)

	CAVH (n=45)	CVVH (n=54)
• Age (years)	3.2±0.8	3.8±0.7
• BW (kg)	13.8±2.7	15.9±2.4
• Sex ratio (M/F)	29/16	36/18
• Diagnosis		
– ARF	5	9
– LCO	16	10
– MOSF	17	30
– Hypervolemia	4	1
– Metabolic crisis	3	4
• Mean arterial pressure (mmHg)	57.9±3.3	56.6±2.3
• Survival rate (%)	60	55
• Duration of CRRT (h)	120±21	147±20

CAVH, continuous arteriovenous hemofiltration; *CVVH*, continuous venovenous hemofiltration; *BW*, body weight; *M*, male; *F*, female; *ARF*, acute renal failure; *LCO*, low cardiac output; *MOSF*, multiple organ system failure; *CRRT*, continuous renal replacement therapy

Continuous arteriovenous hemofiltration

Nineteen neonates, six infants, 11 toddlers, and eight children were treated with CAVH. Operational data during CAVH are given in Table 4. Mean duration of CAVH was 120±21.7 h/patient, ranging from 12 to 720 h. The mean blood flow rates during CAVH ranged from 7±1.2 ml/min (neonates) to 61±11 ml/min (children) and produced ultrafiltration rates ranging from 3.6±0.6 (neonates) to 6.6±1.1 ml/min per square meter (children). The mean hemofilter running time during CAVH was 26.8±2.6 h. The pre-CAVH serum creatinine and urea levels were 2.9±0.4 and 123±11mg/dl, the post-CAVH levels were 2.3±0.2 and 105±6.1 mg/dl, respectively. CAVH was well tolerated by all patients. Frequent clotting of the hemofilter was observed in three neonates with rather low blood flow. Local bleeding at the catheter entrance site was observed in four patients and severe bleeding in two patients. Femoral artery cannulation resulted in transient ischemia of the leg in two neonates. A femoral artery thrombosis necessitated sur-

Table 4. Blood flow and ultrafiltration rates during CAVH in pediatric patients (n=44)

	n	Qb (ml/min)	Qf (ml/min/m^2)	HF exchange (h)	Survival rate (%)
Neonates	19	7.2±1.2	3.6±0.6	26.8±2.6	58
Infants	6	12.7±3.2	3.1±1.0	23.4±4.1	80
Toddlers	11	23.7±5.4	4.9±1.2	24.4±2.9	73
Children	8	61±11	6.6±1.1	28.6±2.3	37.5

Qb, blood flow; *Qf*, ultrafiltration rate; *HF*, hemofilter; *CAVH*, continuous arteriovenous hemofiltration

Table 5. Blood flow and ultrafiltration rates during CVVH in pediatric patients ($n=54$)

	n	Qb (ml/min)	Qf (ml/min/m²)	HF exchange (h)	Survival rate (%)
Neonates	12	22±1.6	10±2.3	57.8±14.1	66
Infants	8	27±4.4	7.5±1.5	66±19	50
Toddlers	19	32±4.2	8.6±1.4	49±5.8	58
Children	15	78±8.9	12±1.1	45±2.2	44

Qb, blood flow; *Qf*, ultrafiltration rate; *HF*, hemofilter; *CVVH*, continuous venovenous hemofiltration

gical revision after 12 days of CAVH in a 1.5-year-old child. The survival rate in neonates, infants, toddlers, and children treated with CAVH was 58%, 80%, 73%, and 37.5%, respectively.

Continuous venovenous hemofiltration

Fifty-four patients were treated with pump-driven hemofiltration. As shown in Table 5 the blood flow and ultrafiltration rates were significantly higher in all age groups during CVVH than during CAVH. The mean hemofilter running time during CVVH ranged from 45±2 to 66±19 h. The pre-CVVH serum creatinine and urea levels were 2.3±0.2 and 117±10mg/dl; the post-CAVH levels were 1.8±0.2 and 96±6.6 mg/dl, respectively. A slight fall in the blood pressure was observed immediately after starting CVVH in patients with severely compromized heart circulation. Blood pressure usually returned to the baseline value within the next 5 min. Complications included partial thrombosis of the vena cava superior or inferior in three patients, hemothorax in one and severe intracranial bleeding in one patient. The survival rate in neonates, infants, toddlers, and children treated with CAVH was 66%, 50%, 58%, and 44%, respectively.

Hemodiafiltration

Table 6 shows the ultrafiltration, urea, and creatinine clearance rates during venovenous hemofiltration and hemodiafiltration using the Miniflow 10 filter in ten neonates/infants. The mean ultrafiltration rates during CVVH were 1.1±0.1 ml/min. Adding a dialysate solution at a rate of 5 ml/min in a countercurrent fashion to blood flow resulted in a significant increase in urea and creatinine clearance with only a minimal change in the ultrafiltration rates.

Six infants were treated with CAVH and continuous arteriovenous hemodiafiltration (CAVHDF) using the Amicon Minifilter and Minifilter plus. During CAVHDF the mean ultrafiltration rates decreased slightly, whereas urea clearances increased significantly by 247% in the Minifilter and by 243% in the Minifilter plus. Simultaneously, the serum urea and creatinine levels fell by 35% and 36%, respectively.

Figure 2 shows the course of serum potassium, urea, and uric acid in a child

Table 6. Operational data during CVVH and CVVHDF using the Hospal Miniflow 10 in ten neonates/infants

	CVVH	CVVHDF	*p*-value
Qb (ml/min)	20±1.4	19.4±1.3	n.s.
Qf (ml/min)	1.1±0.1	1.02±0.1	n.s.
Urea-clearance (ml/min)	1.13±0.13	4.3±0.18	<0.01
Creatinine-clearance (ml/min)	1.08±0.1	4.2±0.16	<0.01
MAP (mmHg)	56±2.7	57±1.9	n.s.

Qb, blood flow; *Qf*, ultrafiltration rate; *Qd*, dialysate flow; *MAP*, mean arterial pressure; *CVVH*, continudes venovenous hemofiltration; *CVVHDF*, continuous venovenous hemodiafiltration

with leukemia and tumor lysis syndrome, resulting in oliguria, azotemia, hyperkalemia and extremely high serum uric acid levels. High volume pump-driven hemodiafiltration enabled rapid normalization of these serum parameters and urinary output revovered within 48 h.

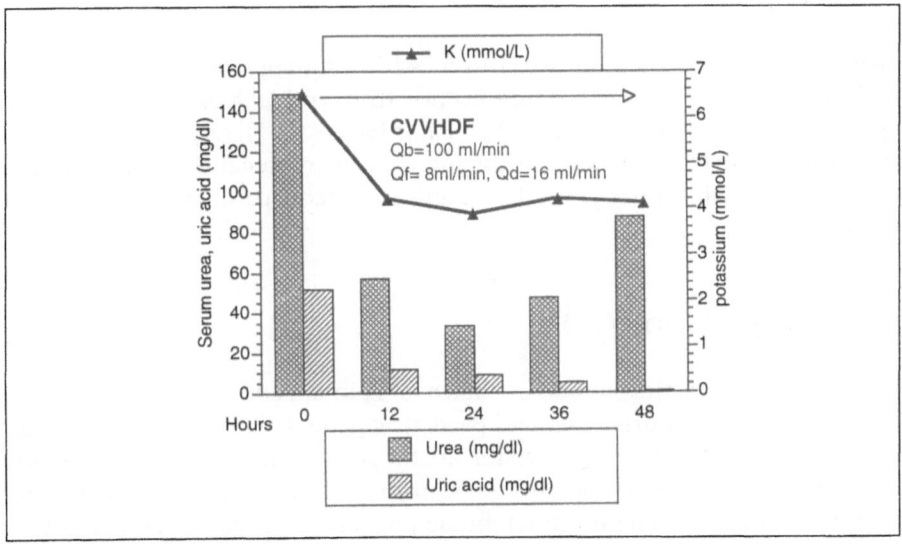

Fig. 2. The course of serum potassium, urea, and uric acid in a 3-year-old child with leukemia and tumor lysis syndrome. *CVVHDF*, continuous venovenous hemodiafiltration; *Qb*, blood flow; *Qf*, ultrafiltration rate; *Qd*, dialysate flow rate

Slow continuous ultrafiltration

SCU is a form of CAVH/CVVH not associated with fluid replacement. We used this technique in 26 infants and children with postoperative low cardiac output and severe hypervolemia unresponsive to conventional treatment. During slow and continuous fluid removal, the haemodynamics improved transiently or permanently in all but four patients. The mean arterial pressure in-

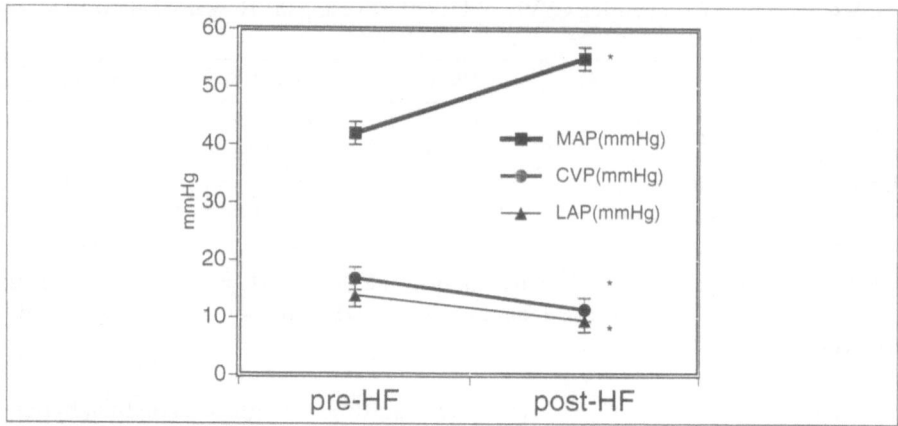

Fig. 3. Hemodynamics pre- and post hemofiltration in infants and children with severe low cardiac output after open heart surgery. *CVP*, central venous pressure; *LAP*, left atrial pressure; *MAP*, mean arterial pressure; *HF*, hemofiltration
* p < 0.01

creased from 41.8±1.4 (pre-SCU) to 55.4±2.8 mmHg (post-SCU) (*p*<0.01) while CVP and LAP decreased significantly from 16.1±0.8 to 11.2±0.7 mmHg (*p*<0.01) and from 14.9±0.7 to 10.1±0.8 mmHg (*p*<0.01), respectively (Fig. 3). In addition, there was a significant increase in oxygenation, and the catecholamine infusion rates could be significantly reduced during the constant fluid removal.

Clinical advances in CRRT

Nowadays, CRRT is the method of choice to maintain adequate metabolic control in critically ill anuric adult and paediatric patients [20-24]. The major determinants for ultrafiltrate production are the surface area and the permeability of the hemofilter membrane and the transmembrane pressure across the hemofilter membrane. The transmembrane pressure depends on the blood flow through the hemofilter device, the colloidosmotic pressure, and the negative pressure on the ultrafiltrate side of the hemofilter created by the distance between the hemofilter and the ultrafiltrate collection bag. The blood flow during CAVH depends on the arteriovenous pressure gradient, length and diameter of blood lines and catheters, and blood viscosity. The advantages of spontaneous CAVH are its simplicity and safety. It allows good control of fluid overload and metabolic imbalances and provides haemodynamic stability. In addition, it allows adequate nutrition and unlimited medication. The risks are bleeding and thrombosis. A disadvantage is its rather low urea clearance, insufficient to control azotemia in hypercatabolic states [25].

In order to improve urea clearance in critically ill patients with multiple organ system failure, CAVHDF and CVVH have recently been introduced [26, 27].

In 1984, Geronemus and Schneider reported that CAVHDF might represent an alternative treatment of acute renal failure in critically ill patients [13]. Using high permeability membranes and a dialysate flow of 16.6 ml/min, urea clearances up to 16.6 ml/min were achieved. During CHDF, the dialysate solution passes on the ultrafiltrate side of the filter countercurrent to blood flow. Thus, diffusion of solutes is added to convective transport and ultrafiltration. The ultrafiltration rates of CAVHDF permit administration of hyperalimentation solutions as well as fluid removal in hypervolemic patients. CAVHDF has the advantages of CAVH in terms of simplicity and sufficient removal of excess plasma water and has the capability of increased solute removal. Rapid volume and osmolar shifts are avoided and haemodynamic stability is provided. Recently, CAVH combined with dialysis has been increasingly used in critically ill adult patients to control azotemia and to provide full nutritional support [28-30]. Bischof et al used continuous hemodiafiltration in four children with acute renal failure and contraindications to hemodialysis or peritoneal dialysis [31]. This treatment mode allowed excellent metabolic control without negative effects on the haemodynamics. In one patient with tumor lysis syndrome CVVH was unable to correct electrolyte disturbances. Initiation of CVVHDF resulted in correction of electrolyte abnormalities and azotemia.

Recently, Gouyon et al reported urea clearance rates during CAVH and CAVHDF in seven anaesthetized adult rabbits which were given urea infusions [32]. For this experiment, a 800 cm^2 polysulfone hemofilter was used. Operational parameters were comparable during CAVH and CAVHDF. Urea clearance increased by 285% during CAVHD. In contrast to our findings they observed an increase in ultrafiltration rates during CAVHDF by 47%. In our experience with polysulfone and polyacrilinitrile filters in small infants, urea clearance improved substantially during CHDF. The simultaneous decrease in ultrafiltration rates might be caused by a pressure increase on the dialysate side, resulting in a lower transmembrane pressure.

CVVH is another extracorporeal renal support system which allows higher ultrafiltration rates and urea clearance [5, 18, 20]. In 1989, Wendon et al. reported that continuous high-volume-pumped venovenous hemofiltration using a double-lumen catheter is an effective method of renal support in catabolic septic adult patients with multiple organ system failure [27]. Inserting a pump into the extracorporeal system means that blood flow and ultrafiltration rates are no longer dependent on the patient's blood pressure.

In 1993 Bellomo et al. published a prospective study on continuous venovenous hemodiafiltration (CVVHDF) in 60 critically ill patients with acute renal failure [33]. The authors concluded that CVVHDF is a very safe approach to renal replacement therapy in critically ill patients. It offers excellent azotemia control and is associated with comparatively favorable outcome.

In a recent study Bellomo et al. compared CAVHDF and CVVHDF in critically ill adult patients [34]. Whereas ultrafiltration rates were significantly higher during the venovenous approach, there was no statistically significant difference in urea and creatinine clearances. The authors noticed a substantial decrease in the number of access-related complications and concluded that CVVHDF may be the treatment of choice for extracorporeal renal support in critically ill patients. In addition, Bellomo et al demonstrated that CVVH with dialysis can remove both TNF-α and IL-1β from the circulation of septic patients [35]. However, the role of inflammatory mediator removal in critically ill patients with multiple organ system failure by CRRT has to be demonstrated in the future.

In our experience blood flow and ultrafiltration rates are significantly higher during pump-driven hemofiltration and hemofilter running time is significantly longer [18]. However, CVVH is technically more difficult, especially in small infants when a double-lumen catheter is used. This problem can be overcome by using two single-lumen catheters and placing the suction catheter in the upper part of the right atrium to optimize drainage of blood into the extracorporeal device.

Recently, Fleming et al. reported that arteriovenous or venovenous hemofiltration offers significant advantages over peritoneal dialysis in paediatric patients after open heart surgery in terms of fluid removal, nutritional support, and control of azotemia [36].

Myocardial damage and a large fluid load during cardiopulmonary bypass may result in low cardiac output with increased blood volume and pulmonary edema. Low cardiac output causes renal hypoperfusion with fluid and sodium retention. When the kidneys become resistant to diuretics, gross edema formation necessitates extracorporeal fluid removal. Slow continuous ultrafiltration allows exact fluid titration to find the optimal filling pressures for best myocardial performance. It improves pulmonary gas exchange and fluid and metabolic balances, resulting in better myocardial performance.

In conclusion, continuous hemofiltration either driven in the arteriovenous or venovenous mode is an effective method of renal support in critically ill infants and children. Both methods allow good control of fluid, electrolyte, and acid-base balances. CAVH requires arterial cannulation and the procedure is blood pressure dependent, resulting in lower ultrafiltration rates and shorter hemofilter running time. The pump-driven mode allows constant blood flow and ultrafiltration rates with excellent control of azotemia even in hypercatabolic states. The use of a pump makes the procedure more complex, but it can be carried out in every paediatric ICU without dialysis-trained staff. The use of CAVHDF substantially increases urea clearances while maintaining the simplicity and safety of the CAVH system. CVVHDF permits the highest urea clearance rates and is indicated in emergency conditions such as severe tumor lysis syndrome or severe metabolic crisis due to an inborn error of metabolism. All techniques allow adequate nutrition and unlimited medication.

Acknowledgement. The authors want to thank the nurses of the paediatric ICU of the Children's Hospital, University of Graz, who enabled this work.

References

1. Fackler JC (1996) Renal, endocrine, and metabolic disorders. In: Rogers MC (ed) Textbook of pediatric intensive care. Williams and Wilkins, Baltimore, pp 1217-1246
2. Schetz M, Lauwers PM, Ferdinande P (1989) Extracorporeal treatment of acute renal failure in the intensive care unit: a critical view. Intensive Care Med 15:349-357
3. Lauer A, Saccaggi A, Ronco C, Belledonne M, Glabman S, Bosch JB (1983) Continuous arteriovenous hemofiltration in the critically ill patient. Ann Intern Med 99:455-460
4. Storck M, Hartl WH, Zimmerer E, Inthorn D (1991) Comparison of pump-driven and spontaneous continuous hemofiltration in postoperative acute renal failure. Lancet 337:452-455
5. Kramer P, Wigger W, Rieger J, Mathaei D, Scheler F (1977) Arteriovenous hemofiltration: new and simple method for the treatment of overhydrated patients resistant to diuretics. Klin Wochenschr 55:1121-1122
6. Lieberman KV (1987) Continuous arteriovenous hemofiltration in children. Pediatr Nephrol 1:330-338
7. Leone MR, Jenkins RD, Golper TA, Alexander SR (1986) Early experience with continuous arteriovenous hemofiltration in critically ill pediatric patients. Crit Care Med 14:1058-1063
8. Lopez-Herce J, Dorao P, Delgado MA, Espinosa L, Ruza F, Martinez MC (1989) Continuous arteriovenous haemofiltration in children. Intensive Care Med 15:224-227
9. Ronco C, Brendolan A, Bragantini L, Chiaramonte S, Feriani M, Fabris A, Dell'Aquila R, La Greca G (1986) Treatment of acute renal failure in newborns by continuous arteriovenous hemofiltration. Kidney Int 29:908-915
10. Ronco C, Parenzan L (1995) Acute renal failure in infancy: treatment by continuous renal replacement therapy. Intensive Care Med 21:490-499
11. Zobel G, Ring E, Müller WD (1989) Continuous arteriovenous hemofiltration in preterm infants. Crit Care Med 17:534-536
12. Zobel G, Ring E, Zobel V (1989) Continuous arteriovenous renal replacement systems for critically ill children. Pediatr Nephrol 3:140-143
13. Geronemus R, Schneider N (1984) Continuous arteriovenous hemodialysis: a new modality of treatment for acute renal failure. J Trans Am Soc Artif Intern Organs 30:610-613
14. Kaplan AA (1985) Pre-vs postdilution for continuous arteriovenous hemofiltration. Trans Am Soc Artif Intern Organs 31:28-31
15. Zobel G, Kuttnig M, Ring E (1990) Continuous arteriovenous hemodialysis in critically ill infants. Child Nephrol Urol 10:196-198
16. Zobel G, Ring E, Trop M, Grubbauer HM (1988) Suction supported continuous arteriovenous hemofiltration in children. Blood Purif 6:37-42
17. Ellis EN, Pearson D, Robinson L, Belsha CW, Wells TG, Berry PL (1993) Pump-assisted hemofiltration in infants with acute renal failure. Pediatr Nephrol 7:434-437
18. Zobel G, Ring E, Kuttnig M, Grubbauer HM (1991) Continuous arteriovenous hemofiltration versus continuous venovenous hemofiltration in critically ill pediatric patients. Contrib Nephrol 93:257-260
19. Jenkins RD, Harrison HL, Jackson EC, Funk JE (1991) Continuous renal replacement in infants and toddlers. Contrib Nephrol 93:245-249
20. Barton IK, Hilton PJ (1993) Veno-venous hemofiltration in the intensive care unit. Clin Intensive Care 4:16-22
21. Bellomo R, Boyce N (1993) Acute continuous hemodiafiltration: a propective study of 110 patients and a review of the literature. Am J Kidney Dis 21:508-518

266   G. Zobel et al.

22. Grootendorst AF, van Bommel EFH (1993) The role of hemofiltration in the critically ill intensive care unit patient: present and future. Blood Purif 11:209-223
23. Ronco C (1993) Continuous renal replacement therapies for the treatment of acute renal failure in intensive care patients. Clin Nephrol 40:187-198
24. Zobel G, Ring E, Kuttnig M, Rödl S (1996) Continuous renal replacement therapy in critically ill pediatric patients. Am J Kidney Dis 28:S28-34
25. Olbricht CJ (1986) Continuous arteriovenous hemofiltration – the control of azotemia in acute renal failure. In: Paganini EP (ed) Acute continuous renal replacement therapy, Nijhoff, Boston, pp 123-141
26. Dickson DM, Brown EA, Kox W (1988) Continuous arteriovenous haemodialysis (CAVHD): a new method of complete renal replacement therapy in the critically ill patient. Intensive Care Med 5:78-80
27. Wendon J, Smithies M, Sheppard M, Bullen K, Tinker J, Bihari D (1989) Continuous high volume veno-venous haemofiltration in acute renal failure. Intensive Care Med 15:358-363
28. Frankenfield DC, Reynolds HN, Wiles CE, Badellino MM, Siegel JH (1994) Urea removal during continuous hemodiafiltration. Crit Care Med 22:407-412
29. Reynolds HN, Borg U, Belzberg H, Wiles CE (1991) Efficacy of continuous arteriovenous hemofiltration with dialyis in patients with acute renal failure. Crit Care Med 19:1387-1394
30. Voerman HJ, Strack-van-Schijndel RJ, Thijs LG (1990) Continuous arterial-venous hemodiafiltration in critically ill patients. Crit Care Med 18:911-914
31. Bischof NA, Welch TR, Strife CF, Ryckman FC (1990) Continuous hemodiafiltration in children. Pediatrics 85:819-823
32. Gouyon JB, Petion AM, Huet F, Lallemant C (1994) Urea removal by hemofiltration and hemodiafiltration. Biol Neonate 65:36-40
33. Bellomo R, Parkin G, Boyce N (1993) Acute renal failure in the critically ill: management by continuous veno-venous hemodiafiltration. J Crit Care 8:140-144
34. Bellomo R, Parkin G, Love J, Boyce N (1993) A prospective comparative study of continuous arteriovenous hemodiafiltration and continuous venovenous hemodiafiltration in critically ill patients. Am J Kidney Dis 21:400-404
35. Bellomo R, Tippling P, Boyce N (1993) Continuous veno-venous hemofiltration with dialysis removes cytokines from the circulation of septic patients. Crit Care Med 21:522-526
36. Fleming F, Bohn D, Edwards H, Cox P, Geary D, McCrindle BW, Williams WG (1995) Renal replacement therapy after repair of congenital heart disease in children. J Thorac Cardiovasc Surg 109:322-331

Chapter 27

Early diagnosis and treatment of life-threatening bacterial infections in neonates and critically ill children

J. FISCHER

In an ideal world specific drugs would effectively kill bacteria without side effects and any risk of selecting resistant strains. These drugs could safely be administered until the patient fully recovers. Bedside tests performed in any symptomatic patient would detect the presence of bacterial infections with the accuracy of HIV testing.

Unfortunately, reality is different. Antimicrobial-resistant microorganisms rapidly emerge and disseminate in hospitals worldwide [1]. Overuse of antibiotics adds selective pressure in microorganisms. The presence of resistant strains in intensive care units forces physicians to administer increasingly potent antimicrobial agents as primary "rule out" therapy. These drugs bear the risk of side effects and further increase the selective pressure in microorganisms [2]. Inappropriate hand disinfection at times of high workload remain an important source of bacterial translocation between patients [3].

Early diagnosis is difficult, too. Some of the widely used laboratory indicators of infection rise with considerable delay compared to the onset of clinical symptoms [4]. White blood cell count, differential or plasma levels of C-reactive protein that successfully differentiate between bacterial infection and other causes of illness in the outpatient setting [5] fail to sustain adequate diagnostic power in paediatric intensive care units. The results of blood cultures usually do not become available until many hours after clinical decisions had to be made. With the small sampling volumes in premature infants and neonates the rate of false-negative cultures is high [6].

Clinical signs lack the desirable sensitivity and specificity to discriminate between infected and uninfected patients. Fever is an all too common symptom, occurring repetitively in most paediatric intensive care patients [7]. In premature infants and neonates symptoms such as tachypnoea, tachycardia, increased gastric residuum, or apnoea may herald the onset of serious nosocomial infection but there is usually a less alarming explanation [8, 9]. The cumulative incidence for a systemic inflammatory response syndrome (SIRS) exceeds 60% in multidisciplinary paediatric ICUs. The incidence of bacterial infection is considerably lower [7].

The high risks associated with untreated infection and the lack of accurate clinical and laboratory prediction models result in a low threshold for initiating empirical antibiotic therapy [10]. To most clinicians, the immediate risks for the patient outweigh the long-term disadvantages of liberal use of antimicrobial treatment [11]. The most promising means of reducing the use of antibiotics without impairing the patient's safety is the early cessation of antibiotic therapy in patients who do not have a bacterial infection.

This paper first briefly reviews the epidemiology and pathophysiology of bacterial infection and then discusses therapeutic and diagnostic strategies. It concludes with recommendations for future research.

Epidemiology

Bacterial infection remains one of the leading causes of death in neonates and children [12]. In industrialized countries the majority of life-threatening bacterial infections are acquired while the patients are under medical care [13]. These nosocomial infections account for additional morbidity, mortality, and treatment costs. Reported nosocomial infection rates vary between 9‰ and 18‰ discharges for newborns and 2‰-17‰ discharges for paediatric patients [14]. Bloodstream infection and pneumonia are the most frequent causes [15]. In extremely low-birth-weight infants the cumulative incidence of microbiologically documented sepsis is higher (250 per 1 000 admissions). Coagulase-negative staphylococci accounted for 55% of the isolates. Nosocomial sepsis was the leading cause of death beyond the first 3 days of life (17% vs 7% for uninfected neonates). In patients who had survived the first 2 weeks the attributable mortality was 45% [16].

Despite major advantages in technology, the mortality of septic shock has not improved much over the last 20 years. In adults, survivors of sepsis have an increased long-term mortality [17]. Similar data are not available for neonates and paediatric patients. The risk of infection correlates with length of stay and device utilization [12]. Other independent risk factors in neonates are fat infusions. Odds ratios between 5.4 and 9.4 have been reported and one study estimated that 85% of all nosocomial infections with coagulase-negative staphylococci in newborns were attributable to parenteral fat administration [18-20].

Isolated pathogens and resistance patterns differ between regions, sites, and patient groups [14]. The majority of infections are caused by gram-positive bacteria, with coagulase-negative staphylococci and *Staphylococcus aureus* accounting for 50%-70% of all positive blood cultures [7, 15, 16]. An increasing proportion of both pathogens is resistant to methicillin. While methicillin resistance complicates treatment, it appears not to increase mortality [21]. Multiresistance enterococci are becoming of increasing concern. In addition to their intrinsic resistance to cephalosporins they are becoming increasingly resistant to aminoglycosides and ampicillin, and in US hospitals to vancomycin (17% in a recent survey) [22]. With gram-negative sepsis, *Escherichia coli* and *Enterobacter* species are the most likely isolates. *Pseudomonas aeroginosa* infections occur particularly in long-term ventilated patients and patients with an impaired host defense system. *Klebsiella pneumoniae* are less so but isolated strains are often multi-resistant. Resistance patterns vary between hospitals.

Important causes of overwhelming sepsis in otherwise healthy neonates are group B streptococci. Sepsis caused by *Neisseria meningitidis* has the highest mortality of all community acquired infections. The disease may rapidly progress to shock with a mortality between 20% and 50%. Other pathogens that are associated with infections requiring admission to intensive care in previously healthy infants are *Haemophilus influenzae* and *Streptococcus pneumoniae*. Resistance to penicillin is frequent (29% of isolates) but does not affect mortality [23]. Fungi account for less than 10% of all bloodstream infections in critically ill children and are usually caused by non-resistant *Candida* species [15].

The importance of rigorous adherence to prevention guidelines cannot be overemphasized. An important source of transmission in intensive care units remain insufficiently disinfected hands of the staff [24]. Currently, Canadian and central European hospitals report much lower resistance rates than US American centers [22]. The available reports suggesting that infections with resistant strains do not increase mortality lead to underestimation of the problem. Patients were saved because other antibiotics were available that did the job. How easily methicillin-resistant *Staphylococcus aureus* (MRSA) spread and the global nature of the problem of multi-resistance were illustrated by an outbreak of MRSA in a Canadian tertiary care hospital. The resistant strain was introduced to western Canada by a patient that had previously been hospitalized for 3 months in India. Shortly after the patient returned to Canada he was admitted to a rural hospital. Subsequently the patient was transferred to a hospital in Vancouver and later to another hospital in Winnipeg. Within 6 weeks of the patient's arrival in Canada, major outbreaks of MRSA occurred at both tertiary centers. Epidemiological typing with a polymerase chain reaction method documented the clonal origin of the strain [25]. It is not unusual that resistant strains become permanent residents of a unit for as long as a decade [26].

Pathophysiology

Potential pathogens do not readily invade the bloodstream of a healthy human organism. Almost impenetrable barriers, potent chemicals such as gastric acid and a plethora of immune-competent cells such as alveolar macrophages guard the body against potential intruders. When bacteria are dislocated into the bloodstream, they are rapidly cleared by phagocytes [27]. This system has withstood the test of evolution and guaranteed the survival of human species.

Medical interventions tilt this balance of powers in favor of microorganisms. The natural barriers in extremely premature infants are much more vulnerable than those in children. Central intravenous lines provide convenient sites for colonization, particularly in patients receiving fat infusions [18]. After cardiac surgery many patients are subject to prolonged periods of compromised circulation with impaired gut perfusion. Inoculation of the patient with pathogens from the hospital can be delayed but rarely be avoided. Patients are at risk of failing to clear bacteremia and to permit systemic dissemination of pathogens. Shock becomes likely and survival is at stake [28].

A brief review of the events naturally occurring with bacteremia and localized infection can help to explain the implications of septic shock. Much of the present knowledge is derived from research into gram-negative infections. Endotoxins are lipopolysaccharide protein complexes of the cell walls of gram-negative bacteria. In human blood, they interact with soluble and surface-bound receptors. An important receptor is the CD14 complex on macrophages and neutrophils. Endotoxins adhere to the surface of endothelial cells [29, 30]. Activated immune cells and activated endothelial cells rapidly excrete a plethora of inflammatory mediators and adhesion molecules [31, 32].

The sequence of increase in plasma levels of these mediators has been studied by many investigators. One study evaluated intravenous administration of 1-4 ng/kg endotoxin to human volunteers [29, 30]. Volunteers developed transient fever that peaked 3-5 h after injection. An initial decrease in the number of peripheral neutrophils over the first 2 h was followed by a pronounced neutrophilia that continued for 24 h. By 1 h after the endotoxin administration plasma levels of tumor necrosis factor α (TNFα) and soluble TNF receptor increased. Ninety min after the injections plasma levels of interleukin-6 (IL-6) and IL-8 began to rise. Shortly thereafter IL-1 receptor antagonist, granulocyte colony-stimulating factor (G-CSF), and granulocyte-macrophage colony-stimulating factor became elevated. Plasma levels of lactoferrin increased at the same time, and an enzyme released by activated neutrophils. G-CSF levels correlated with the amount of injected endotoxin. The rise of plasma G-CSF was temporally associated with the increased neutrophil and band form count. The observed levels (up to 10 000 pg/ml, normal 10-40 pg/ml) peaked at levels comparable to those measured after administration of recombinant human G-CSF to neutropenic patients [33]. Four hours after the endotoxin challenge, levels of soluble E-selectin became elevated, and an adhesion molecule shed from endothelial cells.

At local sites of inflammation the immune response follows a slightly different pattern. The main feature of localized inflammation is massive infiltration of neutrophils within 4-8 h after the insult. Interestingly, neutrophils shed L-selectin from their surface before infiltrating into the peripheral tissue [34]. This adhesion molecule mediates the rolling of neutrophils along vascular endothelium. The cellular response is accompanied by an accumulation of inflammatory mediators. Among them are interferon-γ, IL-6 and IL-8 but surprisingly low amounts of TNFα and interleukin-1β [34]. Neutrophil infiltration into the tissue can be hampered by antibodies to the neutrophil surface antigen CD18 or to the vascular cell adhesion molecule-1 [35, 36].

Endotoxin injection elicits systemic inflammatory response syndrome (SIRS), in an effort to regulate the pro-inflammatory response, a series of anti-inflammatory reactions. The latter have been summarized under the new term compensating anti-inflammatory response syndrome (CARS) [37]. Other assaults to the integrity of the host can lead to a similar sequence of events. The incomplete list of causes includes events such as operation, trauma, burns, or cardiopulmonary bypass [38]. When anti-inflammatory responses dominate, the host's ability to clear bacteria from the bloodstream may be suppressed [37, 39]. A clinician's daily task is to distinguish whether the clinical signs of SIRS (tachypnoea, tachycardia, fever) are explained by non infective causes or whether the observed symptoms result from a proinflammatory reaction to bacteremia.

One of the factors contributing to the task is the difficulty to cultivate viable bacteria from the bloodstream of patients with suspected sepsis. The lack of a gold standard for the diagnosis of sepsis impedes assessment of the true proportion of false-negative cultures. In paediatric patients the rate is unknown [40, 41]. When cultures become positive, the number of colony-forming units per milliliter of collected blood is less than 100 and usually between 1 and 10 [6]. The total bacterial burden calculated from these figures differs from the amount of bacteria required to experimentally induce sepsis by several orders of magnitude. Thus, circulating viable bacteria represent a minute fraction of the true bacterial load. The majority either have adhered to endothelial cells, were absorbed by mononuclear cells, or devitalized by soluble proteins.

When bacteria adhere to the surface of endothelial cells, the vascular layer itself becomes the target organ of the defensive efforts [42, 43]. An in vitro study incubating various strains of Neisseria meningitidis with endothelial cells and human whole blood showed that no damage to the endothelial cells was induced by the organisms alone. The degree of endothelial injury was related to the number of neutrophils that adhered to endothelial cells. Neutrophil activation and likelihood of adherence depended on the characteristics of the bacterial cell wall [44]. However, endothelial injury is not exclusive to septic shock. Other events, such as asphyxia or release of mediators, can also impair endothelial function [43]. Here, different pathways of sepsis and a nonbacterial systemic immune response converge to a single pathophysiological disorder leading to multi-organ dysfunction syndrome [37].

Throughout evolution the instant activation of excessive quantities of neutrophils was crucial to the host's survival. Once the initial mechanisms failed to clear bacteremia, the only chance to defeat the invaders was to take the risk of endothelial injury and to escalate the proinflammatory response [37]. Potent antibiotics assist the host in eradicating bacteria. This stimulates the conceptualization of the attractive strategy of mediating the proinflammatory response before endothelial damage occurs.

Therapeutic strategies

To date, the quest for the miracle drug that reverts septic shock has been disappointing [45]. Based on the hypothesis that checking the proinflammatory immune response would curtail septic organ failure, administration of high-dose corticosteroids were first advocated. High-dose methylprednisolone was dismissed by a carefully conducted prospective cohort trial in 1987 [46]. A recent meta-analysis confirmed these findings. Other agents followed the same course [47-49]. The list contains a wide range from antibodies to TNFα, to antibodies to IL-1, receptor antagonists to platelet-activating factor or IL-1, and monoclonal antibodies against endotoxin. Some studies even suggested harmful effects of the treatment [50]. Many authors have pointed to the fact that some of the failure may be explained by the delayed diagnosis and application of the drug [51]. Endothelial damage may already have occurred at the time the new agents were applied.

A possible solution is to redirect the research effort towards an improved early diagnosis. The Center for Disease Control defines nosocomial infection as a disease that was neither present nor incubating at admission to the hospital. This definition includes all infections acquired during birth. With this definition, almost every case of neonatal sepsis and the vast majority of paediatric sepsis occur in patients under professional care. Even with very virulent pathogens, the clinical course takes several hours from the first nonspecific symptoms to fully established septic shock. Exceptions are meningococcemia or sepsis in severely immune-compromised hosts. A critical review of many cases, however, reveals that the correct diagnosis is often erroneously dismissed for up to 24 h [9]. Early initiation of appropriate empiric therapy is the first step [51].

Empiric therapy usually comprises two or three antimicrobial agents until culture results make it possible to tailor medication according to the resistance pattern. The clinician's reward for effective surveillance is a low incidence of septic shock and increased survival [9]. However, such a policy will inevitably result in many cases of unwarranted medication with the aforementioned disadvantages [24]. An additional problem of unwarranted intravenous antibiotic therapy arises in otherwise healthy neonates that often need to be transferred to another hospital and be separated from their mother.

Successful interventions other than early initiation of antibiotic therapy have been reported from some uncontrolled studies. In one study an improved survival in neutropenic neonates with sepsis after administration of recombinant G-CSF was observed. Patients were compared to a cohort of historical controls [52]. Two drugs may improve the outcome from fulminant meningococcemia. Fibrinolytic therapy with recombinant tissue plasminogen activator appeared to stop the progression of shock and intravascular coagulation [53]. To date, only few cases have been reported in the literature. Treatment with antibodies against human bactericidal/permeability-increasing protein proved efficacious in a phase II trial, and a multicenter phase III trial is now under way [54]. All of these strategies await validation by the scrutiny of prospective randomized trials.

Substantial effort has been directed towards the development of new therapeutic measures in adult patients. Eventually one of the new strategies will prove effective. However, these agents are not cheap. When the monoclonal antibody HA-1A was released in Europe, the costs per dose were priced at US$ 3,000 to 4,000. An estimate for the additional costs per patient with undetected nosocomial sepsis and progression to septic shock in our unit amounted to US$ 15,000, while a US American study accounted the costs as high as US$ 40,000 [55]. This margin leaves ample scope for expenditure on prevention and early diagnosis.

The arduous path to an improved early diagnosis

If nature is unable to discriminate between bacteremia and other noninfective causes of SIRS, the search for biological markers that serve this purpose is in vain. If, however, the immune system can identify the cause with reasonable accuracy, the research task is to identify the molecules mediating the message. A successful strategy is to search for mediators that are elevated in sepsis but not in other causes of SIRS [56]. This requires an evaluation of a cohort of patients with shock caused both by sepsis and non-bacterially. Comparing septic patients to otherwise healthy ICU inhabitants such as extubated premature infants on full enteral nutrition will not produce the answer. Unfortunately, the latter is a preferred research strategy in many studies on new parameters for the diagnosis of sepsis [57-60].

These types of case-control studies suffer from an important selection bias. The exclusion of ambiguously classified patients results in overestimation of the true diagnostic power of the parameter. Such studies underestimate the false-positive rate, propose an erroneously low positivity criterion, and overestimate the sensitivity. Not surprisingly, application of the new parameters in clinical routine fails to reproduce favorable results.

Prospective cohort trials tend to be less elusive. Again, the reader is encouraged to carefully examine the methods section of these papers. Is the population that satisfied inclusion criteria comparable? Is the incidence of nonbacterial SIRS similar to that encountered in the reader's unit? The answer to this question is particularly important since nonbacterial SIRS causes elevations which are similar to those of bacterial sepsis for many parameters. A high incidence rate of SIRS will reduce the diagnostic power of most parameters.

Another important detail is the exact timing of sample collection. Was the sample taken at onset of the first symptoms, many hours later when residents and fellows had agreed on a presumptive diagnosis, or hours after the initiation of therapy? Obviously, samples collected after initiation of antibiotics offer little help to elucidate the potential use in early diagnosis. With the rapid progression of sepsis, delayed sampling increases the chance of any marker to score as true positive. However, such delayed sampling may be appropriate for investigating the potential of new markers to assist in the early termination of unwarranted "rule out" therapy. Samples from different times in relation to onset of symptoms or therapy should therefore not be lumped together in the analysis.

These variations by study design will inevitably add to the natural variability by chance. Thus, the true confidence intervals for any measure of diagnostic accuracy are presumably wider than calculated by statistical software packages. With these considerations in mind, it is easier to interpret the differing results between studies. A good example is plasma levels of procalcitonin. A recently published study on the diagnostic properties of procalcitonin in the early diagnosis of sepsis stated a 100% sensitivity and specificity for late onset sepsis. Some 23 cases of late-onset sepsis were each matched to 92 noninfected NICU patients. The resulting area under the receiver operating characteristic curve is 1.0, indicating a perfect diagnostic tool [58]. In our combined neonatal and paediatric ICU we evaluated the same marker in 345 patients (unpublished data). The case mix was very different, with a high number of infant patients developing a nonbacterial SIRS after cardiac surgery. In this population, procalcitonin performed considerably less well, with a sensitivity of 75% and a specificity of 56%. The resulting area under the receiver operating characteristic curve was 0.74, which differs significantly from the neonatal study.

White blood cell count and differentiation were the first parameters suggested for surveillance of patients at risk of infection. Both marked neutropenia and marked neutrophilia can be associated with bacterial infection [61]. Frequently, the total white blood cell count will remain within the normal range and only a marked increase in the band count indicates an increased utilization of neutrophils. A widely used indicator of severe bacterial infection is the visual inspection of leukocyte morphology. Several authors have addressed the problem to eliminate interpersonal variability in band counts [62]. Furthermore, by the very nature of manual counts wide confidence intervals are yielded. The probability of counts from a given sample follows a Poisson distribution: if the true band count is 15, the 95% confidence interval of a manual count after inspecting 100 cells ranges from 8 to 25.

Throughout Europe surveillance of patients by plasma levels of C-reactive protein (CRP) became routine in many units. The delayed rise of this acute phase protein (up to 24 h after onset of symptoms) limits the sensitivity as to an early diagnosis and has been the cause of many false-negative diagnoses [4]. The frequent rise of CRP in patients with SIRS hampers the specificity. In a recent study at our multidisciplinary ICU, the area under the receiver operating characteristic curve as to the differentiation between sepsis and nonbacterial SIRS was 0.65. Currently, the most promising candidate markers to improve early diagnostic accuracy are plasma levels of IL-6, granulocyte colony-stimulating factor, and procalcitonin [63-68]. Most of the studies reported areas under the curve ranging from 0.8 to 0.9. However, to date no study has been published comparing these markers in the same cohort of patients.

The rapid development of microbiological techniques has lowered the costs of routine cultures. Cultures of tracheal aspirates, urine, blood, or wound secretions are part of routine diagnostic workup in patients with suspected infection. Many units use semiquantitative cultures of tracheal aspirates as part of their routine measures to control infectious diseases. The interpretation of the results remains difficult: Does a negative blood culture in a premature infant with shock born to a febrile mother rule out sepsis? Does a high cultural count for *Klebsiella pneumoniae* from a tracheal aspirate in a subfebrile but otherwise asymptomatic patient after cardiac surgery rule in pneumonia?

A promising strategy is to use new markers for early stopping rules of empiric antibiotic therapy. Such an approach has been tested for the combination of IL-6 and CRP [63, 64].

Recommendations for future research

The goal is to initiate antibiotics in all patients with infection as early as possible and to avoid any unwarranted treatment. Several steps must be taken towards this goal. First, we must elucidate the epidemiology of antibiotic use in neonatal and paediatric ICUs [69]. This will make it possible to identify target areas of unwarranted use. Second, we need clinical prediction rules for nosocomial infection comparable to those suggested for adult patients [70-72] that alert clinicians early in the clinical course. Third, we need to define the risk threshold for initiation or discontinuation of antibiotic therapy in the various subgroups of our patients. Fourth, we need to agree on criteria for the diagnosis of sepsis in symptomatic patients in whom blood cultures fail to grow a pathogen. These definitions should be comparable to those used in studies of sepsis in adult patients. With this information at hand we are then able to test the ability of new diagnostic parameters to assist the decision maker in moving a patient across the threshold for initiation or safe discontinuation of antibiotic therapy. These questions are best addressed in prospective cohort trials, preferably multicenter studies.

If we improve on early diagnosis and stewardship of antibiotic therapy we will arrive at refined guidelines to optimize initiation, selection, dose, and duration of treatment. Prevention of the dissemination of resistant microorganisms will reduce the adverse effects on outcome and their associated increase in costs of health care [73]. Except for some disorders, such as meningococcemia for which additional therapeutic measures are urgently needed, the prevention of delayed diagnosis has the largest potential to improve the outcome of critically ill patients with bacterial infections.

Today, we regard those who save a patient from septic shock as heroes and those who diagnose sepsis early as good clinicians. The real honor should, however, be given to those who prevent nosocomial infection in the first place [74]. Semmelweis introduced rigorous hand disinfection before touching a patient 150 years ago. This brought about one of the largest-ever reductions in morbidity and mortality. Antibiotics are certainly the wrong cure for failures in adhering to Semmelweis' procedure.

References

1. Goldmann DA, Weinstein RA, Wenzel RP, Tablan OC, Duma RJ, Gaynes RP et al (1996) Strategies to prevent and control the emergence and spread of antimicrobial-resistant microorganisms in hospitals. A challenge to hospital leadership. JAMA 275:234-240
2. Pfaller MA, Herwaldt LA (1997) The clinical microbiology laboratory and infection control: emerging pathogens, antimicrobial resistance, and new technology. Clin Infect Dis 25:858-870
3. Sebille V, Valleron AJ (1997) A computer simulation model for the spread of nosocomial infections caused by multidrug-resistant pathogens. Comput Biomed Res 30:307-322

4. Jaye DL, Waites KB (1997) Clinical applications of C-reactive protein in pediatrics. Pediatr Infect Dis J 16:735-747
5. Baker MD, Bell LM, Avner JR (1993) Outpatient management without antibiotics of fever in selected infants. N Engl J Med 329:1437-1441
6. Schelonka RL, Chai MK, Yoder BA, Hensley D, Brockett RM, Ascher DP (1996) Volume of blood required to detect common neonatal pathogens. J Pediatr 129:275-278
7. Proulx F, Fayon M, Farrell CA, Lacroix J, Gauthier M (1996) Epidemiology of sepsis and multiple organ dysfunction syndrome in children. Chest 109:1033-1077
8. Hein HA, Ely JW, Lofgren MA (1998) Neonatal respiratory distress in the community hospital: when to transport, when to keep. J Fam Pract 46:284-289
9. Philip AG, Hewitt JR (1980) Early diagnosis of neonatal sepsis. Pediatrics 65:1036-1041
10. Bhutta ZA (1997) Neonatal infections. Curr Opin Pediatr 9:133-140
11. Timmermans DR, Sprij AJ, de Bel CE (1996) The discrepancy between daily practice and the policy of a decision-analytic model: the management of fever of unknown origin. Med Decis Making 16:357-366
12. Jarvis WR, Edwards JR, Culver DH, Hughes JM, Horan T, Emori TG et al (1991) Nosocomial infection rates in adult and pediatric intensive care units in the United States. National Nosocomial Infections Surveillance System. Am J Med 91:185S-191S
13. Martinot A, Leclerc F, Cremer R, Leteurtre S, Fourier C, Hue V (1997) Sepsis in neonates and children: definitions, epidemiology, and outcome. Pediatr Emerg Care 13:277-281
14. Merritt WT, Green M (1996) Nosocomial infections in the pediatric intensive care unit. In: Rogers M (ed) Textbook of pediatric intensive care. WB Saunders, New York, pp 975-1001
15. Singh-Naz N, Sprague BM, Patel KM, Pollack MM (1996) Risk factors for nosocomial infection in critically ill children: a prospective cohort study. Crit Care Med 24:875-878
16. Stoll B, Gordon T, Korones S, Shankaran S, Tyson J, Bauer C et al (1996) Late-onset sepsis in very low birth weight neonates: a report from the National Institute of Child Health and Human Development Neonatal Research Network. J Pediatr 129:63-71
17. Bates DW, Pruess KE, Lee TH (1995) How bad are bacteremia and sepsis? Outcomes in a cohort with suspected bacteremia. Arch Intern Med 155:593-598
18. Avila-Figueroa C, Goldmann DA, Richardson DK, Gray JE, Ferrari A, Freeman J (1998) Intravenous lipid emulsions are the major determinant of coagulase-negative staphylococcal bacteremia in very low birth weight newborns. Pediatr Infect Dis J 17:10-17
19. Shiro H, Muller E, Takeda S, Tosteson TD, Goldmann DA, Pier GB (1995) Potentiation of Staphylococcus epidermidis catheter-related bacteremia by lipid infusions. J Infect Dis 171:220-224
20. Freeman J, Goldmann DA, Smith NE, Sidebottom DG, Epstein MF, Platt R (1990) Association of intravenous lipid emulsion and coagulase-negative staphylococcal bacteremia in neonatal intensive care units. N Engl J Med 323:301-308
21. Harbarth S, Rutschmann O, Sudre P, Pittet D (1998) Impact of methicillin resistance on the outcome of patients with bacteremia caused by Staphylococcus aureus. Arch Intern Med 158:182-189
22. Pfaller MA, Jones RN, Doern GV, Kugler K (1998) Bacterial pathogens isolated from patients with bloodstream infection: frequencies of occurrence and antimicrobial susceptibility patterns from the SENTRY antimicrobial surveillance program (United States and Canada, 1997). Antimicrob Agents Chemother 42:1762-1770
23. Pallares R, Linares J, Vadillo M, Cabellos C, Manresa F, Viladrich PF et al (1995) Resistance to penicillin and cephalosporin and mortality from severe pneumococcal pneumonia in Barcelona, Spain. N Engl J Med 333:474-480
24. Goldmann DA, Huskins WC (1997) Control of nosocomial antimicrobial-resistant bacteria: a strategic priority for hospitals worldwide. Clin Infect Dis 24(Suppl 1):S139-145

25. Roman RS, Smith J, Walker M, Byrne S, Ramotar K, Dyck B et al (1997) Rapid geographic spread of a methicillin-resistant Staphylococcus aureus strain. Clin Infect Dis 25:698-705
26. Huebner J, Pier GB, Maslow JN, Muller E, Shiro H, Parent M et al (1994) Endemic nosocomial transmission of Staphylococcus epidermidis bacteremia isolates in a neonatal intensive care unit over 10 years. J Infect Dis 169:526-531
27. Parrillo JE (1993) Pathogenetic mechanisms of septic shock. N Engl J Med 328:1471-1477
28. Bone RC (1996) The sepsis syndrome. Definition and general approach to management. Clin Chest Med 17:175-181
29. Tennenberg SD, Weller JJ (1997) Endotoxin-induced, neutrophil-mediated endothelial cytotoxicity is enhanced by T-lymphocytes. J Surg Res 69:11-13
30. Kuhns DB, Alvord WG, Gallin JI (1995) Increased circulating cytokines, cytokine antagonists, and E-selectin after intravenous administration of endotoxin in humans. J Infect Dis 171:145-152
31. Shanley TP, Warner RL, Ward PA (1995) The role of cytokines and adhesion molecules in the development of inflammatory injury. Mol Med Today 1:40-45
32. Bone RC (1996) Toward a theory regarding the pathogenesis of the systemic inflammatory response syndrome: what we do and do not know about cytokine regulation. Crit Care Med 24:163-172
33. Welte K, Gabrilove J, Bronchud M, Platzer E, Morstyn G (1996) Filgastrim (r-metHuG-CSF): the first 10 years. Blood 88:1907-1929
34. Kuhns DB, DeCarlo E, Hawk DM, Gallin JI (1992) Dynamics of the cellular and humoral components of the inflammatory response elicited in skin blisters in humans. J Clin Invest 89:1734-1740
35. Essani NA, Bajt ML, Farhood A, Vonderfecht SL, Jaeschke H (1997) Transcriptional activation of vascular cell adhesion molecule-1 gene in vivo and its role in the pathophysiology of neutrophil-induced liver injury in murine endotoxin shock. J Immunol 158:5941-5948
36. Mercer-Jones MA, Heinzelmann M, Peyton JC, Wickel D, Cook M, Cheadle WG (1997) Inhibition of neutrophil migration at the site of infection increases remote organ neutrophil sequestration and injury. Shock 8:193-199
37. Bone RC (1996) Immunologic dissonance: a continuing evolution in our understanding of the systemic inflammatory response syndrome (SIRS) and the multiple organ dysfunction syndrome (MODS). Ann Intern Med 125:680-687
38. Davies MG, Hagen PO (1997) Systemic inflammatory response syndrome. Br J Surg 84:920-935
39. Bone RC, Grodzin CJ, Balk RA (1997) Sepsis: a new hypothesis for pathogenesis of the disease process. Chest 112:235-243
40. Jawaheer G, Neal TJ, Shaw NJ (1997) Blood culture volume and detection of coagulase negative staphylococcal septicaemia in neonates. Arch Dis Child Fetal Neonatal Ed 76:F57-F58
41. Laforgia N, Coppola B, Carbone R, Grassi A, Mautone A, Iolascon A (1997) Rapid detection of neonatal sepsis using polymerase chain reaction. Acta Paediatr 86:1097-1099
42. Gill EA, Imaizumi T, Carveth H, Topham MK, Tarbet EB, McIntyre TM et al (1998) Bacterial lipopolysaccharide induces endothelial cells to synthesize a degranulating factor for neutrophils. FASEB J 12:673-684
43. Chen X, Christou NV (1996) Relative contribution of endothelial cell and polymorphonuclear neutrophil activation in their interactions in systemic inflammatory response syndrome. Arch Surg 131:1148-1154

44. Klein NJ, Ison CA, Peakman M, Levin M, Hammerschmidt S, Frosch M et al (1996) The influence of capsulation and lipooligosaccharide structure on neutrophil adhesion molecule expression and endothelial injury by Neisseria meningitidis. J Infect Dis 173:172-179

45. Bone RC (1996) Why sepsis trials fail. JAMA 276:565-566

46. Bone RC, Fisher CJ Jr, Clemmer TP, Slotman GJ, Metz CA, Balk RA (1987) A controlled clinical trial of high-dose methylprednisolone in the treatment of severe sepsis and septic shock. N Engl J Med 317:653-658

47. Ziegler EJ, Fisher CJ Jr, Sprung CL, Straube RC, Sadoff JC, Foulke GE et al (1991) Treatment of gram-negative bacteremia and septic shock with HA-1A human monoclonal antibody against endotoxin. A randomized, double-blind, placebo-controlled trial. The HA-1A Sepsis Study Group. N Engl J Med 324:429-436

48. Bernard GR, Wheeler AP, Russell JA, Schein R, Summer WR, Steinberg KP et al (1997) The effects of ibuprofen on the physiology and survival of patients with sepsis. The Ibuprofen in Sepsis Study Group. N Engl J Med 336:912-918

49. Fisher CJ Jr, Agosti JM, Opal SM, Lowry SF, Balk RA, Sadoff JC et al (1996) Treatment of septic shock with the tumor necrosis factor receptor: Fc fusion protein. The Soluble TNF Receptor Sepsis Study Group. N Engl J Med 334:1697-1702

50. Stephenson J (1996) Reflecting and regrouping after failed trials, sepsis researchers forge on. JAMA 275:823-824

51. Perez EM, Weisman LE (1997) Novel approaches to the prevention and therapy of neonatal bacterial sepsis. Clin Perinatol 24:213-229

52. Kocherlakota P, Gamma EFL (1997) Human granulocyte colony-stimulating factor may improve outcome attributable to neonatal sepsis complicated by neutropenia. Pediatrics 100:E6

53. Zenz W, Muntean W, Gallistl S, Zobel G, Grubbauer HM (1995) Recombinant tissue plasminogen activator treatment in two infants with fulminant meningococcemia. Pediatrics 96:44-48

54. Giroir BP, Quint PA, Barton P, Kirsch EA, Kitchen L, Goldstein B et al (1997) Preliminary evaluation of recombinant amino-terminal fragment of human bactericidal/permeability-increasing protein in children with severe meningococcal sepsis. Lancet 350:1439-1443

55. Pittet D, Tarara D, Wenzel RP (1994) Nosocomial bloodstream infection in critically ill patients. Excess length of stay, extra costs, and attributable mortality. JAMA 271:1598-1601

56. Fischer J, Fanconi S (1996) Systemic inflammatory response syndrome (SIRS) in pediatric patients. In: Tibboel D, van der Voort E (eds) Intensive care in childhood. A challenge to the future. Springer-Verlag, Berlin Heidelberg New York, pp 239-254

57. Doughty LA, Kaplan SS, Carcillo JA (1996) Inflammatory cytokine and nitric oxide responses in pediatric sepsis and organ failure. Crit Care Med 24:1137-1143

58. Chiesa C, Panero A, Rossi N, Stegagno M, De Giusti M, Osborn JF et al (1998) Reliability of procalcitonin concentrations for the diagnosis of sepsis in critically ill neonates. Clin Infect Dis 26:664-672

59. Berger C, Uehlinger J, Ghelfi D, Blau N, Fanconi S (1995) Comparison of C-reactive protein and white blood cell count with differential in neonates at risk for septicaemia. Eur J Pediatr 154:138-144

60. Grant HW, Hadley GP (1997) Prediction of neonatal sepsis by thromboelastography. Pediatr Surg Int 12:289-292

61. Charache S, Nelson L, Saw D, Keyser E, Wingfield S (1992) Accuracy and utility of differential white blood cell count in the neonatal intensive care unit. Am J Clin Pathol 97:338-344

62. Schelonka RL, Yoder BA, desJardins SE, Hall RB, Butler J (1994) Peripheral leukocyte count and leukocyte indexes in healthy newborn term infants. J Pediatr 125:603-606

63. Ng PC, Cheng SH, Chui KM, Fok TF, Wong MY, Wong W et al (1997) Diagnosis of late onset neonatal sepsis with cytokines, adhesion molecule, and C-reactive protein in preterm very low birthweight infants. Arch Dis Child Fetal Neonatal Ed 77:F221-F227

64. Doellner H, Arntzen KJ, Haereid PE, Aag S, Austgulen R (1998) Interleukin-6 concentrations in neonates evaluated for sepsis. J Pediatr 132:295-299

65. Gendrel D, Assicot M, Raymond J, Moulin F, Francoual C, Badoual J et al (1996) Procalcitonin as a marker for the early diagnosis of neonatal infection. J Pediatr 128:570-573

66. Messer J, Eyer D, Donato L, Gallati H, Matis J, Simeoni U (1996) Evaluation of interleukin-6 and soluble receptors of tumor necrosis factor for early diagnosis of neonatal infection. J Pediatr 129:574-580

67. Kennon C, Overturf G, Bessman S, Sierra E, Smith KJ, Brann B (1996) Granulocyte colony-stimulating factor as a marker for bacterial infection in neonates. J Pediatr 128:765-769

68. Assicot M, Gendrel D, Carsin H, Raymond J, Guilbaud J, Bohuon C (1993) High serum procalcitonin concentrations in patients with sepsis and infection. Lancet 341:515-518

69. Archibald LK, Gaynes RP (1997) Hospital-acquired infections in the United States. The importance of interhospital comparisons. Infect Dis Clin North Am 11:245-255

70. Bates DW, Cook EF, Goldman L, Lee TH (1990) Predicting bacteremia in hospitalized patients. A prospectively validated model. Ann Intern Med 113:495-500

71. Bates DW, Sands K, Miller E, Lanken PN, Hibberd PL, Graman PS et al (1997) Predicting bacteremia in patients with sepsis syndrome. Academic Medical Center Consortium Sepsis Project Working Group. J Infect Dis 176:1538-1551

72. Pittet D, Thievent B, Wenzel RP, Li N, Auckenthaler R, Suter PM (1996) Bedside prediction of mortality from bacteremic sepsis. A dynamic analysis of ICU patients. Am J Respir Crit Care Med 153:684-693

73. Shlaes DM, Gerding DN, John JF Jr, Craig WA, Bornstein DL, Duncan RA et al (1997) Society for Healthcare Epidemiology of America and Infectious Diseases Society of America Joint Committee on the Prevention of Antimicrobial Resistance: guidelines for the prevention of antimicrobial resistance in hospitals. Clin Infect Dis 25:584-599

74. Goldmann D, Larson E (1992) Hand-washing and nosocomial infections. N Engl J Med 327:120-122

Chapter 28

Clinical severity scores in neonates

M. Orzalesi, A. Dotta, G. Seganti

Neonatal morbidity and mortality rates may vary greatly among countries and, within the same country, among different centers. Such rates are often utilized as indicators of the quality of care. However, they are also influenced by other variables and/or risk factors unrelated to the type of treatment. It is well known that some biological variables (such as birth weight, BW, gestational age, GA, sex, etc.) and/or socio-economic variables (such as social class, annual income, parental education, etc.) may exert a strong influence on the short- and/or the long-term prognosis of newly born infants [1, 2]. The variability of the above-mentioned factors and the differences in type and severity of the disease states make the newborn infant a very heterogeneous patient. Such heterogeneity persists even when considering apparently "homogeneous" groups of babies, such as those defined as very low birth weight (VLBW) infants (i.e. with a BW ≤1500 g and/or a GA ≤32 weeks).

For the evaluation of the quality of care it is necessary to distinguish the variability in outcome related to the diagnostic and/or therapeutic interventions from that derived from the intrinsic characteristics of the patients under our care (case mix) [3, 4]. The so-called clinical severity scores (CSS) have been introduced into clinical practice for the identification and classification of homogeneous groups of patients, with clinical conditions of comparable severity and similar expected prognosis or outcome [1, 5-8]. The independent effects of treatment on the final expected outcome could then be better evaluated in such homogeneous populations of patients.

CSS in neonatology

Initially, CSS have been utilized in the newborn only for single disease entities. Such scores, better defined as "specific discriminants", have been useful in guiding and evaluating innovative treatments for some common pathological conditions: for example, the use of exchange-transfusion and/or phototherapy in neonatal jaundice; the application of some forms of mechanical ventilation or exogenous surfactant in respiratory distress syndrome (RDS) in preterm infants;

Supported by a grant from the Italian Ministry of Health.

and the utilization of extracorporeal membrane oxygenation (ECMO) in infants with severe cardio-pulmonary insufficiency.

The recent literature has seen the introduction and validation of more "global" clinical scores which can be applied in the evaluation of more extensive and more heterogeneous groups of babies admitted in neonatal intensive care units (NICU) (Table 1). These new clinical scores have been derived from the experience obtained in adult patients and/or older children requiring intensive care.

In general, such scores are calculated by recording biological, clinical, and laboratory variables and then ranking them numerically according to their degree of deviation from normality and to their prognostic significance. The final score represents the algebric sum of the values given to each single variable. The higher the numerical value of the total score, the worse the expected outcome.

Some of the clinical scores, such as the Neonatale Therapeutic Intervention Scoring System (nTISS), are extremely sophysticated and complex [5, 7]. They include a high number of variables and can be employed for the sequential evaluation of the clinical conditions as well as for the evaluation of the intensity of care and the use of resources. Other scores, such as the Score for Acute Neonatal Physiology (SNAP) and the SNAP-PE (SNAP-perinatal extension), are simpler and include a reduced number of variables [1, 5, 6, 8, 9]. They are obtained within the first few hours of admission to the hospital (generally within 24 h) and are employed essentially for prognostic purposes.

Among the various scores proposed for the newborn, the so-called CRIB (Clinical Risk Index for Babies), based on only six variables obtained within 12 h of admission, has gained wide acceptance since it is simple and yet reliable [2, 8-10]. The six variables included in the score are easily obtainable in any neonatal unit, which of course facilitates the possibility of comparing the performance of different centers [2, 11-14] (Table 2).

The reduction in the number of variables makes the recording more complete

Table 1. Clinical severity scores in the newborn

nTISS	Neonatal Therapeutic Intervention Scoring System 62 variables, points from 0 to 4, on admission and sequential
SNAP	Score for Neonatal Acute Physiology 26 variables, points from 0 to 5, within 24 h of admission
SNAP-PE	SNAP-Perinatal Extension 29 variables, as above + 3 perinatal variables, within 24 h of admission
CRIB	Clinical Risk Index for Babies 6 variables, points from 0 to 7, only VLBW infants, within 12 h of admission

VLBW, very low birth weight

Table 2. Clinical risk index for babies (CRIB)

Variable	Score
Birth weight (g)	
• >1 350	0
• 851-1 350	1
• 701-850	4
• ≤700	7
Gestational Age (weeks)	
• >24	0
• ≤24	1
Congenital malformations[a]	
• None	0
• Without acute life risk	1
• With acute life risk	3
Worse base deficit within first 12 h (mmol/L)[b]	
• >−7.0	0
• −7.0 to −9.0	1
• −10.0 to −14.9	2
• ≤−15.0	3
Appropriate FiO_2 - minimal value within first 12 h[c]	
• ≤0.40	0
• 0.41-0.80	2
• 0.81-0.90	3
• 0.91-1.00	4
Appropriate FiO_2 - maximal value within first 12 h[c]	
• ≤0.40	0
• 0.41-0.80	1
• 0.81-0.90	3
• 0.91-1.00	5

[a] With the exclusion of inevitably lethal malformations (i.e., anencephaly)
[b] For example 3.0 mmol/L: score 0; 16.0 mmol/L: score 3
[c] To obtain a PO_2 (transcutaneous or arterial) >50 mmHg and/or O_2 saturation (transcutaneous) >90%

and the percentage of missing data is greatly reduced [9, 10]. Furthermore, the shortening of the initial period of recording (from 24 to 12 h after admission) makes the score more "specific" since the variables recorded are less influenced by therapeutic interventions and truly reflect the "initial" severity of the clinical condition. Notwithstanding its simplicity the CRIB score has demonstrated a specificity, sensitivity, and predictive value similar to scores based on a greater number of variables.

The CRIB score has been validated exclusively in VLBW infants (BW≤1500 g) and only in a limited number of centers or geographic contexts, mainly Anglo-saxons. A recent multicenter study in the Lazio region in Italy has confirmed the validity of the CRIB score in the Italian context as well [16]. This study, performed in VLBW infants (BW≤1500 g and/or GA≤32weeks), has shown that in-hospital neonatal mortality increases progressively and significantly with increasing CRIB values and has confirmed that the predictive value of the CRIB score is significantly better than that of BW or GA alone. The area under the receiving operator curve (ROC) was: for CRIB=0.87 (S.E. 0.02); for BW=0.78 (SE 0.02); and for GA=0.71 (S.E. 0.03) [16].

Practical applications of CRIB

The CRIB score can be used to compare the performance of different centers or, within the same center, different treatment routines (Table 3).

Indeed, a higher neonatal mortality rate in a given center is not necessarily the expression of poor performance and/or low quality of care. It could be entirely due to a more severely affected populations of patients: in other words, to a case mix with a worse initial prognosis. With the CRIB scores one can adjust the mortality according to the initial severity of the patients treated and then make a fair comparison of the quality of care using the adjusted rates [16].

The CRIB score also allows a better description of the case mix of any given center in comparison to that of other centers and/or of the whole geographical area where the center is located.

For example, the mean value of the CRIB score of VLBW infants admitted to our NICU in the past 2 years was 4.54, compared with a mean value of 3.85 for the whole region. The percentage of VLBW infants with a CRIB score ≥7 was also higher (30.4% vs 22.4%). It is, therefore, no surprise that the in-hospital mortality for VLBW infants in our unit was slightly higher than the mean regional value (27.4% vs 22.4%). However, when appropriate adjustments were made

Table 3. Relative risk of death in VLBW infants admitted to seven NICU centers in the Lazio region (years 1994-1995): raw risk and risk adjusted according to CRIB score [16]

Center n.	Raw relative risk	Center n.	Adjusted relative risk[a]
0[b]	1.00	0[b]	1.00
1	1.08	4	0.98
2	0.90	5	0.91
3	0.81	6	0.79
4	0.78	3	0.81
5	0.64	1	0.52[c]
6	0.55[c]	2	0.52[c]

VLBW, very low birth weight; CRIB, clinical risk index for babies
[a] Adjusted for CRIB according to Cox model
[b] NICU with the highest number of babies both inborn and outborn
[c] Significantly lower than 1 ($p<0.05$)

according to the CRIB score our mortality was actually slightly lower than the regional standard.

Other authors have demonstrated that the CRIB score can also be utilized in a single center or area to monitor the changes in performance and outcome with time or following the introduction of new treatments [17].

Limitations of the CRIB score

The CRIB, like other CSS, has some limitations and disadvantages [15, 16, 18, 19]. The first limitation is related to the subjectivity of some variables utilized, for example, the minimal or maximal FiO_2 which is necessary to obtain a "good" or "appropriate" oxygenation of the baby. The level of oxygenation considered "appropriate" may vary from unit to unit and, within the same unit, from doctor to doctor and, for the same doctor, from patient to patient. Consequently the minimal and/or maximal FiO_2 can also vary considerably and be very subjective.

A second drawback derives from the redundancy of variables included in the score.

For example, BW and GA are, to a certain extent, superimposable as indices of maturity and therefore as prognostic discriminants.

Finally, the CRIB score does not include some variables that have important and significant discriminant prognostic value.

Indeed, in the already mentioned multicenter Italian study for the validation of the CRIB score, a total of 13 possibly significant variables were recorded for each baby, including those utilized for the CRIB score. When the data were analyzed according to the COX model, only six of the 13 variables were significantly able to discriminate for mortality and only two of the six were among those included in the CRIB score [16] (Table 4).

These data suggest that the association of mortality with some biological variables (sex, GA) can be almost entirely accounted for by BW. Also, among many variables descriptive of clinical condition on admission, only the 5-min Apgar score, blood pH and maximal FiO_2 are really significant. Finally, the lack of prenatal steroid prophylaxis and the absence of NICU in the hospital of birth are also important risk factors for a poor prognosis.

These observations emphasize once more the importance of "in utero" transport of VLBW infants within a well-organized regionalization of perinatal care and the need for more extensive use of prenatal steroids in women at risk of preterm labor and delivery.

Conclusions

CSS are useful for the identification of homogeneous neonatal "populations", with some homogeneity regarding prognosis, outcome, and resource utilization. Furthermore, since they correlate with mortality and, according to one study, al-

Table 4. Analysis[a] of determinants of in-hospital neonatal mortality of VLBW infants in a mulcenter study of seven NICU of the Lazio region (years 1994-1995)[16]

	Relative risk	95% C.I.
Apgar score at 5° min.		
• 7-10		
• 4-6	2.19	1.36-3.52
• 0-3	1.74	0.94-3.21
• Intubated	2.75	1.63-4.64
Birth weight (g)		
• ≤999		
• 1 000-1 499	0.38	0.25-0.56
• ≥1 500	0.30	0.13-0.66
pH on admission		
• ≥7.30		
• 7.20-7.29	1.24	0.80-1.94
• <7.20	1.50	0.89-2.52
Unknown	3.37	1.95-5.84
Place of birth		
• "Inborn"		
• "Outborn"	1.87	1.28-2.73
Prenatal steroids		
• Yes		
• No	2.01	1.32-3.06
• Unknown	1.43	0.72-2.85
FiO$_2$ max. within first 12 h		
• ≤0.40		
• 0.41-0.60	1.75	1.02-2.99
• 0.61-1.00	2.38	1.41-4.01

[a] The analysis was performed according to the Cox model on the six variables of the CRIB score and on the following seven variables chosen for their possible prognostic value: place of birth, sex, treatment with prenatal steroids, Apgar score at 5 min, presence of spontaneous respiration on admission, rectal temperature and pH on admission

so to long-term morbidity, they could be useful for the evaluation of new diagnostic and/or therapeutic strategies. They can also be utilized for comparing the performance of different centers and for auditing the performance of a single NICU [20].

There is a good correlation among the different CSS that have been proposed and validated in the neonate (SNAP, SNAP-PE, CRIB). However, since the CRIB score is equally reliable and much simpler, it is preferred in clinical practice.

The discriminant power of the CRIB score may be further improved by an integration with some other variables presently not included that are strongly associated with the risk of mortality in VLBW infants.

The problem of CSS in the neonate is still being investigated and evolving rapidly. Further studies are needed for the identification and validation of an optimal CSS that could possibly be used also in groups of babies other than VLBW infants [9, 10, 14, 16, 18-20].

Acknowledgment. We thank Mrs A. Piro for her assistance in this paper.

References

1. Richardson DK, Gray JE, McCormick MC, Workman K, Goldmann DA (1993) Score for neonatal acute physiology: a physiologic severity index for neonatal intensive care. Pediatrics 91:617-623
2. Hughes-Davies TH (1993) The CRIB score. Letter to the Editor. Lancet 342:938
3. Pedrotti D (1992) Valutazione dell'assistenza ostetrico-neonatale su base territoriale. L'esperienza della provincia di Trento. Neonatologica 3:158-164
4. Bracci R (1994) La terapia intensiva oggi. Neonatologica 1:61-69
5. Gancia GP, Stronati M, Avanzini A, Ferrari G, Rondini G (1992) Proposta di un sistema di classificazione dei neonati in Terapia Intensiva. Neonatologica 1:53-58
6. Richardson DK, Gray JE, McCormick MC, Workman K, Goldmann DA (1993) Birth Weight and Illness Severity: Indipendent Predictors of Neonatal Mortality. Pediatrics 91:969-975
7. Gray JE, Richardson DK, McCormick MC, Workman-Daniels K, Goldmann DA (1992) Neonatal therapeutic intervention scoring system: a therapy-based severity-of-illness index. Pediatrics 90:561-567
8. The International Neonatal Network (1993) The CRIB (clinical risk for babies) score: a tool for assessing initial neonatal risk and comparing performance of neonatal intensive care units. Lancet 342:193-198
9. Rautonen J, Makela A, Boyd H, Apajasalo M, Pohjavuori M (1994) CRIB and SNAP: assessing the risk of death for preterm neonates. Lancet 343:1272-1273
10. Bard H (1993) Assessing neonatal risk: CRIB vs SNAP. Lancet 342:449-450
11. Grant JM, Fenton AC, Field DJ, Solimano A, Annich G, Ehrhardt P, Tarnow-Mordi W, Cooke R, Parry G, Ogston S (1993) The CRIB score. Letter to the Editor. Lancet 342:612-613
12. Tarnow-Mordi W, Parry G (1993) The CRIB score. Letter to the editor. Lancet 342:1365
13. Sepkowitz S (1993) The CRIB score. Letter to the editor. Lancet 342:938
14. De Courcy-Wheeler RHB, Wolfe CDA, Fitzgerald A, Spencer M, Goodman IDS, Gamsu HR (1995) Use of the CRIB (clinical risk index for babies) score in prediction of neonatal mortality and morbidity. Arch Dis Child (Fetal and Neonatal Edition) 73:F32-F36
15. Zullini MT, Bonati M (1993) Geographical bias of prognostic scoring systems? Lancet 342:1115
16. Studio Multicentrico Laziale (1997) Validazione ed utilizzo di un punteggio di gravità clinica per i neonati di peso e/o età gestazionale molto basso assistiti nei reparti di Terapia Intensiva Neonatale. Oss Epidem Regione Lazio, Roma
17. Kaaresen P, Dohlen G, Fundingsrund HP, Dahl LB (1998) The use of CRIB (Clinical Risk Index for Babies) score in auditing the performance of one neonatal intensive care unit. Acta Paediatr 87:195-200
18. Hope P (1995) CRIB, son of APGAR, brother to APACHE. Arch Dis Child (Fetal and Neonatal Edition) 72:F81-F83

19. Seganti G, Latini M, Orzalesi M (1996) Indici di gravità e valutazione delle cure neonatali. Aggiornamenti in Neonatologia 4(1-2):195
20. Richardson DK, Tarnow-Mordi W (1998) Neonatal Illness Severity and the new insights into perinatal audit. Acta Paediatri 87:134-135

Chapter 29

Epidemiology and management of sepsis in neonates

B. Urlesberger, B. Resch, E. Gradnitzer, W. Müller

Epidemiology

Introduction

The term neonatal sepsis refers to invasive bacterial infections that involve primarily the bloodstream in infants during the first month of life. As a "compromised host", the neonate does not localize infections well. Two patterns of disease have been associated with systemic bacterial infections: early-onset and late-onset sepsis. Early-onset disease presents as a fulminant, multisystemic illness within the first 96 h of life; it is associated with a high mortality rate (15%-50%). Whereas late-onset sepsis, occurring later than 4 days of postnatal age, usually presents as a slowly progressive illness with focal infection (most often meningitis), it is associated with a lower mortality rate (10%-20%)[1]. Some organisms, such as *Escherichia coli, group B Streptococcus,* and *Listeria monocytogenes,* may be responsible for both early-onset and late-onset sepsis, whereas others, such as *Staphylococcus aureus* and *Pseudomonas aeruginosa,* are usually only associated with late-onset disease.

The incidence of neonatal sepsis varies from 1 to 10 cases per 1 000 live births. The incidence and mortality of neonatal sepsis at the Graz Neonatal Intensive Care Unit (NICU) in the last 10 years is shown in Table 1. Spreading from the bloodstream to the meninges is frequent during the first month of life, occurring in 25%-30% of cases [1].

There are two principal sources of newborn infection: the mother and the nursery environment. Infection may be acquired from the mother in utero, during delivery, or in the postnatal period. Infections manifesting in the first week

Table 1. Total number of all admitted infants and number of infants with neonatal sepsis. Data represent sepsis with positive culture and clinical sepsis (Graz NICU, from 1988 to 1997)

Infants	Total admitted	Sepsis	Incidence %	Mortality %
<1 500g	514	102	19.8	23
1 500-2 500g	863	117	13.6	11
>2 500g	1 981	200	10	6
Total	3 364	423	12.6	12

of life are usually due to microorganisms of maternal origin; infections presenting later can have a maternal or environmental source (i.e., nursery personnel, respiratory equipment, or indwelling lines).

Pathogenesis

The developing fetus is quite well protected from the microbial flora of the mother. Initial colonization in the neonate usually takes place after rupture of the maternal membranes. In most cases the infant is infected from the microflora of the birth canal during delivery. If delivery is delayed, however, vaginal bacteria may ascend and produce inflammation of the fetal membranes, umbilical cord, and placenta. Fetal infection may then result from aspiration of infected amniotic fluid. Nevertheless, transplacental hematogenous infection during or shortly before delivery is possible, too. Microorganisms acquired by the infant during birth colonize in the skin and mucosa, including nasopharynx, oropharynx, and conjunctivae. Transient bacteremia may accompany procedures that traumatize mucosal membranes, such as endotracheal suctioning. Metastatic foci of infection may follow bacteriemia and may involve the lungs, kidneys, spleen, bones, and central nervous system. Microbial factors, such as inoculum size and virulence of the organism, are undoubtedly significant. Fetal hypoxia and acidosis may impede certain host defense mechanisms or allow localization of organisms in necrotic tissue.

Bacteriology

The pattern of bacterial pathogens responsible for neonatal sepsis has changed over time. In the United States, gram-positive cocci were the most common pathogens before introduction of antibiotics. This predominance shifted to gram-negative enteric bacilli after antimicrobial agents came into common use. In the years 1950-1960, *Staphylococcus aureus* and *Escherichia coli* were the most common organisms isolated. Since the late 1960s a predominance of group B streptococci has developed, followed by *E.coli* and *Staphylococcus epidermidis* [1, 2] (Table 2).

Table 2. Most common bacteria isolated in neonatal sepsis and meningitis since 1980 [1, 2] and own data from 1988 to 1997 (162 patients with positive blood culture)

Isolate	Sepsis max %	Meningitis max %	Own data (sepsis) %
Group B *streptococcus*	34	52	54
Escherichia coli	17	47	2
Staphylococcus epidermidis	14	4	25
Klebsiella-Enterobacter species	9	12	4
Staphylococcus aureus	19	16	5
Enterococcus species	8	12	4

Group B streptococci (GBS) have been isolated from the genital or lower gastrointestinal tract cultures or both of 5%-41% of pregnant women [3]. Regardless of whether the genital or gastrointestinal mucosa is the primary site for GBS colonization in women, it is well documented that the presence of GBS in the maternal genital tract at delivery is a significant determinant of infection in the neonate, whether asymptomatic, as occurs in the majority, or symptomatic (sepsis, pneumonia, or meningitis). The risk of neonates acquiring GBS infection by a vertical route has been directly correlated to the intensity of maternal genital infection (inoculum size). Because sepsis develops in only one of 50 to 100 colonized infants, identification of the carrier mother is not a reliable predictor of neonatal sepsis. The attack rates for GBS early-onset sepsis varied from 0.7 to 3.7 per 1000 live births, whereas the attack rates for GBS late-onset sepsis ranged from 0.5 to 1.8 per 1000 [3].

Similar rates of colonization and disease have been reported for K1 *E.coli*, the strains of *E.coli* most often associated with neonatal sepsis and meningitis. Similar to GBS, *E.coli* infection may result in early-onset as well as late-onset sepsis.

Further important pathogens for neonatal sepsis are *S.aureus* and *S.epidermidis*. Most episodes of sepsis due to *S.aureus* are hospital acquired, with low birth weight as the most important risk factor. The apparent increased incidence in *S.epidermidis* sepsis has been associated with increased survival of very small, premature infants with immature immune systems and with the increase in invasive procedures, including the long-term vascular access devices used in neonatal intensive care. *S.epidermidis* can adhere to and grow on the surface of the synthetic polymers used for catheters. Various strains may produce a mucoid substance that stimulates adherence of microcolonies to various surfaces. In addition to an adhesive function, this mucoid substance may protect staphylococci against antibiotics.

The incidence of neonatal sepsis caused by anaerobic bacteria remains uncertain, but data are available from some surveys: the proportion of bacterial sepsis related to anaerobes was 7.5%-23% [4, 5].

The pathogens associated with neonatal sepsis also vary geographically. In the United States the pattern is similar to that in western Europe, as described above. In Latin American countries, however, gram-negative enteric bacilli are the most commonly isolated microorganisms, and GBS is rare.

Risk factors

Many studies have demonstrated that infants who develop sepsis, particularly early-onset disease, usually have a history of one or more significant risk factors associated with the pregnancy and delivery.

Obstetric risk factors

Many maternal factors may influence the development of systemic bacterial infection. Among these are prolonged rupture of membranes, maternal fever during delivery, and colonization of the maternal lower genital tract with either subclinical or clinical infection. Myriad aerobic and anaerobic bacteria, mycoplasmas, chlamydiae, fungi, viruses, and protozoa can be found in the maternal genital tract. Some of these organisms pose little threat to the newborn infant, and others are infrequent causes of neonatal disease. Much research has been conducted on GBS colonization in pregnant women, because this group of organisms has most often been associated with neonatal septicemia in Europe and the United States of America since the 1970s. In several studies GBS have been isolated from genital or lower gastrointestinal tract cultures or both of 5%-40% of pregnant women [3]. Colonization during the third trimester without any complications of pregnancy carries a risk of infection of the newborn of about 1%. This risk is increased, however, if colonization is associated with prematurity, maternal fever, or prolonged rupture of membranes.

In several reports, the incidence of prolonged rupture of membranes has ranged from 4%-7% of total deliveries [6]. In addition to being a possible cause of premature labor, subclinical infection may be a cause of prolonged rupture of membranes. Acute inflammation of the placental membranes is twice as common when membranes rupture within 4 h before labor than when they rupture after onset of labor [6]. The risk of neonatal infection is increased fourfold in association with coexistence of prolonged rupture of membranes and chorioamnionitis [7].

Among the peripartum risk factors are untreated or incompletely treated focal infections of the mother, such as urinary tract, vaginal, or cervical infections, as well as systemic infections, such as maternal septicemia, and maternal fever without a focus. Another peripartum risk factor is the use of fetal scalp electrodes.

Furthermore, there are some diffuse factors. Among these are socioeconomic factors, race, and geographic factors.

Neonatal risk factors

The factor associated most significantly with bacterial sepsis and meningitis is low birth weight. The smaller the infant at birth, the higher the incidence of sepsis. The smallest infants (weighing 1000-1500 g) have a sepsis rate almost twice as high as that of larger infants (1500-200 g), and almost eight times that of infants weighing 2000 g or more [1]. Infants with a birth weight of less than 1000 g who survived the problems of the first 5 days of intensive care treatment often died of late-onset sepsis, so late-onset infection has been an important factor in late mortality of the smallest infants. Furthermore, severely depressed respiratory function requiring intubation and resuscitation increases the risk for neonatal sepsis [8]. Prolonged rupture of membranes associated with perinatal asphyxia increases the risk for neonatal sepsis [7]. Fetal hypoxia and acidosis may impede certain host defense mechanisms or allow localization of organisms in necrotic tissue. Neonates with galactosemia are at risk of developing neonatal sepsis caused by gram-negative enteric bacilli [9], probably as a consequence of impaired neutrophilic function caused by elevated galactose concentrations.

Susceptibility to infection is also increased in the neonate with: a) a defect in host defenses, including immunologic deficits; b) absence of viscera related to defense against infection (i.e., congenital asplenia); c) defects of integrity of the skin or mucosa.

Other risk factors

Newborn infants in intensive care units show a high rate of sepsis. As these centers care for a selected group of very sick infants, organisms may be transferred from infant to infant by the hands of the nursery personnel. Factors that may increase nosocomial neonatal infection include the presence of foreign materials such as endotracheal tubes, indwelling arterial and venous lines, and ventriculoperitoneal shunts, previous antimicrobal use, prolonged hospitalization, and a high infant-to-nurse ratio in the NICU. Furthermore, contaminated parenteral fluids and oral formula as well as the frequent use of lipid emulsions have been associated with systemic infections. Regular parenteral nutrition with lipid emulsion, administered through a venous catheter with organisms adherent to the catheter, provides nutrients for the growth of bacteria with subsequent invasion of the bloodstream.

Management

Diagnosis

Clinical manifestations

The neonate who presents with signs of infection should be promptly examined. The initial signs may be minimal and are often nonspecific. Temperature instability (hyperthermia more common than hypothermia) occurs in two thirds of infants with sepsis [1, 10]. Respiratory distress (apnea, cyanosis, tachypnea, grunting, flaring, and retractions) occurs in one-half of infants with sepsis. Feeding intolerance (anorexia, vomiting, ileus, or abdominal distension) is often associated with neonatal sepsis. Glucoregulation is altered during sepsis in newborn infants, and so the development of lactic acidosis and increased glucose requirements may be early markers of sepsis [11]. Seizures, hepatomegaly, and jaundice have also been associated with neonatal sepsis.

Cultures

Prior to administration of antibiotics, appropriate cultures must be obtained from the neonate. A positive blood culture is extremely important for the definitive diagnosis of neonatal sepsis. The optimal number of blood cultures and volume of blood per culture has not been established for neonates; however, minimum of 0.5 ml of blood per bottle is recommended [12]. It is important to know that blood cultures can be sterile in about 20% of infants with sepsis [13].

Analysis of the cerebrospinal fluid (CSF) is an important part of the evaluation for sepsis. This procedure may be postponed if the infant is haemodynamically unstable or demonstrates thrombocytopenia. The potential risks of a lumbar puncture, especially in preterm infants less than 24 h of age without historical risk factors, clinical signs, or positive blood cultures, may exceed the diagnostic benefit of the procedure. CSF should be examined in the laboratory for cell count, differential cell analysis, and chemical analysis, as well as for gram stain and culture [14].

Urine should be obtained in a sterile manner. Urine cultures may be positive in infants with sepsis in the absence of primary urinary tract infection, but generally the yield for positive urine cultures is low. It is imperative, however, that urine culture is obtained in all infants for late-onset disease [15].

Antigen tests

Latex particle agglutination (LPA) is the most commonly reported rapid immunologic assay for the detection of GBS [16]. It can be used to detect GBS antigen in blood and CSF, although concentrated urine is the specimen of choice. The sensitivity, specificity, positive predictive accuracy, and negative predictive accuracy have been reported to be 88%, 98%, 79%, and 99%, respectively [17]; however, several studies have demonstrated high false-positive rates for urine LPA test [18]. Due to the high false-positive rate, asymptomatic infants should not be screened for sepsis with LPA in the setting of maternal colonization and pretreatment with antibiotics.

Hematologic tests

A complete blood count with differential cell analysis is the cornerstone in the detection of sepsis in most neonatal wards. Leukocytosis or leukopenia, defined as more than 30 000/mm^3 and fewer than 9 000/mm^3, respectively, within the first 24 h of life were initially thought to be reliable indicators of infection, but now are known to be insensitive and nonspecific [19, 20]. Manroe et al. [20] established reference ranges for the absolute total neutrophil count (ATN), total immature neutrophil count, and the ratio of immature to total neutrophils (I/T) for neonates. Of these neutrophil indices, the I/T ratio is the single most sensitive and specific indicator of bacterial infection in neonates. The maximal I/T ratio in uninfected term infants is 0.16 in the first 24 h, decreasing to 0.12 by 60 h postnatal age. The upper limit for healthy neonates of 32 weeks gestation or less is slightly higher, at 0.2.

In 10%-60%, platelet counts of less than 100 000/mm^3 were observed during neonatal sepsis. The duration of thrombocytopenia was about 1 week and may last as long as 3 weeks [21].

Acute-phase reactants

Acute-phase reactants are nonspecific, primitive proteins produced by hepatocytes in response to cellular degeneration, infection, and trauma. Unfortunately, acute-phase reactants do not distinguish between infectious and noninfectious causes of inflammation. There are many different acute-phase reactants, including C-reactive protein (CRP), fibrinogen, C3 complement, α_1-acid glycoprotein, α_1-antitrypsin, orosomucoid, transferrin, prealbumin, ceruloplasmin, and elastase α_1-proteinase inhibitor. CRP is the most common acute-phase reactant used in clinical practice. It is a globulin so named because it forms a precipitate in the presence of the C-polysaccharide of *S.pneumoniae*. Its function is not entirely clear, but it is thought to be a carrier protein involved in removing potentially toxic material. There is minimal, if any, transplacental passage of maternal CRP, and concentrations are unaffected by gestational age. An increasing CRP value is usually detectable within 6 to 18 h, and the peak CRP is seen at 8-60 h after onset of inflammation. CRP is significantly elevated at the time of the initial evaluation in 50%-90% of infants with systemic bacterial infections. Pourcyrous et al. [22] showed that serial determinations of CRP at 12-h intervals after the onset of clinical signs of sepsis increased the sensitivity of CRP in detecting sepsis. This illustrates well one disadvantage of CRP: it requires some time before it can be detected. Another disadvantage is the low specifity of the test, since elevated CRP levels can be observed after birth asphyxia or noninfectious processes such as meconium aspiration pneumonitis.

Cytokines

Although cytokine kinetics have not been thoroughly investigated in neonates, it is felt by many that measuring cytokine concentrations can be helpful in early diagnosis of neonatal sepsis. Girardin et al. [23] found elevated levels of serum tumor necrosis factor (TNF-α) in eight of nine infants with systemic infection, whereas only one of 60 noninfected infants had an elevated value. Buck et al. [24] evaluated prospectively the use of interleukin-6 (IL-6) and CRP measurements in the diagnosis of sepsis in 222 neonates. Elevated IL-6 concentrations were observed in 73% of newborns with culture-positive infection and in 87% of infants with a clinical diagnosis of sepsis but negative cultures.

Procalcitonin

Procalcitonin (PCT), which is the key precursor of calcitonin, has been reported to be a specific marker of bacterial infections. Gendrel et al. [25] showed that procalcitonin levels were significantly higher in nonpremature neonates with sepsis than in uninfected symptomatic neonates and healthy newborns. Chiesa et al. [26] conducted a prospective study on the reliability of PCT serum concentrations for the diagnosis of early- and late-onset sepsis. They showed that PCT had a sensitivity of 86% in the initial test and of 100% in the next one. They concluded that PCT might be a promising marker for diagnosis of neonatal sepsis.

Diagnosis

In the absence of either subtle or overt signs of sepsis, the clinician must deduce from the maternal history and neonatal course whether the fetus is at risk for sepsis and/or the newborn infant is significantly susceptible to the development of bacteremia or septicemia. Because the signs and symptoms of neonatal sepsis are nonspecific, noninfectious etiologies should be considered in the differential diagnosis.

Fowlie and Schmidt [27] determined the clinical value of common diagnostic tests for bacterial infections in early life by a systematic review of 194 studies. They found a generally poor methodological quality, an enormous variation in test accuracy, and limited value in the diagnosis of infection in this population. If the blood culture is negative, the sepsis score introduced by Töllner [28] may be helpful for early detection of septicemia, including clinical and haematologic symptoms and certain historical factors associated with increased risk for infection. A modified, but similar sepsis screening was used by Chiesa et al. [26] consisting of white blood count, absolute neutrophil count, I/T-ratio, and CRP level. If any two or more of the four test results are abnormal, this may indicate possible infection (see Table 3).

Table 3. Sepsis screening in the neonatal period (pathological leukocyte indices according to Manroe et al [20] and Avery et al [19])

Pathologic Criteria	<24 hours of age	>72 hours
• WBC	<9 000/mm³	<5 000/mm³
(Leukopenia/ leukocytosis)	>30 000/mm³	>20 000/mm³
• Absolute neutrophil count	<7 800/mm³	<1 750/mm³
(neutropenia/neutrophilia)	>14 500/mm³	>5 400/mm³
• I/T-ratio	>0.16 (0.2)	>0.12
• CRP	>6 mg/L	>6 mg/L

WBC, white blood count; I/T-ratio, immature to total neutrophils ratio; CRP, C-reactive protein; positive score: two or more pathological findings of the four criteria indicate possible septicemia

Therapy

Antimicrobial therapy

Initial therapy of an infant with presumed sepsis during the first days of life (early-onset disease) must cover gram-positive cocci, particularly GBS, and gram-negative enteric bacilli. Treatment of infants with presumed late-onset sepsis may need to cover hospital-acquired organisms such as S.aureus, S.epidermidis, and gram-negative enteric bacilli such as Pseudomonas species.

GBS are uniformly sensitive to penicillins and cephalosporins. Group D streptococci vary in susceptibility to penicillins; optimal therapy for diseases related to enterococci includes penicillin and aminoglycoside. Most strains of *S.aureus* produce β-lactamase and are thereby resistant to penicillin G, ampicillin, carbenicillin, and ticaricillin. The use of penicillase-resistant penicillins and selected cephalosporins must be considered when staphylococcal disease is known or suspected. As bacterial resistance must be considered when therapy fails, a switch to vancomycin may be necessary. Most strains are sensitive to vancomycin. Especially with the use of intravascular catheters or ventriculoperitoneal shunts, *S.epidermidis* may be the cause of infection. As many strains are resistant to penicillinase-resistant penicillins and cephalosporins, the initial choice may be vancomycin in this case. Furthermore, removal of the device is often necessary to effect a cure. *Listeria monocytogenes* is resistant to cephalosporins but is susceptible to penicillin G and ampicillin; the latter is first choice in cases of proven or suspected infection. The choice of antibiotics for infection with gram-negative bacteria depends on the particular pattern of susceptibility in the hospital. In general, most aminoglycosides are highly effective against most strains of *E.coli, Enterobacter, Klebsiella, Proteus* species, and *Pseudomonas aeruginosa*. Carbapenems (imipenem and meropenem) may be a good choice as well. Carbapenems have an extremely broad spectrum of activity against gram-positive and gram-negative bacteria, including anaerobes. Third-generation cephalosporins may be good choice in that case, too, especially in cases of a combination of sepsis and meningitis. The rapid development of resistance of gram-negative enteric bacilli with the use of third-generation cephalosporins as standard regimen should be considered.

Supportive therapy

Although appropiate antimicrobal therapy is crucial, supportive care is equally important. Ventilatory support may be necessary, particularly for infants with fulminant early-onset sepsis. Particularly in the neonate, GBS infections may cause acute respiratory distress syndrome due to surfactant depletion. It has been shown that surfactant replacement therapy improved gas exchange [29]. However, the response to surfactant is rather slow, and so repeated and probably higher doses of surfactant are often necessary. Intravenous hydration and, often, parenteral nutrition with close monitoring of glucose and electrolytes are necessary. Septic shock, if present, often needs to be treated appropriately with fluids and inotropes, as indicated by the clinical situation. In patients with meningitis, prompt seizure control is required to achieve proper oxygenation, decrease metabolic demands, and prevent additional cerebral edema. Attention to details of urine output and electrolyte balance and osmolality may be necessary to detect and manage the early complications of meningitis, such as inappropriate secretion of antidiuretic hormone and increased intracranial pressure.

Extracorporeal membrane oxygenation (ECMO) has been used as rescue therapy for newborns with overwhelming early-onset GBS sepsis with distinct hypotension due to septic shock, and/or persistent pulmonary hypertension.

Despite ECMO, the prognosis of severe sepsis remains uncertain. The survival rate of neonatal sepsis on ECMO is, at about 60%, low as compared to 90% in meconium aspiration syndrome [30].

Immunotherapy

The newborn's immune system is compromised in many aspects, including the neutrophilic chemotactic response to pathogens, T-cell production of proin-flammatory lymphokines, and functional complement activity. Preterm infants are further compromised by hypogammaglobulinemia, as maternal transfer of IgG to the fetus occurs predominantly after 32 weeks' gestation. The average IgG concentration in a premature infant is 400 mg/dl, whereas in the term infant it is 1 000 mg/dl. With the increased risk of overwhelming bacterial infection in the preterm infant, trials for improving treatment of neonatal sepsis with the use of intravenous immune globulin (IVIG) were conducted. Multiple studies have been published concerning the use of IVIG in preventing neonatal infection in high-risk infants. The studies are difficult to compare, but the authors who attempted to do so came to the conclusion that there was no clear evidence that the prophylactic use of IVIG was beneficial for preterm infants [31, 32].

Fewer studies have been published concerning the use of IVIG as an adjunctive therapy. The meta-analysis of Baley and Fanaroff [33] demonstrated that IVIG therapy, in conjunction with antibiotics, resulted in a significant decrease in mortality. But they also concluded that these results should be interpreted with caution because they represent only a small number of patients. Therefore, the use of IVIG is still a matter of controversy and further studies are needed. If IVIG is used, current data suggest that 500 to 1 000 mg/kg/dose would be appropriate for treatment.

Fresh frozen plasma contains antibody, complement, fibronectin, and other proteins that help to protect against infection and have been found to be deficient in the neonate. Fresh frozen plasma infusions are sometimes given to neonates with hypotension and are well tolerated.

Adjunctive therapy

The use of recombinant human granulocyte colony-stimulating factor (rhG-CSF) as an adjunctive therapy in the treatment of septic neutropenic neonates has been reported recently. Preliminary data seem promising. Gillian et al. [34], in their randomized placebo-controlled study, demonstrated the efficacy of rhG-CSF in producing neutrophilia. rhG-CSF produced a significant increase in absolute neutrophil concentrations, in the peripheral and bone marrow and the induced C3bi expression. No acute toxicity was recognized. In a 2-year follow-up rhG-CSF treatment was not associated with any long-term adverse hematologic, immunologic, or developmental effects [35].

Other adjunctive strategies include granulocyte transfusions, exchange transfusions, on-line plasma exchange, and continuous hemofiltration. Some of these strategies are considered to be experimental, but none is clinically relevant at the moment.

References

1. Klein JO, Marcy SM (1995) Bacterial sepsis and meningitis. In: Remington JS, Klein JO (eds) Infectious diseases of the fetus and newborn infant. WB Saunders, Philadelphia, pp 835-890
2. Mustafa MM, HcCracken GH Jr (1992) Perinatal bacterial diseases. In: Feign RD, Cherry JD (eds) Textbook of paediatric infectious diseases. WB Saunders, Philadelphia, pp 891-924
3. Baker CJ, Edwards Ms (1995) Group B Streptococcal Infections. In: Remington JS, Klein JO (eds) Infectious diseases of the fetus and newborn infant. WB Saunders, Philadelphia, pp 980-1054
4. Dunkle LM, Brotherton TJ, Feigen RD (1976) Anaerobic infections in children: a prospective study. Paediatrics 57:311
5. Spector SA, Ticknor W, Grossman M (1981) Study of the usefulness of clinical and hematologic findings in the diagnosis of neonatal bacterial infections. Clin Paediatr 20:385
6. Gibbs RS (1995) Obstetric factors associated with infections of the fetus and newborn infant. In: Remington JS, Klein JO (eds) Infectious diseases of the fetus and newborn infant. WB Saunders, Philadelphia, pp 1241-1263
7. St.Geme JW Jr, Murray DL, Carter JA et al (1984) Perinatal infection after prolonged rupture of membranes: an analysis of risk and management. J Paediatr 104:608
8. Gluck L, Wood HF, Fousek MD (1966) Septicemia of the newborn. Paediatr Clin North Am 13:1131
9. Kelly S (1971) Septicemia in galactosemia. JAMA 216:330
10. Voora S, Srinivasan G, Lilien LD et al (1982) Fever in full term newborns in the first four days of life. Paediatrics 69:40
11. Fitzgerald MJ, Goto M, Myers TF et al (1992) Early metabolic effects of sepsis in the preterm infant: lactic acidosis and increased glucose requirements. J Paediatr 121:951
12. Hickey SM, McCracken G Jr (1997) Postnatal bacterial infections In: Fanaroff AA, Martin RJ (eds) Neonatal-perinatal medicine. Diseases of the fetus and infant. Mosby, St.Louis, pp 717-800
13. Squire EN, Favara B, Todd J (1979) Diagnosis of neonatal bacterial infection: hematologic and pathologic findings in fatal and nonfatal cases. Paediatrics 64:60
14. Visser VE, Hall RT (1980) Lumbar puncture in the evaluation of suspected neonatal sepsis. J Paediatr 96:1063
15. Visser VE, Hall RT (1979) Urine culture in the evaluation of suspected neonatal sepsis. J Paediatr 94:635
16. Baker CJ, Rench MA (1983) Commercial latex particle agglutination for detection of group B streptococcal antigen in body fluids. J Paediatr 102:393
17. McIntosh EDG, Jeffrey HE (1992) Clinical application of urine antigen detection in early onset group B streptococcal disease. Arch Dis Child 67:1198
18. Sanchez PJ, Siegel JD, Cushion NB et al (1990) Significance of a positive urine group B streptococcal latex agglutination test in neonates. J Paediatr 116:601
19. Avery GB, Fletcher MA, MacDonald MG (1994) The leucocyte count and the differential count during the first 2 weeks of life. In: Avery GB, Fletcher MA, MacDonald MG (eds)

300   B. Urlesberger et al.

Neonatology-pathophysiology and management of the newborn. Lippincott, Philadelphia, p 1399

20. Manroe BL, Weinberg AG, Rosenfeld CR et al (1979) The neonatal blood count in health and disease. I. Reference values for neutrophilic cells. J Paediatr 95:89

21. Powell KR, Marcy SM (1995) Laboratory aids for diagnosis of neonatal sepsis. In: Remington JS, Klein JO (eds) Infectious diseases of the fetus and newborn infant. WB Saunders, Philadelphia, pp 1223-1240

22. Pourcyrous M, Bada HS, Korones SB et al (1993) Significance of serial C-reactive protein response in neonatal infection and other disorders. Paediatrics 92:431

23. Girardin EP, Berner ME, Grauge H et al (1990) Serum tumor necrosis factor in newborns at risk for infections. Eur J Paediatr 149:645

24. Buck C, Bundschuh J, Gallati H et al (1994) Interleukin-6: a sensitive parameter for the early diagnosis of neonatal bacterial infection. Paediatrics 93:54

25. Gendrel D, Assicot M, Raymond J et al (1996) Procalcitonin as a marker for the early diagnosis of neonatal infection. J Paediatr 128:570

26. Chiesa C, Panero A, Rossi N et al (1998) Reliability of procalcitonin concentrations for the diagnosis of sepsis in critically ill neonates. Clin Inf Dis 26:664

27. Fowlie PW, Schmidt B (1998) Diagnostic tests for bacterial infection from the birth to 90 days-a systematic review. Arch Dis Child Fetal Neonatal Ed 78:F92

28. Töllner U (1982) Early diagnosis of septicemia in the newborn. Eur J Paediatr 138:331

29. Herting E, Harms K, Gefeller O et al (1997) Surfactant treatment of respiratory failure in neonatal group B streptococcal infections: first results of a european retrospective trial. Biol Neonate 71:67

30. Zobel G, Kuttnig-Haim M, Dacar D et al (1995) Die extrakorporale Membranoxygenierung bei Neugeborenen und Kindern. Wien Klin Wochenschr 107/14:427

31. Lacey J, Ohlsson A (1995) Administration of intravenous immunglobulins for prophylaxis or treatment of infection in preterm infants: meta-analysis. Arch Dis Child 72:151

32. Weisman L, Cruess DF, Fischer GW et al (1993) Standard versus hyperimmune intravenous immunoglobulin preventing or treating neonatal infections. Clin Perinatol 20:211

33. Baley J, Fanaroff A (1992) Neonatal infections: II. Specific infectous diseases and therapies. In: Sinclair J, Bracken M (eds) Effective care of the newborn infant. Oxford University Press, Oxford, pp 496-506

34. Gillian E, Christensen RD, Suen Y et al (1994) A randomized, placebo controlled trial of recombinant human granulocyte colony-stimulating factor administration in newborn infants with presumed sepsis: significant induction of peripherial and bone marrow neutrophilia. Blood 84:1427

35. Rosenthal J, Healey T, Ellis R et al (1996) A two-year follow-up of neonates with presumed sepsis treated with recombinant human granulocyte colony-stimulating factor during first week of life. J Paediatr 128:135

Main symbols

AOP	Airway Occlusion Pressure
ARDS	Acute Respiratory Distress Syndrome
BPD	Bronchopulmonary Dysplasia
CARS	Compensating Anti-Inflammatory Response Syndrome
CAVH	Continuous Arteriovenous Hemofiltration
CDH	Congenital Diaphragmatic Hernia
CHDF	Continuous Hemodiafiltration
CMV	Controlled Mechanical Ventilation
CPAP	Continuous Positive Airway Pressure
CRIB	Clinical Risk Index for Babies
CROP	Complicance, Rate, Oxygenation and Pressure
CRP	C-reactive protein
CRRT	Continuous Renal Replacement Therapy
CSF	Cerebrospinal fluid
CVP	Central Venous Pressure
CVVH	Continuous Venovenous Hemfiltration
DIC	Disseminated Intravascular Coagulation
ECF	Extracellular Fluids
ECLS	Extracorporeal Life Support
ECMO	Extracorporeal Membrane Oxygenation
EPCA	Epidural Patient-Controlled Analgesia
FRC	Functional Residual Capacity
GBS	Group B Streptococci
HFJV	High Frequency Jet Ventilation
HFOV	High Frequency Oscillation
HFOV	High Frequency Oscillatory Ventilation
HFV	High-Frequency Ventilation
HIE	Hypoxic-Ischemic Encephalopathy
HLHS	Hypoplastic Left Heart Syndrome
HMD	Hyaline Membrane Disease
ICF	Intracellular Fluids
ILV	Independent Lung Ventilation
IMV	Intermittent Mandatory Ventilation
iNO	Inhaled Nitric Oxide
IVIG	Intravenous Immune Globulin
KMC	Kangaroo-Mother Care
LMA	Laryngeal Mask Airway
LPA	Latex Particle Agglutination

MAC	Minimum Alveolar Concentration
MIP	Maximal Inspiratory Pressure
MRSA	Methicillin-Resistant Staphylococcus Aureus
MV	Minute Volume
NCPAP	Nasal Continuous Positive Airway Pressure
NICU	Neonatal Intensive Care Units
NSAIDs	Nonsteroidal Anti-Inflammatory Drugs
nTISS	Neonatal Therapeutic Intervention Scoring System
P0.1	Inspiratory drive
PCA	Patient-Controlled Analgesia
PCT	Procalcitonin
PEEP	Positive End Expiratory Pressure
PFC	Persistent Fetal Circulation
PICU	Paediatric Intensive Care Unit
PIP	Peak Inflation Pressure
PLV	Partial Liquid Ventilation
PONV	Postoperative Nausea and Vomiting
PPHN	Persistent Pulmonary Hypertension of the Newborn
PRISM	Paediatric Risk of Mortality
PRVC	Pressure-Regulated Volume Control
PSV	Pressure Support Ventilation
PTT	Partial Thromboplastin Time
PTV	Patient-Triggered Ventilation
RDS	Respiratory Distress Syndrome
rhG-CSF	Recombinant Human Granulocyte Colony-Stimulating Factor
RSB	Rapid Shallow Breathing
SCU	Slow Continuous Ultrafiltration
SIMV	Synchronized Intermittent Mandatory Ventilation
SIRS	Systemic Inflammatory Response Syndrome
SNAP	Score for Neonatal Acute Physiology
SOD	Superoxide Dismutase
TLV	Total Liquid Ventilation
URI	Upper Respiratory Infection
VC	Vital Capacity
VLBW	Very Low Birth Weight
VSV	Volume Support Ventilation

Subject index